THE PHILOSOPHY OF

PSYCHIATRY

INTERNATIONAL PERSPECTIVES ON

PHILOSOPHY AND PSYCHIATRY

Series Editors:

K. W. M. (Bill) Fulford, University of Warwick and University of Oxford
Katherine J. Morris, University of Oxford
John Z. Sadler, University of Texas Southwestern Medical Center
Giovanni Stanghellini, University of Florence

Published in the Series:

Nature and Narrative: An Introduction to the New Philosophy of Psychiatry
Edited by the Series Editors

The Philosophy of Psychiatry: A Companion
Edited by Jennifer Radden

THE PHILOSOPHY OF

PSYCHIATRY

A Companion

Edited by

JENNIFER RADDEN

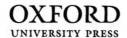

OXFORD

UNIVERSITY PRESS

OXFORD
UNIVERSITY PRESS

Oxford University Press, Inc., publishes works that further
Oxford University's objective of excellence
in research, scholarship, and education.

Oxford   New York
Auckland   Cape Town   Dar es Salaam   Hong Kong   Karachi
Kuala Lumpur   Madrid   Melbourne   Mexico City   Nairobi
New Delhi   Shanghai   Taipei   Toronto

With offices in
Argentina   Austria   Brazil   Chile   Czech Republic   France   Greece
Guatemala   Hungary   Italy   Japan   Poland   Portugal   Singapore
South Korea   Switzerland   Thailand   Turkey   Ukraine   Vietnam

Copyright © 2004 by Oxford University Press, Inc.

Published by Oxford University Press, Inc.
198 Madison Avenue, New York, New York 10016

www.oup.com

First issued as an Oxford University Press paperback, 2007

Oxford is a registered trademark of Oxford University Press

Library of Congress Cataloging-in-Publication Data
The philosophy of psychiatry : a companion / edited by Jennifer Radden.
p. cm.
Includes bibliographical references and index.

ISBN-13 978-0-19-531327-7 (pbk.)
1. Psychiatry—Philosophy. 2. Psychiatry—Moral and ethical aspects.
3. Psychology and philosophy. I. Radden, Jennifer.
RC437.5.P4376 2004
616.89'001—dc21   2003053094

Printed in the United States of America
on acid-free paper

To FTK and TNRK, with love.

FOREWORD

....

DOUBT is a scarce commodity in psychiatry today. Propeled by advances in diagnostic reliability, epidemiologic methods, genetic analyses, and neuroimaging, with ever more effective pharmacologic and psychotherapeutic treatments at hand, psychiatry appears to be on the verge of resolving the mysteries of mental illness that frustrated generations of our psychiatric forebears. Every issue of our journals trumpets new findings on the etiology, pathophysiology, and genetics of psychiatric disorders. New, improved medications appear each year, as if on cue. It is, in all, a wonderful time to be a psychiatrist.

Of course, that is what many of our psychiatric progenitors thought as well. When moral treatment was introduced in the late eighteenth and early nineteenth centuries, its proponents had no doubt of either its theoretical basis or its therapeutic efficacy. Nor did the champions of the mental hygiene movement at the turn of the twentieth century, or the practitioners of lobotomy and other psychosurgical procedures in the wake of World War II. Community psychiatrists of the 1960s were persuaded not only that they could effectively treat mental disorders, assuming that they were detected at an early enough stage, but that by altering the social environment, they could prevent the development of psychopathology as well. As a field, we were certain—serially, recidivistically certain—that the enigma of mental illness had at least been dispelled. If only we had been right.

Might it be different this time? Yes, it might. One need not be ensnared by the fallacies of scientism to believe that progress is being made in explaining the basis of mental disorders or to recognize that we can treat symptoms today against which we were largely powerless even a few decades ago. But the dangers of hubris still lurk. Psychiatrists now in midcareer will recall having witnessed the rise and fall of the norepinephrine hypotheses of depression in the 1970s, multiple presumed genetic loci in psychiatric disorders in the 1980s, and the epidemic of multiple personality disorder in the 1990s. The atypical antipsychotic medications that were so enthusiastically embraced as more efficacious and less harmful than their predecessors are now recognized as having substantial therapeutic limitations and often problematic side effects of their own.

Which brings me to the importance of the philosophical study of our complex field. Philosophers excel precisely at the task we need them most to do: to challenge the presumed verities by which we lead our professional lives. However reassuring it is to reflect on the advances in psychiatry, it is only by focusing on the weaknesses of our theories, the holes in our knowledge, and the errors in our practices that further progress becomes possible. Hence, though I almost never leave a piece of philosophical writing on some aspect of psychiatry without feeling less certain than I did at the outset of what I believed to be correct, I find this experience uplifting rather than demoralizing. What a marvelous corrective to so much of the remainder of our professional literature in which, buffeted by the combined force of theory and data, we join in the pretense that doubt has been vanquished.

The thoughtful collection of inquiries into the philosophy of psychiatry presented in this volume nicely demonstrates the many areas in which philosophical analyses can contribute to clarity of thought—not by removing doubt but by introducing it. The phenomenological tradition of careful description of mental function and dysfunction often reveals unexpected diversity among presentations grouped under a common rubric and raises questions regarding theories of etiology. Both of these enterprises may have direct, practical implications for diagnosis and treatment. Similarly, from long philosophical experience with the development of typologies come important critiques of the dominant diagnostic schemata, especially regarding the difficult task of defining the boundary between the pathologic and the normal.

Ethics is probably the most familiar area of philosophical activity for the average clinician, encompassing such everyday dilemmas as determining decisional competence and assigning responsibility for criminal acts. At its best, ethical analysis undercuts facile judgment based on unspoken assumptions and makes evident a range of options available for the resolution of moral quandaries. But at a time of neurobiologic hegemony in the construction of models of mental disorder, it may be the critique that careful analysis can bring to this modeling process and the refusal to abandon alternative explanatory constructs that may be philosophy's most valuable contribution. Whether or not mental phenomena will ever be reducible to cellular interactions in the brain, and hence explicable at the molecular level, it is clear that a premature reductionism is one of the greatest threats to progress in our field.

Though I can speak firsthand about the value of philosophy for the psychiatrist, I must rely on the judgments of my philosopher-friends regarding the usefulness of the study of psychiatric disorders for the philosopher. They tell me that the phenomenology of mental disorders, the complex ethical issues that arise, and the dilemmas inherent in the line-drawing process of diagnosis provide challenging opportunities to test and refine philosophical theories. A focus on psychiatry also offers philosophers the chance to make real contributions to the welfare of a society that must somehow cope with the pain and perturbations of the social order evoked by mental illness.

Perhaps that is why so many of the chapters in this book are cowritten by philosophers and clinicians, and why philosophy and psychiatry has become such an active field of investigation, with its own journals, societies, and meetings. As psychiatrists, we cannot but be better off for this intellectual ferment and challenge. What is true for us as individuals applies as well to our field, and ultimately to those whose benefit we seek by our efforts. When it comes to casting doubt where doubt is called for, the philosophical study of psychiatry renders great service to us all.

Paul S. Appelbaum, M.D.
A. F. Zeleznik Distinguished Professor and Chair of Psychiatry
Director, Law and Psychiatry Program
University of Massachusetts Medical School

ACKNOWLEDGMENTS

So many people helped in the conception and preparation of this book that I cannot hope to name them all. But particular thanks and appreciation are due to the group of my friends and colleagues from the Association for the Advancement of Philosophy and Psychiatry who, at the University of Louisville in October 2000, offered decisive suggestions about the volume's organizational schema: Jerry Kroll, Don Mender, Marilyn Nissim-Sabat, Jim Phillips, John Sadler, Louis Sass, Osborne Wiggins, and Melvin Woody. As I sought authors to cover all the subfields represented in that schema, George Graham gave generously of his unmatched "who's Who" knowledge of this field, and I appreciate this assistance. For valuable philosophical and editorial help with my own written contributions to the *Companion*, I owe particular thanks to the members of PHAEDRA: Jane Roland Martin, Ann Diller, Barbara Houston, Beatrice Kipp Nelson, Janet Farrell Smith, and Susan Douglas Franzosa. For support in my quest for a suitable image for the dust jacket, which proved a quest indeed, I am grateful to Barbara Baum Pollans, Beatrice Radden Keefe, and Patrick Radden Keefe. As well as those I have already named, I want to acknowledge my splendid authors, who deserve so much credit for their efforts. Throughout this process, I benefited from the unobtrusive help, intelligent and thoughtful interest, and encouragement of my editor Peter Ohlin; from the unfailing support of series editors Bill Fullford and John Sadler; and from the understanding and appreciation of my husband Frank Keefe.

CONTENTS

Foreword, vii
Paul S. Appelbaum

Contributors, xvii

Introduction, 3

PART I: PSYCHOPATHOLOGY AND NORMALCY

1. Cognition: Brain Pain: Psychotic Cognition, Hallucination
   and Delusions, 21
   Grant Gillett

2. Affectivity: Depression and Mania, 36
   Jennifer Hansen

3. Desire: Paraphilia and Distress in DSM-IV, 54
   Alan G. Soble

4. Character: Moral Treatment and the Personality Disorders, 64
   Louis C. Charland

5. Action: Volitional Disorder and Addiction, 78
   Alfred R. Mele

6. Self-ascription: Thought Insertion, 89
   George Graham

7. Memory: The Nature and Significance of Dissociation, 106
   Stephen E. Braude

8. Body: Disorders of Embodiment, 118
   Shaun Gallagher and Mette Vaever

9. Identity: Personal Identity, Characterization Identity and Mental Disorder, 133
Jennifer Radden

10. Development: Disorders of Childhood and Youth, 147
Christian Perring

PART II: ANTINOMIES OF PRACTICE

11. Diagnosis/Antidiagnosis, 163
John Z. Sadler

12. Understanding/Explanation, 180
James Phillips

13. Reductionism/Antireductionism, 191
Tim Thornton

14. Facts/Values: Ten Principles of Values-Based Medicine, 205
K. W. M. (Bill) Fulford

PART III: NORMS, VALUES, AND ETHICS

15. Gender, 237
Nancy Potter

16. Race and Culture, 244
Marilyn Nissim-Sabat

17. Competence, 258
Charles M. Culver and Bernard Gert

18. Dangerousness: "The General Duty to All the World," 271
Daniel N. Robinson

19. Treatment and Research Ethics, 282
Ruth Chadwick and Gordon Aindow

20. Criminal Responsibility, 296
Simon Wilson and Gwen Adshead

21. Religion, 312
    Brooke Hopkins and Margaret P. Battin

PART IV: THEORETICAL MODELS

22. Darwinian Models of Psychopathology, 329
    Dominic Murphy

23. Psychoanalytic Models: Freud's Debt to Philosophy and His
    Copernican Revolution, 338
    Bettina Bergo

24. Phenomenological and Hermeneutic Models: Understanding
    and Interpretation in Psychiatry, 351
    Michael Alan Schwartz and Osborne P. Wiggins

25. Neurobiological Models: An Unnecessary Divide — Neural
    Models in Psychiatry, 364
    Andrew Garnar and Valerie Gray Hardcastle

26. Cognitive-Behavioral Models: Cognitive-Behavior Therapy, 381
    Edward Erwin

27. Social Constructionist Models: Making Order out of Disorder —
    On the Social Construction of Madness, 393
    Jennifer Church

PART V: CIRCUMSCRIBING MENTAL DISORDER

28. Setting Benchmarks for Psychiatric Concepts, 409
    Rom Harré

29. Defining Mental Disorder, 415
    Bernard Gert and Charles M. Culver

30. Mental Health and Its Limits, 426
    Carl Elliott

    Index, 437

Contributors

GWEN ADSHEAD is a forensic psychiatrist and psychotherapist at Broadmoor Hospital, U.K. She has a master's degree in medical law and ethics and is involved in teaching and writing about ethics in psychiatry. She is currently involved in a project with Jonathan Glover (Professor of Moral Philosophy at Kings College, London) to study moral reasoning in antisocial personality disorder.

GORDON AINDOW is Senior Lecturer in Mental Health Nursing at St Martin's College, Lancaster, U.K. He has worked in several areas of mental health nursing practice, including forensic mental health and acute psychiatric in-patient care and as a community psychiatric nurse.

MARGARET (PEGGY) P. BATTIN is Distinguished Professor of Philosophy and Adjunct Professor of Internal Medicine, Division of Medical Ethics, at the University of Utah. A graduate of Bryn Mawr College, she holds an M.F.A. in fiction writing, as well as a Ph.D. in philosophy, from the University of California, Irvine. She writes extensively on end-of-life issues, and many of her pieces are incorporated in *The Least Worst Death: Essays in Bioethics on the End of Life* (Oxford University Press, 1994). She has also worked on applied-ethics issues in religion: she is the author of *Ethics in the Sanctuary: Examining the Practices of Organized Religion* (1990) and co-author of *Praying for a Cure: When Medical and Religious Practices Conflict* (1999).

BETTINA BERGO is Assistant Professor of Philosophy at Duquesne University. She has worked on contemporary Jewish and continental thought. She is researching the history of anxiety in nineteenth-century philosophy and psychoanalysis.

STEPHEN E. BRAUDE is Chair and Professor of Philosophy at The University of Maryland Baltimore County. He has been writing on the topic of dissociation for the past 15 years, and he is the author of numerous articles and four books, including *The Limits of Influence: Psychokinesis and the Philosophy of Science; First Person Plural: Multiple Personality and the Philosophy of Mind;* and *Immortal Remains: The Evidence for Life after Death.*

RUTH CHADWICK is Professor of Bioethics and Director of the ESRC Centre for Economic and Social Aspects of Genomics, Lancaster University. She has coordinated a number of projects funded by the European Commission, including the Euroscreen projects (1994–96 and 1996–99) and coedits the journal *Bioethics.* She is a member of the Human Genome Organisation (HUGO) Ethics Committee, the Advisory

Committee on Novel Foods and Processes, and the Medical Research Council Advisory Committee on Scientific Advances in Genetics. She was editor in chief of the award-winning *Encyclopedia of Applied Ethics* (1998).

LOUIS C. CHARLAND holds a joint appointment in the Department of Philosophy and the Faculty of Health Sciences at The University of Western Ontario in London, Canada. His main areas of research are the philosophy of emotion and the philosophy of psychiatry.

JENNIFER CHURCH is Professor of Philosophy at Vassar College. She has published articles on irrationality, the emotions, consciousness and the unconscious, imagination, and ownership and the body.

CHARLES M. CULVER, M.D., Ph.D., is a Professor of Medical Education at Barry University in Miami Shores, Florida, where he also serves as Associate Director of the Physician Assistant Program. Dr. Culver has written extensively on topics in bioethics and the philosophy of medicine.

CARL ELLIOTT teaches philosophy and bioethics at the University of Minnesota. His books include *A Philosophical Disease: Bioethics Culture and Identity* (1999), *Slow Cures and Bad Philosophers: Essays on Wittgenstein, Medicine and Bioethics* (2001), and *Better Than Well: American Medicine Meets the American Dream* (2003).

EDWARD ERWIN is a Professor of Philosophy at the University of Miami. He is the editor of the recently published *Freud Encyclopedia: Theory, Therapy, and Culture* (2002) and is the author of *Behavior Therapy: Scientific, Philosophical, and Moral Foundations* (1978), *A Final Accounting: Philosophical and Empirical Issues in Freudian Psychology* (1996), and *Philosophy and Psychotherapy: Razing the Troubles of the Brain* (1997).

K. W. M. (BILL) FULFORD, D. Phil., is Professor of Philosophy and Mental Health at the University of Warwick and Honorary Consultant Psychiatrist, University of Oxford. He is author of many articles and books in the philosophy of psychiatry and serves as series coeditor of Oxford University Press's International Perspectives in the Philosophy of Psychiatry. His recent publications include *Moral Theory and Medical Practice* (1989, reprinted 1999), "Spiritual Experience and Psychopathology" (with M. Jackson, 1997), "Teleology without Tears: Naturalism, Neo-Naturalism and Evaluationism in the Analysis of Function Statements in Biology (and a Bet on the Twenty-first Century)" (2000), and "Report to the Chair of the DSM-VI Task Force from the Editors of PPP on 'Contentious and Noncontentious Evaluative Language in Psychiatric Diagnosis (Dateline 2010)' " (2002).

SHAUN GALLAGHER is Professor of Philosophy and Director of the Cognitive Science Program at Canisius College in Buffalo, New York. He is editor of the journal *Phenomenology and the Cognitive Sciences*. His research focuses on the philosophy and phenomenology of mind and the cognitive sciences. His most recent book is *The Inordinance of Time* (1998).

ANDREW GARNAR is an instructor in philosophy and a Ph.D. candidate in the Science and Technology Program at Virginia Tech. He is concerned with the social, cultural, and technological dimensions of mental health and mental disorders.

BERNARD GERT is Stone Professor of Intellectual and Moral Philosophy, Dartmouth College, and Adjunct Professor of Psychiatry, Dartmouth Medical School. He is first author of *Morality and the New Genetics* (1996) and *Bioethics: A Return to Fundamentals* (1997), and author of *Morality: Its Nature and Justification* (1998).

GRANT GILLETT is Professor of Medical Ethics at the University of Otago in Dunedin, New Zealand. He is also a practicing neurosurgeon. His main philosophical work is in the philosophy of mind and psychiatry, though he also writes on topics in bioethics. His most recent books are *The Mind and Its Discontents* (Oxford University Press, 1999), and he has co-authored *Medical Ethics* and *Consciousness and Intentionality*. He is interested in postmodern and traditional analytic approaches to bioethics, mind and language, and psychiatry.

GEORGE GRAHAM is A. C. Reid Professor of Philosophy at Wake Forest University in Winston-Salem, North Carolina. His research focuses on philosophy of mind, philosophical psychopathology, and cognitive science. With G. Lynn Stephens, Graham is the co-author of *When Self-Consciousness Breaks* (2000).

JENNIFER HANSEN is an Assistant Professor of Philosophy at Gettysburg College. She edits the journal *Studies in Practical Philosophy* and does research in the areas of philosophy of psychiatry, feminist theory, and aesthetics.

VALERIE GRAY HARDCASTLE is Professor of Philosophy and Director of the Science and Technology Studies Program at Virginia Tech. Her area of research expertise concerns what the intersection of cognitive science, neuroscience, psychology, and psychiatry is like and what it should be like. Her most recent books are *The Myth of Pain* (1999) and *Constructing Selves* (forthcoming).

ROM HARRÉ began his academic career in mathematics, later turning to philosophy and psychology. He is Emeritus Fellow of Linacre College, Oxford, and currently is teaching at Georgetown and American Universities in Washington, D.C. His most recent publication is *Cognitive Science: A Philosophical Introduction* (2002).

BROOKE HOPKINS is a Professor of English at the University of Utah. His B.A. and Ph.D. are from Harvard University, where he taught for five years. He has published several papers on the relationship between psychoanalysis and religion in *The International Journal of Psychoanalysis*, as well as numerous essays in literary criticism and related topics.

ALFRED R. MELE is the William H. and Lucyle T. Werkmeister Professor of Philosophy at Florida State University. He is the author of *Irrationality* (1987), *Springs of Action* (1992), *Autonomous Agents* (1995), *Self-Deception Unmasked* (2001), and *Motivation and Agency* (2002). He also is the editor of *The Philosophy of Action* (1997), co-editor (with John Heil) of *Mental Causation* (1993), and co-editor (with J. Piers Rawling) *of Handbook of Rationality* (forthcoming). (All are published by Oxford University Press except for *Self-Deception Unmasked.*)

DOMINIC MURPHY is Assistant Professor of Philosophy at the California Institute of Technology. He works on the philosophy of the cognitive and social sciences and is currently finishing a book on explanation and classification in psychiatry.

MARILYN NISSIM-SABAT, Ph.D., M.S.W., is Professor Emeritus and Adjunct Professor of Philosophy, Lewis University, Romeoville, Illinois, and a clinical social worker practicing psychoanalytic psychotherapy in Chicago. Dr. Nissim-Sabat has many publications on the interrelations among Husserlian phenomenology, psychoanalysis, feminism, and critical race theory.

CHRISTIAN PERRING is Chair of the Department of Philosophy at Dowling College, New York. He received his Ph.D. from Princeton University. His main research interests are in the philosophy of psychiatry, medical ethics, and moral psychology. He is also the editor of *Metapsychology Online Review.*

JAMES PHILLIPS is in the private practice of psychiatry and is Associate Clinical Professor of Psychiatry in the Yale School of Medicine. He is interested in the interface of philosophy and psychiatry and has written on hermeneutic theory in psychiatry and psychoanalysis, on the role of narrativity in psychiatric theory, and on technical reason in psychiatry. He is editor of the *Bulletin of the Association for the Advancement of Philosophy and Psychiatry.*

NANCY POTTER is an Associate Professor of Philosophy at the University of Louisville. Her research interests include ethics, philosophies of peace, and, in philosophy of psychiatry, the diagnosis and treatment of borderline personality disorder. She has published articles in *Philosophy, Psychiatry, and Psychology* and *Hypatia* and the book *How Can I Be Trusted? A Virtue Theory of Trustworthiness.*

JENNIFER RADDEN is Professor and Chair of the Philosophy Department at the University of Massachusetts, Boston Campus. She is author of many publications within the philosophy of psychiatry, including *Madness and Reason* (1985), *Divided Minds and Successive Selves: Ethical Issues in Disorders of Identity and Personality* (1996), and (as editor) *The Nature of Melancholy: From Aristotle to Kristeva* (2000). Between 1997 and 2002 she was president of the Association for the Advancement of Philosophy and Psychiatry.

DANIEL N. ROBINSON is Distinguished Research Professor Emeritus, Georgetown University, Adjunct Professor of Psychology at Columbia University, and a member of the Philosophy Faculty at Oxford University. Prof. Robinson's many books include *Wild Beasts and Idle Humours: The Insanity Defense from Antiquity to the Present* (1996) and *The Mind: An Oxford Reader* (Oxford University Press, 1998). His most recent book is *Praise and Blame: Moral Realism and Its Applications* (2002). Prof. Robinson's principle interests are in history and philosophy of psychology, philosophy of mind, and philosophy of law.

JOHN Z. SADLER, M.D., is Professor of Psychiatry and Director of Undergraduate Psychiatric Education at the University of Texas Southwestern Medical Center, Dallas. He has coedited (with K. W. M. Fulford) the journal *Philosophy, Psychiatry, and Psychology* since its inception in 1994. His most recent book, *Descriptions and Prescriptions: Values, Mental Disorders, and the DSMs* (2002) reflects his ongoing fascination with the philosophical aspects of psychiatric diagnosis and classification.

MICHAEL ALAN SCHWARTZ, M.D., is founding president of the Association for the Advancement of Philosophy and Psychiatry and Clinical Professor of Psychiatry at Case Western Reserve University School of Medicine. Together with Osborne Wiggins, Dr. Schwartz is recipient of the Dr. Margrit Egner-Stiftung Prize, for "contributing with their work to a more human world in which the human being with its mental needs stands in the center."

ALAN G. SOBLE is University Research Professor and Professor of Philosophy at the University of New Orleans. Among his books are *Sexual Investigations* (1996) and *Pornography, Sex, and Feminism* (2002). He has written journal articles on sex and love, most recently on Kant's notion of sexual perversion (2003) and on St. Augustine's sex life (2002). Some of his articles have been translated into French, German, Hungarian, and Italian, and some can be found on his web site at http://www.uno.edu/asoble/essays.htm.

TIM THORNTON is Lecturer in Philosophy at the University of Warwick and Manager of the Philosophy and Ethics of Mental Health Programme. In addition to philosophy of psychiatry, his research interests are philosophy of thought and language, metaphysics, philosophy of science and philosophy of mind, Wittgenstein, Davidson, and McDowell.

METTE VAEVER is currently in a clinical psychology traineeship at the University of Copenhagen. Her research interests include thought disorder and phenomenology of the schizophrenia spectrum disorders. She is also affiliated with the Cognitive Research Unit at the Department of Psychiatry, Hvidovre Hospital, in Copenhagen, where she is conducting a follow-up study of children of schizophrenic mothers, with a special focus on neurocognitive developmental trajectories.

OSBORNE P. WIGGINS, Ph.D., is Professor and Chair of Philosophy at the University of Louisville, in Louisville, Kentucky. He has published essays on phenomenology, psychiatry, and ethics. He is a recipient of the Dr. Margrit Egner-Stiftung Prize for his work in philosophy and psychiatry.

SIMON WILSON, B.Sc., M.B. Ch.B., M.A., M.R.C.Psych, is Consultant Forensic Psychiatrist at HM Prison Brixton, London, and assistant editor of the *Journal of Forensic Psychiatry*.

THE PHILOSOPHY OF
PSYCHIATRY

INTRODUCTION

CLINICAL practice, psychiatric theorizing and research, mental health policy, and the economics and politics of mental health care each ineluctably engage philosophical ideas. Disease, health, and disability are moral and metaphysical categories as much as they are social and legal descriptions. Conceptions of rationality, personhood, and autonomy, the preeminent philosophical ideas and ideals grounding modern-day liberal and humanistic societies such as ours, also frame our understanding of mental disorder and rationales for its social, clinical, and legal treatment. Philosophical questions of evidence, reality, truth, science, and values give meaning to each of the social institutions and practices concerned with mental health and unhealth. The psyche, the mind and its relation to the body, subjectivity and consciousness, personal identity and character, thought, will, memory, and what Descartes called the passions of the soul — these are the stuff equally of traditional philosophical inquiry and of the psychiatric enterprise.

Psychiatry, it seems fair to say, is a branch of medicine and a healing practice with a subject matter and presuppositions that are deeply and unavoidably philosophical. Recognition of this has spawned a new research field, the philosophy of psychiatry, and provides the raison d'être for the following work.

Mental disorder and mental health care not only engage philosophical ideas but also are part of the fabric of our everyday lives. Though stigma, shame, and silence still often shroud its manifestations, the "ordinary everydayness" of mental disorder is inescapable. By whatever index, its incidence in the population is significant; by some indices, at least, it is growing rapidly. Increasingly, conditions like depression and schizophrenia are recognized to impose a burden that is not only personal and societal but economic. (Depression alone will soon replace heart disease as the leading cause of morbidity worldwide, according to studies that estimate the global and national costs of diseases.)

Acknowledgment of the profound social and political importance of mental health care has increased correspondingly, and with it has come some acknowledgment of the social values and philosophical principles to which psychiatric theory and practice owe allegiance. Psychiatry still cleaves to its traditional self-conception as a biological science and medical subspecialty, however, and one purpose of this book is to expose the philosophical presuppositions within psychiatry and to spotlight the need for philosophical approaches to this branch of medicine.

Each of the essays that follows testifies to and goes some way toward satisfying this need. To illustrate its urgency in this preliminary discussion, the case of delusional thinking will serve. Delusional thinking is a standard criterion for identifying severe mental disorder—a mainstay in diagnosis, research, treatment, and mental health policy. Yet delusion is far from the simple, descriptive category this suggests. Despite its undeniable importance, the loose characterizations of delusional thinking employed within psychiatry for decades, all insufficient, went largely unquestioned. It had been maintained that delusions were false beliefs, though not all false beliefs are delusions (we all mistakenly believe something untrue on occasion) and not all delusions are false (sometimes your wife is truly cheating on you); it had been held that delusions were fixed beliefs, though not all fixed beliefs are delusional (religious and moral beliefs are often unshakably fixed, yet they are not usually designated delusions) and not all delusions are held with such tenacity. Delusion is a complex, nuanced category, recent systematic attention has revealed, with both normative and descriptive elements. Its definition calls for sophisticated philosophical tools and a refined understanding of language and epistemology.

As the category of delusion also makes clear, descriptions of psychopathological symptoms and the very idea of mental disorder must contain abiding interest for the philosophically minded. How could a philosopher fail to be intrigued by the following first-person description, introduced in chapter 1: "I simply don't have any body sensation any more, no feeling of the body still belonging to me. I sense that I'm sitting here, but it is an alien feeling"? Or by the remark of a patient (also described by Grant Gillett) who, upon noticing three marble tables in a cafe, was suddenly convinced that the end of the world was imminent? The lucid, the rational, the coherent, and the self-controlled have been subject to enduring Western philosophical inquiry, speculation, and theorizing. As their antitheses, delusional and disordered states ought to form part of that inquiry. The point was made by Wittgenstein. If in life we are surrounded by death, he remarks, so, too, "in the health of our intellect we are surrounded by madness" (1977: 44).

BACKGROUND

The philosophy of psychiatry has attracted the attention of some of the ablest thinkers and most compelling writers of the past hundred years, among them William James, Sigmund Freud, Karl Jaspers, and Thomas Szasz. Apart from luminous discussions by such thinkers, however, the field remained largely neglected, as much by those within philosophy as by most within psychiatry, until the last couple of decades of the twentieth century. During the 1970s, controversial critiques of orthodox medical psychiatry mounted by R. D. Laing, Szasz, and Michel Foucault piqued a broad cultural interest in the philosophical assumptions that underlie psychiatric theory and practice. Pioneering philosophical writing by Tristram Englehardt Jr., Christopher Boorse, Charles Culver, and Bernard Gert also emerged during that period. Philosophy itself changed and broadened with the last quarter of the twentieth century. From the inward-looking and narrowed discipline of the previous decades, it expanded, applying its methodology to new subjects such as history, social science, and medicine. The 1980s saw growing appreciation that philosophical analyses were called for in psychiatry and that clinicians, as well as philosophers, must contribute to this research — an appreciation due in no small part to the interdisciplinary efforts of the Association for the Advancement of Philosophy and Psychiatry in the United States and its fellow organizations elsewhere, including the Philosophy Group of the Royal College of Psychiatrists in London, the Nordic Network of Philosophy and Mental Health in the Scandinavian countries, and, most recently, the 2002 inauguration of the International Network for Philosophy and Psychiatry (INPP). Spurred by international conferences, meetings, discussion groups, and seminars, and by the 1993 inauguration of the specialized journal PPP (*Philosophy, Psychiatry and Psychology*), philosophers and philosophically trained psychiatrists have belatedly begun a series of vital cross-disciplinary exchanges.

This volume introduces some fruit of those exchanges. Original discussions by leading thinkers in this area are not only expository and critical but also a reflection of their authors' distinctive and often powerful and imaginative viewpoints and theories. Together, these discussions constitute a significant new exploration, definition, and mapping of the borderland where philosophy and psychiatry meet.

One of the most attractive aspects of the emerging philosophy of psychiatry lies in its acknowledgment of the value of both phenomenological and analytical approaches to the examination of psychiatric theory and practice. This may in part be a result of the powerful influence of Jaspers's phenomenological work: the great two-volume *General Psychopathology*, from 1959, is still read today as a model of psychiatric method and analysis. As well as Jaspers's important legacy, the centrality to psychiatric practice of subjective, first-person narrative and the attention paid to meaning and symbolism in traditional notions of psychotherapy deriving from Freudian and post-Freudian psychoanalysis have predisposed those who engage in philosophical analyses to acknowledge, respect, and even privilege phenomenological niceties. Both analytic and phenomenological methodologies and traditions are represented in the chapters that follow, and this eclectic mix immeasurably enhances the resultant multistranded whole.

Cross-disciplinary research yields unexpected insights and fresh connections. Some of its distinctive, synergic vitality derives from differences of approach between the disciplines involved, and several of these can be identified in research represented here. Goals and emphases differ. Philosophers approach the phenomena of psychopathology with a focus on clarification and definition that sets their inquiries apart from the emphasis on describing, understanding, and healing that are common in mainstream psychiatry, for example. Methods differ, also. Less wedded to observational approaches, the philosophically trained enhance their theorizing with the imaginative appeal to counterfactuals known as thought experiments, for example. (See chapter 25.) Most obviously, those who work at the perimeter of disciplinary boundaries — such as philosophers writing about psychiatry — tap a literature and traditions rarely encountered in writing that is closer to the disciplinary core. Wittgensteinian theories of language help us understand psychosis in the following pages; efforts to define volitional disorder are illuminated by perplexities over weakness of will tracing back to Plato's writing, and critical race theory allows us to recognize how race intersects with psychiatry. Such interdisciplinary riches occur throughout this volume.

DIAGNOSTIC CLASSIFICATIONS

Casting a long shadow over most of the essays here are nosologies such as the American Psychiatric Association's Diagnostic and Statistical Manuals (DSMs) and the World Health Organization's International Classifications of Diseases (ICDs). Whether framed as flawed science or as repositories of dangerous social power, these documents — particularly the DSMs — have been subject to unrelenting critique, much of it by philosophers, since the 1970s and 1980s. Whatever flaws they contain, however, the presence and influence of these classifications are evident in every facet of the research field represented here. From DSM definitions of particular symptoms and distinct disorders, to the DSMs' account of mental disorder, to their "evidence-based" methodology and findings, to the changes they have undergone with new editions, these documents represent a unique portrait of current psychiatric understanding. As such, they are acknowledged, but also challenged, throughout the present volume.

MAPPING THE RESEARCH FIELD

The research represented here clusters around five kinds of inquiry (introduced later in this chapter) and engages most of the branches of philosophy, including the philosophy of mind, epistemology and metaphysics, ethics, the philosophy of science, and methodology and analysis.

Like any broad research endeavor, the philosophy of psychiatry has proliferated in piecemeal fashion. Discussions of philosophical psychopathology have taken place at some remove from the more obviously practical and evaluative contexts in which treatment and research ethics and mental health norms and policies are introduced. And a similar de facto separation has divided discussions of clinical practice from those that are more, or are solely, theoretical. The breadth, depth, and unifying themes of the field are concealed by such artificial separations, however, and another goal of this volume is to emphasize the interconnections between these separate inquiries and the coherence of the philosophy of psychiatry conceived as a single body of research.

That this is rightly construed as one field rather than several is easily demonstrated. Theoretical and more purely philosophical discussions have powerful and far-reaching implications for practical contexts and evaluative considerations. But they are also affected by praxis. The case of dissociation and dissociated states illustrates these inherent interconnections particularly well. Metaphysical theories of personal identity and even responsibility alter the way we understand and conceptualize dissociation: certain theories require that, however dissociated, all states are nonetheless ascribed to a unitary self, for example. Moreover, because of ties between theories of personal identity and personal responsibility, aspects of practice with dissociated patients are directly affected by those theories. (See chapter 9.) Thus, the decision to attribute responsibility to a person whose wrongdoing took place during a dissociated state, for example, may presuppose the unitary self-conception of personal identity outlined earlier. The treatment decision to override an earlier established advance care directive might reflect a "multiple selves" metaphysics. Any analysis of dissociation will have metaphysical, moral, practical, and ethical implications and will be incomplete to the extent that these implications—and their interconnections—remain unexplored.

Summing up, then, the philosophy of psychiatry is here understood to encompass the philosophical assumptions and ideas that arise from, and the application of philosophical method to, not only psychopathology but also psychiatric theorizing, mental health categories, clinical practice, and psychiatric research. The five sections into which the present volume is arranged represent the interconnected parts of what is emphatically one field of study, not several. A brief summary of the chapters in the order in which they occur is provided at the end of this introduction.

PART I: PSYCHOPATHOLOGY AND NORMALCY

It has become something of a truism to point out that philosophy can learn as much or more from states of mental disorder as it contributes to our understanding of those states. Nowhere is this more apparent than in the symptom descriptions that constitute psychopathology—the vivid, strange, and puzzling phenomenology of delusion, dissociation, and compulsion and the ruptures between thought and desire, willing and doing, mood and belief that are revealed through fine-grained clinical description. At least in Western philosophical traditions, our conceptions of agency, personhood, self-identity, memory, desire, affectivity, character, and rationality are rooted in, and presuppose, certain psychological and social norms concerning subjectivity and behavior: these are the norms of mental health. Psychopathology exposes these norms, their incumbent limitations — their very normativity — and the gaps in our understanding that result from those limitations. It reveals divisions in states hitherto supposed seamless and exceptions to relations earlier believed internal. A critical analysis of these mental health norms is a recurring goal of the research undertaken here. That said, an appeal to psychopathology to extend our understanding of normal psychology requires an exacting methodology, which can easily be misused, as illustrated by the foregoing research. Reports of "thought insertion" (the denial by a patient of ownership of a conscious thought or experience) appear at first sight to require us to adjust our conviction that the only thoughts we know are our own and that we know these without the possibility of error. When we look closer, however, it seems more likely that first-person reports of inserted thoughts may be equivocal. (See chapter 6.) Similarly, the temptation to derive a nonunitary view of the normal self from the apparently divided minds that occur in dissociation has been shown to rest on faulty reasoning. (See chapter 7.)

Psychiatry boasts an impressive tradition of meticulous clinical description. In some instances this has been inspired by a thoroughgoing application of empirical method, in others by phenomenological assumptions, and in yet others by no more — or less — than a remarkable ear for meaning and nuance in spoken and unspoken expression. Nonetheless, philosophical analysis has drawn attention to conceptual confusions and unclarities, inadequate definitions and unexplored assumptions in psychiatric lore about symptoms. Recent critical work — including some in this volume — on delusion, hallucination, thought disorder, dissociation, and volitional disorder has begun to remedy these omissions.

The influence of the DSMs is nowhere more evident than in the discussion of psychopathology; indeed, the category of psychopathology itself, defined as the symptom expression of a disorder or disease in the individual, derives from these classifications. But philosophical approaches to psychopathology in the following pages sometimes separate themselves from the structuring of the psychiatric classifications. In analyzing personality or character disorders, for example, it may prove pertinent to ask not what disorder afflicts personality but what treatment heals these conditions. This approach leads to the radical conclusion that, *pace* DSM, personality disorders are moral, not medical, conditions. (See chapter 4.) Similarly, DSM assumptions about the attribution of mental disorders to children and youth can be exposed and, once exposed, challenged. Instead of seeing these disorders as "in" the young, it is arguable that, because the influence of psychological maturation on diagnosis renders the same behavior a symptom at one time and a normal response at another, children's symptoms are best seen not as in them but as relational attributes. (See chapter 10.)

Strictly psychiatric symptomatology seems to shade off into other, closely related states in neurological disorders and in religious experience. When manifested solely in terms of psychological (including behavioral) dysfunction, psychological disorders used to be distinguished as "functional" in contrast to "organic," and this feature regularly separated psychiatry, which treats functional conditions, from neurology, with its focus on organic ones. Today's classifications are not structured to give this distinction salience, however, and theorizing increasingly hazards causal accounts for "functional" conditions like schizophrenia and bipolar disorder, even though the actual etiology of such conditions is not fully understood. Epistemologically, functional and organic disorders remain significantly distinct. Yet symptom similarities sometimes invite a disregard for the division separating functional from organic disorders and, by extension, psychiatry from neurology even in philosophical analyses. To take one example: in disorders of agency, the patient complains of doing things without the usual sense of ownership and agency. Similar symptom descriptions are attributed at times to schizophrenia, a functional disorder, and at other times to frontal lobe damage, an organic condition. Should philosophical psychopathology disregard these differences? An understanding of organic disease and damage to the brain has stimulated a rich vein of recent research and theorizing, and, because of symptom similarities, some philosophical work in the field usefully extends to neurology. In the following pages, the topic of embodiment is approached this way: the recent studies on body image and body schema come from both organic and from functional pathology. (See chapter 8.)

If neurology represents one boundary of psychopathology, religious experience provides us with another. How to conceptualize this boundary, though, is itself a complex philosophical matter, as James's well-known discussion of the relationship between psychiatric symptoms and religious experiences in *The Varieties of Religious Experience* illustrates. Consider the case, introduced in chapter 21, of a man diagnosed with schizophrenia who, on hearing a loud and repeated creaking in the walls, concluded it was God telling him what he was doing was wrong. Were these sounds delusions? Medieval and early modern interpretations often portrayed "disorders of the imagination" like these as the result of supernatural forces: they were delusions and also from God. But if they were sent by God, could we allow that the sounds were still delusions? And could a religious man's beliefs clarify the meaning of his delusions, even if they were not from God?

Part II: Antinomies of Practice

Epistemological issues arise with some of the greatest urgency in psychiatric practice, where the conceptions of knowing and knowledge on which that practice depends reveal themselves in apparent antitheses. Diagnosis seems central to psychiatric practice, for example. One impulse is to describe and classify, sort and label. Yet we are wary of the false concreteness, resist the inherent artificiality, and fear the social and psychological consequences of such labeling. Or, another example: reductionism seeks to equate the mind with the brain. We are drawn to believe that the disordered mind reflects, and perhaps is nothing but, a disordered brain. Yet the patient is a person, his actions and responses the manifestations of something more than—and quite different from—a brain. Dilthey decreed that we can *explain* nature, not understand it, but we *understand* psychic life, and such understanding does not explain. Yet the demands of practice make this ostensible incompatibility deeply unsatisfying. Psychiatric practice calls for both understanding of the human sufferer we treat *and* an explanation of the source of that suffering. Several of these tensions are almost antinomies, those apparent contradictions that Kant thought arose when reason attempted to use categories completely divorced from experience. And, indeed, several of the contrasts mentioned seem to echo and exemplify Kant's Fourth Antinomy: "There is freedom in man, versus there is no freedom, only the necessity of nature."

Aspects of knowledge and belief, but also fundamental ontological questions of meaning and reality, are raised in the practice-based tension between diagnosis and antidiagnosis, as they are in the tenets of antireductionism understood within the practice context, in the methodological contrast between explanation and interpretation as it applies to psychopathology and mental disorder, and in the complex intertwining of fact and value.

PART III: NORMS, VALUES, AND ETHICS

Mental disorder affects the person in ways that reach to the very core of traditional Western values, as has been noted already. Rational autonomy and competence, responsibility and unified personhood are some of the qualities that make us human, inspire our reverence, and guide and explain ethical and cultural practices. By eroding those attributes that are most importantly definitive of personhood itself, mental disorder places its sufferers at risk of stigma, discrimination, ill treatment, and neglect and has stood for centuries as an emblem of negativity.

Policies and practices pertaining to the treatment and care of the mentally ill by others, such as the involuntary commitment of those dangerous to others or themselves, seem to be particularly polarizing and irreconcilably contested. An underlying tension sets apart the liberal values that emphasize individual freedom and permit adults to determine their own fate, however self-destructive, from the values of a paternalism or "parentalism" that emphasizes the social nature of individuals and the responsibilities of others to care for, protect, and promote the well-being and best interests of those individuals.

In the arena of treatment and research ethics, the special vulnerability of mental patients, the effect of their condition on their capacity to defend themselves against exploitation, and the harm they risk due to negative social attitudes—all call for special constraints on those who treat them. The attention, confidentiality, respect, patience, and integrity patients deserve from caregivers and researchers alike suggest that treatment and research ethics involve certain niceties and require the cultivation of certain virtues not as essential in other professional or even other medical settings.

Efforts to identify and define criminal insanity highlight the place of responsibility concepts in psychiatry. The guiding tenet—that when mental disorder brings about wrongful actions, it serves to exculpate—reveals the deeply metaphysical attitudes at work here and the close links with theories of self, personhood, and free will, (never far from the surface in discussions of responsibility), that complicate conclusions and alter intuitions in this area.

Although cultural categories such as gender and race are pertinent to every illness, the many-stranded Western cultural associations that link gender and race to madness have had an especially profound influence on psychiatry. As forms of otherness, madness and blackness, for example, and madness and the feminine have both been entwined in cultural tropes that influence diagnosis, perceptions of mental health, and aspects of psychiatric treatment. To give one example: gender affects the way we come to form and express conceptions of identity and selfhood at the center of the therapeutic enterprise of self-transformation. In a culture in which these classifications have such prominence, my therapeutic goal is to be a more mentally healthy woman as much as to be a more mentally healthy person.

Part IV: Theoretical Models

Since its inception with Greek medicine—when the condition of the four humors of blood, phlegm, yellow bile, and black bile was believed to explain all abnormal as well as normal states—theorizing about madness, melancholia, and mental disorder has been elaborate and all-encompassing. With the decline of humoral accounts and the emergence of a discipline recognizable as early psychiatry came new, contradictory, and strongly contested theories and theorizing. By the first decades of the twentieth century, Darwinism, psychoanalysis, behaviorism, and phenomenology (together with something closer to today's biomedical psychiatry) each proffered competing theories and theoretical models in their efforts to explain and treat mental disorder. The fortunes of these different models have waxed and waned, and each has been subject to significant refinement and reformulation; so transformed, each of these alternative theoretical frameworks has its supporters today. And to these explanatory theories have been added, in the last quarter of the twentieth century, social constructionist analyses.

Most influential in contemporary biological psychiatry, the neurobiological model offers us a seamlessly naturalistic explanation. Merely because the patient is a person—his actions and responses the manifestations of something more than a brain—we may be dissatisfied by the implicit reductionism in this account. But close philosophical analysis also reveals problems internal to the naturalistic system. (See chapter 25.) And the analyses undertaken here identify somewhat comparable flaws in each of the explanatory models enumerated, including the suggestive, but incomplete, social constructionist hypothesis.

Moreover, the composite "biopsychosocial" theory, which attempts an amalgam of several of these types of explanation, has fared no better when subject to a careful analysis; it is not a model in any scientific sense (McLaren 1998).

The quest for explanation in psychiatry appears to be far from ended. Yet the importance of finding a successful explanatory model or explanatory models for psychiatry can hardly be overestimated. Remarkable advances have been made in an "evidence-based" measurement of mental disorder and its treatment, advances that account for increasingly precise and extensive predictive knowledge. But only a complete understanding of etiology can permit the targeted treatment, prevention, and even cure that must be the fervently sought goal of all. Painstaking and impeccable empirical research grounded in coherent and precise theorizing is the only likely path toward that understanding.

PART V: CIRCUMSCRIBING MENTAL DISORDER

Two discussions in the philosophy of psychiatry stand out for their far-reaching moral and social policy implications, of which one, noted earlier, centers on the category of delusion. The other concerns the category of mental disorder itself and the presumption that, while not easily captured in a covering definition, such a category usefully unites the many and various psychological and behavioral "syndromes" collected in, for example, the DSMs and ICDs (Diagnostic and Statistical Manuals and International Classification of Diseases). Important philosophical aspects of this issue include the extension and intension of the expression "mental disorder." Attempts to define mental disorder such as Wakefield's well-known account, which combines a value term ("harmful") with a scientific one ("disfunction") to yield a hybrid definition of mental disorder as harmful disfunction, appear to be flawed, much recent philosophical analysis has suggested. (See chapter 29.) An alternative definition is examined and defended here.

As vigorously debated as the intensional definition of mental disorder are the reasons why, rather than representing a stable phenomenon the way other medical conditions generally do, mental disorders appear to multiply and mutate at a confusing and even a suspicious rate. Now at more than 800 pages, the most recent edition of the DSM is swollen with new diagnostic categories, and startling increases are today reported in other disorders that once were believed rare. These changes in diagnosis are sometimes attributed to previous underdiagnosis and misdiagnosis. At other times, they are attributed to changes in epidemiology. The latter interpretation seems to presuppose causes for mental disorder that are as much social, political, and broadly cultural as internal and biological, or even more so—a position for which there is considerable, and unsettling, support. The part allegedly played by the psychopharmacology industry in psychiatric research and the apparently growing "medicalization" of aspects of human behavior are trends with profound moral and philosophical implications. These implications, and the politics and economics of psychiatry, call for unswerving and disinterested investigation.

This is a book that should be of equal interest to philosophers, psychiatrists, and psychologists; to theorists and practitioners; and, not least, to those whose troubling mental states are its central concern.

Overview of the Chapters in This Volume

Chapter 1—Grant Gillett explores the clinical phenomenology of symptoms such as hallucination, delusion, loosened associations, and pressure of thought that collectively make up what is sometimes termed a "loss of contact with reality." Employing the presuppositions of his influential narrative theory of the mind, Gillett shows the implications of these deficiencies in a creature that depends, as we humans do, on epistemological foundations secured intersubjectively through convergence with others in judgment, affirmation, and validation. On this analysis, psychotic thinking results from a loss of attunement, as Gillett puts it, between the cognitive skills of the psychotic person and those of others.

Chapter 2—In a comprehensive review of recent philosophical interest in depression and manic depression, Jennifer Hansen distinguishes three broad approaches: the moral one, which explores the effect of depression on moral psychology, particularly self-knowledge; the medical one, which seeks to clarify whether depression is a natural kind or a discrete disease entity; and the social/political one, which asks, as she puts it, what depression reveals about how modernity and its political and social forces press upon humanity. This thoughtful discussion concludes with the observation that philosophers and other creative people are "doomed to muse about depression as long as they muse about anything."

Chapter 3—Alan Soble takes as his topic the psychiatric disorder category of paraphilia, hitherto known by the perjorative label "sexual perversion." In a close analysis of changes between the third edition of the DSM, with its landmark omission of homosexuality from the category of paraphilias, and the current fourth edition, Soble explores the heavy conceptual reliance on a criterion of subjective distress over sexuality, whether homosexual or heterosexual, and points to serious vulnerabilities incumbent in that reliance which suggest that apparent progress on this subject may be illusory.

Chapter 4—Louis Charland explores the normative concept of character that underlies the conditions known as personality disorders. In an innovative analysis, Charland argues that these conditions are moral, not medical, entities, characterized in terms of moral traits. As such, he argues, they are best approached through moral treatment reminiscent of the concept of moral treatment employed in nineteenth-century practice. Through a nuanced and historically sensitive discussion, Charland illustrates the presence of evaluative elements alongside the descriptive elements within psychiatric categories and theorizing.

Chapter 5—Weakness of will has perplexed philosophers since Plato. In this new analysis, Al Mele approaches the definition of volitional disorders by trying to draw a line between the commonplace though puzzling condition known to philosophers as weakness of will and volitional disorder. Key here is the notion of the irresistability and resistability of pertinent desires, which Mele explores in relation to George Ainslie's work on the ability to make and adhere to personal rules.

Chapter 6—The strange phenomenon of thought insertion appears to tell us something important about all human subjectivity. Building on his earlier, influential work in this field, George Graham here argues that, although descriptions of thought insertion at first sight provide counterexamples that require us to adjust our principle of ascription immunity by which present-tense ascription of one's thoughts is immune from ascription error, when we look closer, it proves more plausible to see first-person reports of inserted thoughts as equivocal.

Chapter 7—The literature on dissociation provides many opportunities for clarification and analysis. Following his earlier groundbreaking work on dissociation, Stephen Braude offers a criterion for attributing dissociation that corrects lacunae and errors in the standard definitions. Using that analysis, he critiques the debate over whether dissociation constitutes one or several distinct phenomena and comments on its apparent significance for philosophical assertions about the unity of the self.

Chapter 8—Disorders of embodiment, in this illuminating and original discussion by Shaun Gallagher and Mette Vaever, are disorders in which the body is not only the cause of the problem but the locus or theme of symptomatology—depersonalization, anorexia nervosa, and unilateral neglect, for example. Appealing to phenomenological accounts of embodied action, these authors focus on how disorders of embodiment can affect the "minimal self," a precondition for more sophisticated forms of cognition and action, and its corresponding form of self-awareness.

Chapter 9—Mental disorder disrupts the continuity that unites earlier and later parts of ourselves and constitutes personal identity; because these ideas also implicate categories such as agency and responsibility, moreover, the challenges to personal identity inherent in mental disorder provide some guide to the practical and policy issues concerning the mentally ill. Jennifer Radden shows how characterization identity, constituted by the content of a person's self-concept, plays an important part in practice, as well as in diagnostic categories such as Gender Identity Disorder, a diagnosis that has been the subject of recent, vehement critique.

Chapter 10—Thus far, Christian Perring points out, philosophers have paid scant attention to the several ethical, conceptual, metaphysical, and epistemological issues raised by psychopathology in children and adolescents. This is a rich field of inquiry, though, with distinctive and pressing ethical concerns over, for example, consent to treatment. Theories of child development have been the focus of philosophical attention since Greek theories of innate knowledge. Today, Perring illustrates, child development is central to debates over the "theory" theory of mind, feminist critiques of Freud's psychosexual theories, and sociological theorizing about the effects of culture.

Chapter 11—In his discussion of diagnosis, John Sadler emphasizes that this most apparently scientific activity of sorting and labeling disorders is imbued with moral, social, and political meaning, and he explores diagnosis as characterization, as disclosure, as relevance, as privilege, as rationality, and as ritual. For Sadler, at least, diagnosis is a way of life and a language game of the greatest cultural significance: it cannot be reduced to the labeling practices that its critics have so vociferously decried.

Chapter 12—Exploring Dilthy's decree that we *understand* rather than explain psychic life, James Phillips asks not simply what we gain and lose if we substitute causal, disease-oriented explanations for interpretive understanding of meaning structures in psychiatry but how we might transcend their apparent incompatibilities to employ both methodologies together. He explores these in relation to a richly described clinical case, that of Mrs. D., who suffers from clinical depression.

Chapter 13—Philosophical naturalism and the doctrine of the unity of science, Tim Thornton illustrates, have provided a powerful impetus for a sweeping reductionism by which the mind, including the disordered mind, is nothing more than the brain. But, as Thornton goes on to point out in a creative and original discussion, there is a long tradition that can be traced from Jaspers through Wittgenstein to the contemporary philosopher John McDowell's contrast between the space of reasons and the realm of law, in which mind, meaning and mental content, and mental disorder, are importantly irreducible.

Chapter 14—That values are inextricably tied to facts throughout psychiatry—as, indeed, throughout all medicine—is incontrovertible today; so is the fact that values represent an irreducible plurality. In a path-breaking development on these two points, Bill Fulford has delineated the ten principles that make up what he terms Values-Based Medicine (VBM): the theory and practice of effective health-care decision making in situations in which diverse and potentially incompatible values perspectives are present.

Chapter 15—Arguing for an acknowledgment of (and a resolve to better understand the central place of) gender in psychiatric practice, Nancy Potter emphasizes that gender differences are partly marked and constituted by the very words we utter. And so fundamental is this gendering of language that we may need to search for another language for psychiatric practice with women, a language that will "allow women to situate themselves as subjects, not in dominant discourse but in an alternative discourse of their own making." Moreover, because of its links with gender and power, Potter illustrates that trust and building trust must be part of all therapeutic engagement.

Chapter 16—In an important and compelling discussion, Marilyn Nissim-Sabat exposes the influence of race and culture within psychiatry, using the ideas of thinkers who have shaped race theory. The categories of race and culture are linked, Nissim-Sabat argues, in and through the historical and material character of race as a cultural construct and through "raciation," the process of cultural production that perpetuates racism and all its incumbent suffering. The work of Michel Foucault, Frantz Fanon, and E. V. Wolfenstein is presented and subjected to careful critique in this far-reaching analysis.

Chapter 17—Charles Culver and Bernard Gert here analyze the definition of consent and its application in particular cases. No concept is more central to mental health law and bioethics than is competence to consent, and this discussion possesses significant practical implications. Culver and Gert propose going beyond the "understanding plus appreciation" definition, sometimes employed with counterintuitive results. A person is competent to make a particular medical decision on Culver and Gert's definition if and only if she has the ability to make a rational decision of the particular kind involved.

Chapter 18—Daniel Robinson cites case law and public policy in his thorough discussion of the important moral and legal concept of dangerousness as it applies to mental disorder. His account highlights the uneasy balance between ensuring safety for those endangered when their actions pose a threat (to self or others) and respecting individual rights. In the end, he concludes, the fulcrum that would seek to balance these conflicting goals should be set at a point that is clearly advantageous to the rights of the individual over the collective.

Chapter 19—Ruth Chadwick and Gordon Aindow provide an illuminating analysis and taxonomy of the myriad ethical issues that arise in psychiatric treatment and research settings. These range from enduring concerns over compulsory treatment and the questions of consent that occur in treatment and research settings alike to recently encountered dilemmas over drug treatment and psychiatric genetics. Chadwick and Aindow also explore broader questions, including the appropriate ethical framework for treatment and research ethics, the relationship between psychiatric and other biomedical ethics, and the current dominance of the autonomy principle.

Chapter 20—The history of efforts to identify and define criminal insanity, elegantly reviewed by Simon Wilson and Gwen Adshead, illustrates the intertwining of methodological, metaphysical, and moral theorizing in this area. The links with personhood and theories of free will complicate conclusions and alter intuitions, these authors illustrate, as do psychiatry's moves between physical and intentional explanations for bad intentions.

Chapter 21 — In a controversial and intriguing discussion, Brooke Hopkins and Margaret Battin ask whether the medical model of psychiatric illness might leave room for other, more religiously based approaches to mental suffering. In developing an answer to this broad question about the compatibility between religion and psychiatry, these authors compare religious experience with psychiatric symptoms and investigate the relationships between religion and such symptoms and between religion and psychiatry understood as institutions.

Chapter 22 — Mental disorders are likely not all explained the same way from an evolutionary perspective. But agreement over evolutionary psychiatry and its significance, Dominic Murphy illustrates, is limited to an acceptance of the basic model wherein at least some mental disorders are understood as failures of domain-specific modules to perform their evolutionary function. Beyond that, he shows, different and incompatible theories can be sorted into two strategies: one that seeks to identify a once adaptive trait that is no longer adaptive; the other arguing that mental disorders are inevitable by-products of normally adaptive traits.

Chapter 23 — The psychoanalytic model delineated by Freud reflects the extent to which Freud was a philosophical thinker, Bettina Bergo emphasizes, aware both of the antecedents and of the philosophical implications of his metapsychology. Freud's own great philosophical contribution, which forms the basis of that model not just for abnormal psychology but for all psychotherapeutic endeavor, is the notion of the unconsciousness, and Bergo provides us with a meticulous and illuminating account of the philosophical context for that category. In addition, she shows how hysteria, the emblematic condition of Freudian psychopathology, upset fundamental philosophical assumptions — about mind and body, the experiential and the speculative, and even the masculine and the feminine.

Chapter 24 — Michael Schwartz and Osborne Wiggins argue that an exclusive employment of the methodologies of "evidence-based" psychiatry and neurobiology, neither applicable to psychopathology and psychotherapy, forfeits, as they say, a large part of the understanding of mental disorders. While insisting that there cannot be an all-inclusive theory of mental disorders, these authors detail and discuss the "laws of psychological understanding" enunciated by Karl Jaspers and emphasize the neglected value of understanding and interpretation in an essential and complementary explanatory model.

Chapter 25 — In considering the neurobiological model that is so influential in contemporary psychiatry, Andrew Garnar and Valerie Hardcastle identify an unacknowledged assumption, the concept of "soma," on which the model appears to rest. Soma is compared to a Sellarsian "given," at once a transcendental abstraction and an imminant particular. The identification of "soma" within the neurobiological model is one of several challenges to the completeness and orientation of that model put forward in this controversial and arresting analysis.

Chapter 26 — In his discussion of cognitive-behavioral models for therapy, Edwin Erwin portrays a field deeply divided over such fundamental questions as the causal role of cognitions and the effectiveness of the cognitive therapies (Albert Ellis's Rational Emotive Behavior Therapy and Aaron Beck's cognitive therapy, for example).

Disagreements also persist, he illustrates, about a wide range of less immediately practical questions, including postulating unobservables, the goals of science, epiphenomenalism, and the nature of truth, logic, explanation, and causation.

Chapter 27 — Reviewing contemporary social constructionist models, Jennifer Church remarks that these are exciting, but also exasperating. In her even-handed analysis of social constructionist accounts of mental disorder, Church points out that there is no reason to suppose a socially constructed mental disorder would be any easier to change than a naturally constituted disorder, or that such a change is even desirable. But this new theory has strengths also, eliciting more imaginative responses from us and making us less inclined to seek consensus.

Chapter 28 — What Rom Harré calls the "benchmark problem" is the problem of determining a diagnostic benchmark beyond which the ordinary (or normal) becomes extraordinary (or abnormal). Through an exploration of three diagnoses, Chronic Fatigue Syndrome, schizophrenia, and Tourette's syndrome, Harré shows the extent to which psychiatric diagnosis involves what philosophers have called essentially contested concepts. When discernible physically abnormal states are absent, he shows, benchmarks for normality and tolerability are intrinsically unstable and arbitrary.

Chapter 29 — In order to reach those who treat mental disorders, Bernard Gert and Charles Culver focus their discussion on the "official" definition of mental disorders found in the current edition of the DSM, a definition that these authors have been instrumental in formulating and refining. Gert and Culver explain the DSM definition, defending it against criticisms and showing its virtues in contrast to Wakefield's influential alternative definition of mental disorder.

Chapter 30 — Carl Elliott takes as his topic the significance of what studies suggest is "an epidemic of psychopathology." His explanation is multifaceted and far-reaching, pointing to the ascendency of biomedicine and to psychodynamic theory, the development of psychopharmacology, the blurred boundaries of diagnostic categories, and the collusion of patients and patient groups, among other factors. The pervasive influence of biomedicine, Elliott concludes, has come to affect the way we all describe our mental lives.

REFERENCES

McLaren, N. (1998) "A Critical Review of the Biopsychosocial Model." *Australian and New Zealand Journal of Psychiatry* 32: 86–92.
Wittgenstein, L. (1977) *Culture and Value*. Oxford: Blackwell.

PART I

PSYCHOPATHOLOGY
AND NORMALCY

CHAPTER 1

COGNITION

Brain Pain: Psychotic Cognition, Hallucinations, and Delusions

GRANT GILLETT

THE psychoses, which normally are taken to include schizophrenia and major mood disorders, present clinicians with dramatic examples of thought disorder. Patients with these conditions are prone to hallucinations, delusions, pressure of thought, and thought insertion, along with disorganized speech, flattening of affect, and social or occupational dysfunction (American Psychiatric Association 1994: 285). Each of these represents a major departure from the natural and assured patterns of thought and feeling exhibited by normal people such that the key cognitive symptoms have been collectively termed "loss of contact with reality." Exploration of the clinical phenomenology of these symptoms yields a vivid picture of psychotic thought disorder and allows us to sketch a synthetic understanding of the breakdown in cognition that occurs and the suffering that marks these most severe of psychiatric disorders.

DELUSIONS

James was admitted to the emergency psychiatric assessment unit because his roommates were alarmed by his behavior and conversation. He said he knew of a serious conspiracy. He had signed up while still a student to be part of military intelligence, and, in the course of his service, he had come across some revealing evidence. He had noticed that people were shadowing him on campus and in the streets and had applied for a firearm license to protect himself. He was really on edge because, he said, the conspirators were actively placing people close to him, sometimes disguised as friends and acquaintances, and he believed they wanted to have him killed.

Delusions are usually conceptualized as false beliefs, and James's delusions are typical examples of the phenomenon. However, it has long been recognized that the contents of some delusions are not the sort of thing that is straightforwardly true or false and that some can (by any test) be true — the famous Othello delusion is a case in point. A characteristic type of this sort of indeterminate delusion is the conviction that one is totally corrupt and verminous and, because of this mortal corruption, already destined for eternal damnation. The conceptual problem posed by defining what counts as a delusion has motivated attempts to find a definition that includes all thoroughgoing examples of psychotic delusions but not other things such as over-valued ideas. Jaspers claims that delusions are *so implausible as to be incomprehensible*, but others say that they are incorrigible and therefore unresponsive to evidence. However, the conceptual problems persist. For instance, psychotic patients are *not* unresponsive to evidence; rather, they tend to accommodate it into their paranoid thought in a way that defies credibility. Imagine that James (in our example) is given evidence that his roommates have been totally supportive and that, in fact, some of them have been friends for years. He agrees but responds by arguing that part of the plot involves the substitution of secret agents who look exactly like his closest friends for the real friends (Capgras syndrome; Gelder et al. 1983: 15).

The nature of psychotic irrationality and the cognitive dynamics of a psychotic break in the sense of self are both hotly debated. In entering this debate, it seems obvious that any account of these phenomena in the context of psychosis ought to draw on an adequate understanding of our normal thinking and its role in informing our contact with the world.

Our prereflective theory of knowledge locates the individual in a community of socially embodied creatures who share a perspective on the world and jointly come to know what their surroundings are like. But philosophical reflection on these common-sense cognitive skills often begins by supposing that the individual has only the clues provided by perception to work with and that those clues derive only from the sensory excitations of our receptor surfaces and nerve endings. Ulrich Neisser, a cognitive psychologist, comments on the difficult task of perception, as seen through this model. He notes that the subject has to figure out what the world is really like from a retinal image that is "upside-down, foreshortened, and the wrong size" (1976: 16). Even a short walk along this garden path encourages one to question the traditional empiricist view and to try to relate cognition directly to the real world of public objects and other people. Such an account would, in the present context, turn the philosophical gaze on the cognitive skills that go wrong when the mind evinces "a gross impairment in reality testing" (American Psychiatric Association 1994: 273).

HALLUCINATIONS

Most psychotic hallucinations are auditory and involve voices. The voices may be unpleasant and accusatory or just offer commentary and asides on the situation in which the person finds himself. DSM IV states that psychotic "voices" are "perceived as distinct from the person's own thoughts" (American Psychiatric Association 1994: 275), and Jaynes observes that hallucinations in hospitalized patients have certain common characteristics, such as suddenness of onset, religious themes, conflicting messages, and a critical tone (1990: 160). He also notes that verbal hallucinations are in fact common in disparate groups, including homeless people in New York City, normal college students, children, and nonverbal populations such as patients with cerebral palsy. He argues that verbal hallucinations, which are often admonitory, are residues of verbal interactions that are improperly integrated into the consciousness of the subject and represent a reversion to a preconscious form of mentality (1990: 170). I will pursue this strand of thought in the theoretical framework for psychotic thought that emerges from a post-Kantian approach to epistemology and the philosophy of mind.

THOUGHT DISORDER: LOOSENING OF ASSOCIATIONS

> In my mind I have gold and jewels but I must give them away because I'll get lost in the maddening wine. I give you a million spherical dreams. The jewels of friends. Halley's comet is in the sky and it's the sign of a new rock and roll song of a new generation while the conflict between the person I should have been and the person I am reverberates down the echo chambers of my mind. The last book has rolled into place. (Gates and Hammond 1993: 178)

As in many examples of psychotic thought, one has the impression that there is a train of thought here, despite the distortions and distractions, able to be followed and interpreted. The illusion that one has almost got a clear view of a mental will-o'-the-wisp is a revealing phenomenological feature about psychotic thinking. It indicates that the thoughts are connected but the connections are slippery; they elude one's cognitive grasp, and the illusion of meaningfulness is like that found in a blurred or shifting puzzle picture the content of which seems to change as you try to define it or get it in focus.

The incoherence seems to result, at least in part, from a loosening of associations or dysfunction at a neurocognitive level. Most regard this as a causal, extraconscious, or biological factor in the genesis of psychotic thought patterns (somewhat similar to the motor effects commonly seen in psychosis; Manschrek 1992). The effects of this associational disorder in the brain are manifold and include such things as flight of ideas (the tendency for thoughts to rapidly shift from one idiosyncratic and haphazard theme to another often linked only in a tenuous or fanciful way), incoherent thought, pressure of speech (the impression that the patient's words are jostling to be spoken and form a forced, unstoppable flow of conversation), clang associations ("thanks" — "banks"; "extensive" — "intensive"; "Holy Grail" — "wailing wall"). These are collectively designated *Zerfahrenheit*, or loss of the internal and external connectedness of those series of ideas that, for most of us, form trains of thought. *Zerfahrenheit* indicates a detachment of thinking from the framework of everyday knowledge, common sense, and practical relevance and comprises "paralogies, neologisms, bizarreness, mannerisms, stereotypies, perseverations, iterations, verbigerations, viscosity" and other abnormalities evident in psychotic thought (Sass 1992). For example, "one of Gruhle's patients, in a specific affective state, noticed three marble tables in a cafe and was suddenly convinced that the end of the world was imminent" (1992: 153). One can only speculate why a thought of the end of the world might attach itself to this perception, but, once it has done so, as Gruhle and Sass both remark, the idea becomes imbued with the same direct certainty as the perception of the tables.

Recent experimental work confirms that purely incidental or meaningless connections occur more frequently in schizophrenic patients (Spitzer 1992). Gruhle's example brings out the fact that the psychotic treats such connections as if they have the same epistemic status as those that underpin normal beliefs. The idea of associational promiscuity and attempts to investigate it are not new; Jung investigated word associations in healthy people under normal conditions and noticed that conceptually driven associations decreased while clang associations increased when attention was artificially disengaged by distraction from the task in hand (Spitzer 1992: 170). Jung's explanation centered on the nature of attention as a device serving "the purpose of maintaining a particular idea within consciousness and stabilizing its direction or goal" (Spitzer 1992: 171). More recent work on lexical decision making and semantic priming in psychosis reveals "a larger semantic priming effect in thought disordered schizophrenic patients" which reverts to normal as the acute disorders of thought are brought under control (Spitzer 1992: 186–87). On studying the patterns of loosening of associations, Spitzer concludes:

> Inhibitory processes by which irrelevant associations are normally excluded from consciousness are defective in schizophrenic patients. As the maintenance of an organized sequence of thought and of organized language utterance requires the operation of a goal-directed organization of thoughts . . . it can only be accomplished by active inhibition (exclusion) of associations that are irrelevant to the intended utterance. (187)

Spitzer and psychiatrists such as Jung, Kraepelin, and Jaspers use their understanding of the nature of the mind to illuminate the disorders found in psychotic thinking. In contemporary psychiatric literature, disorders of thought form, and content (such as delusion, hallucination, and flight of ideas) are often studied empirically by some sort of counting. But, when we look at the mental phenomena of psychotic consciousness more phenomenologically, we begin to lay bare the true suffering of psychosis.

Attentional Disorder

Luria, the Russian neuropsychologist, thought deeply about cognitive functions and the brain mechanisms that subserved them, sometimes with surprising results. For instance, he concluded that the training of the skills of attention is a social function and that its adult form was as much a social as a biological product (Luria 1973: 262). He argued that the direction of cognitive resources toward selected environmental targets is a skill that is shaped in children by adults and maintained by the culture in which a thinker is embedded.

The idea of intersubjectivity as a significant medium for the development of cognitive skills (such as the ability to make warranted judgments and come to justified beliefs) is found in both Kant (1789 [1929]) and Wittgenstein (1953: #242). Both argue that a grasp of the rules that govern the use of a concept (its applications and its internal role in thought sequences) is shaped by modeling the actions of fellow human beings and responding to their corrective responses. The idea is that one learns to make certain judgments, such as <that is red>, <that dog is running>, and so on, from others and achieves congruence with them. The structure and coherence of one's mental world therefore reflects, in part, the cumulative result of using skills developed in human forms of life, rather than the functioning of a set of mechanistic cognitive operations working (solipsistically) on the stimulations falling on receptor surfaces.

On this view, which we could call "discursive naturalism," the mind is fluid, dynamic, and open to interpersonal effects, its operations governed by informal (prescriptive) norms imparted through discourse. As a result of relationships between persons *qua* persons who think and act, we configure each others' cognitive networks to work in congruent ways in relation to a shared environment. Thus, human individuals normally (in the sense of a "normal function," as discussed by Millikan 1993) communicate and cooperate in a way that crucially involves mutual comprehension. This is the secret of our success as members of a collectively adapted species who both equip one another and learn from one another so as to form a social order comprised of complementary empowering discourses. Discourses embed what Wittgenstein called language games, and it is in these that patterns of activity and explanation (where ideas such as expectation, hope, commitment, and so on) can arise, forming a consistent context for interpersonal behavior. R. D. Laing has argued (famously or notoriously, depending on your point of view) that these normal features of human intercourse may be suspended in the Kafkaesque world of certain institutional settings and in some families (1966).

The norms that shape discourse are pervasive, governing judgments about the contents of an experience, techniques of belief formation, and the conduct of mental life in general. Thus, individual mental life—forming an autobiographical consciousness—is built on techniques that are informal and intersubjective, and human beings latch onto these techniques by participating in situations and relationships where linguistic terms or signs mark certain ways of responding to the world (Gillett 1992). Note that, on this view, any given individual does not choose the techniques that underpin the use of a concept; she obeys shared prescriptive norms and in grasping those norms must appreciate that there are right and wrong ways of organizing her thoughts about the relevant experiences. In this sense, the normative (Husserl—"noematic"; Wittgenstein—"grammatical") permeates the actual world of human discourse affecting individual functioning and generates an adequate set of cognitive skills.

SELF-KNOWLEDGE

The discursive approach also elucidates the problem of self-reflexive thought. A thinker learns to shape her own use of concepts according to the normative reactions of others to her judgments, as when she says, "That is a car," and they say, "No, it is a van." But, just as she can learn to imitate their responses to objects of mutual attention, so she can learn to mimic their corrective responses toward herself as a thinker. Thus, in the process of mastering concepts, a thinker also masters the ability to judge of herself whether she is doing it right. Lewis observes "with every mental activity—or act—there is an observing or registering of its apprehended quality apart from the material upon which the function in question is being exercised" (1934: 19). Regarding self as an object of one's own judgments (which the existentialists and phenomenologists call "reflective consciousness") is often called "internalization" of, inter alia, the fact that others regard self as such an object. Freud, in fact, focused on the moral or conative role of self-reflexive judgment when he discussed the formation of the superego. On the present account, this is a complex task in which the subject focuses on his own response and assays a normative assessment of that response according to parental, social, and cultural residues. The techniques we are talking about are pervasive and allow one to formulate, as it were, a normative commentary that implicitly relates one's own judgments to the judgments of others. They are also multifaceted, with evaluative and epistemic overtones that, one imagines, might plausibly become intertwined, especially in light of the fact that belonging to a well-adapted human group is so fundamental in the human motivational structure.

Reflective techniques are, as one would expect, a little more difficult to master than the ability to make straightforward judgments about external states of affairs, and the judgments are much more loaded with emotive, conative, or evaluative nuances and implications. It is, therefore, understandable that self-knowledge — or the set of abilities gathered under the term "insight" — is highly prone to disruption by disorders of thought and judgment. That disruption is exaggerated greatly when the individual is attentionally "out of synch" with others because of internal neurocognitive disfunction or a context of disordered or pathological interpersonal discourse.

Human beings learn a set of focused and directed intentional skills that fix the conditions sufficient to ground a given conceptualization and then use this directed activity to organize and guide their behavior. We learn these skills from others by building a repertoire of well-honed normative and rule-governed techniques that structure our cognitive engagement with the social and natural world. However, it seems that psychosis is marked by a crucial inability to screen stimuli and develop selective attentional skills, an impairment that is explained by a neurophysiological or psychological disfunction (Hemsley 1977). Studies of attention, perception, and cognition in schizophrenic patients lead Hemsley to conclude that "schizophrenia is characterized by a weakening of the influence of regularities of previous input on current perception" (1992: 236). We might therefore expect the schizophrenic patient to be alienated from a world in which others feel secure and assured in their mental life and are cognitively supported by concurrence in judgment with others. This loneliness is a source not only of confusion and the thought disorders characteristic of schizophrenia but also of the suffering that results from the feeling of isolation and the loss of one's place in the world.

The impaired operation of socially attuned attentional mechanisms might also be expected to explain the hyperacuity of schizophrenic patients, who sometimes notice all sorts of things about their therapist and appear to "look right through" the many little strategies the therapist and normal people have for hiding their imperfections or disaffections in a conversation. It seems that the strategies of self-presentation, designed to distract people well attuned to prevalent social conventions, do not have that effect in someone who is not so attuned and who may be hyperattentive to incidental and "irrelevant" stimulus cues.

A fundamental neurochemical disorder responsible for loosening of associations may also be discerned in the motor disorders commonly seen in schizophrenia. The most frequent disorders seem maximally to affect practiced rhythmic activities in which a normal subject would use the inherent redundancy of the task to allow it to be performed in a more or less automatic mode (Manschrek 1992). When we look for a related disorder in thought, it seems that the rhythmic background of cognitive processing that attunes a human being to the normal flow of interpersonal and ecological information is disrupted and to thereby throw the patient "out of synch" with others.

In fact, a great deal of work was done on attention in the 1960s that both prefigured and inspired recent experiments. The thrust of the work was that selective attention processes are disabled in psychosis (McGhie 1969: 44–45). A number of first-person reports from patients support this suggestion:

> I take more time to do things because I am always conscious of what I am doing.
> If I could just stop noticing what I am doing, I would get things done a lot faster.
>   My trouble is that I've got too many thoughts. You might think about something, let's say that ashtray and just think, oh yes, that's for putting my cigarette in, but I would think of it and then I would think of a dozen different things connected with it at the same time. (48)

The suggested role of attention in thought and experience is directly reminiscent of remarks by Luria and the phenomenologists to the effect that we categorize the information that reaches us from the environment in light of past experience so as to organize and interpret the otherwise chaotic flow of information available to consciousness (49). Selective attention and techniques of judgment that underpin the content of consciousness produce the autobiographical narrative that is lived personal identity. The posited disorders of attention would have serious and diverse effects on the thought life of the psychotic patient, creating significant dislocation between his cognitive world and the world of others.

McGhie differentiates between two types of cognitive disorder in psychosis: one characterized by disintegration and fragmentation of experience and narrative consciousness and the other a focused paranoid type of psychosis in which attention is intensified and constrained by a delusional system or systems. In either case, there is a loss of the normal balance between flexibility and focus of cognition. Thought develops a schizoid quality (characterized by shyness, oversensitivity, conflict, and contradiction), which denies the psychotic mind the practiced adaptive interaction between mind and world that most people enjoy. Attentional mechanisms organize this normal engagement so that the exploration of novelty and the focused attention on what is familiar are combined in the exercise of successful behavioral strategies. The "schizoid gap" results from a breakdown of attentional synchrony with other human beings. This is a rift both between the subject and the world and between the psychotic and others with whom they share that world so that even ordinary conversation can become difficult:

> When people talk to me now it's like a different kind of language. It's too much to
> hold at once. My head is overloaded and I can't understand what they say. It
> makes you forget what you've just heard because you can't get hearing it long
> enough. It's all in different bits which you have to put together again in your head —
> just words in the air unless you can figure it out from their faces. (62)

This conversational disorder seems related to the schizophrenic patient's inability to use the normal contextual, structural, and rhythmic clues and the redundancies and stimulus parsing that normal subjects use to disambiguate the flow of linguistic information (63). Again we see the disruption of an often overlooked cognitive task that is pivotal in maintaining mental contact between human beings in relation to their shared environment. Given the sensitive two-way connection between language and thought and the role of language in training and maintaining the skills used in thinking about what is happening to oneself and others, the malfunction of these mechanisms is seriously maladaptive and deeply threatening to one's sense of who one is and the significance of events around one.

McGhie's work has stimulated ongoing experimentation on links between attentional mechanisms and schizophrenia to examine whether psychotic thought is disrupted because of "flooding by excessive and poorly inhibited enteroceptive and exteroceptive stimuli leading to cognitive fragmentation" (Venables 1960: 78). It emerges that information-processing deficits at least correlate with, and may have a causal relationship to, thought disorder (Perry and Braff 1994). For instance, the ego-impairment index examines the consistency with which subjects deploy categories or "internal constructs to interpret exteroceptive stimuli" (366). Poor scores on this index are correlated with impaired prepulse inhibition of auditory startle responses, which is a measure of experiential effects on responses to novel stimuli (startle responses can be diminished by giving the subject a warning stimulus before the unexpected stimulus is delivered). What is more, severe social dysfunction in schizophrenic patients is correlated with greater defects on selected attentional tasks (Carter et al. 1992). Taken together, these findings support the hypothesis that there are defects in inhibition and attentional screening of information that interfere with the adaptation of the psychotic patient in ordinary society. This is as one would expect if, as cognitive psychologists suggest, normal subjects are continually creating and refining expectations that allow them to deal with the flux of stimuli that bombards them in the everyday world.

This set of studies and the appeal to Luria's remark that attention is a social rather than a biological mechanism emphasizes the fact that psychosis involves a defect in the skills that enable an integrated and holistically functioning psychosomatic reality. Psychotics think and move in strange ways, sketching and filling in their perceptual worlds differently from those of us who march to the beat of the shared cognitive drum. This difference alienates them from the rest of us, and they experience the confusion and distress of being apparently abandoned in a world that has not only lost its familiarity but in which they are cast adrift from the guides that would normally sustain their participation in it. Thus, the thesis that we actively construct consciousness and self-knowledge in and through the experience of life among others has profound implications for our understanding of psychotic experience.

THE NARRATIVE SELF AND ITS INTEGRITY

I have, at diverse times and places, suggested a narrative theory of the conscious mind of the type indicated here (Gillett 1997, 1999, 2000, 2001). According to this view, we make discursive and narrative sense of ourselves as persons who live and move and have our being among others. The narrative is constructed out of the events that befall persons as detected by their information-gathering systems and rendered meaningful by their conceptual skills. The resulting story shapes holistic patterns of brain activity and thereby affects the neurophysiological stream that constitutes the proximal effect of one's doings in the world. In making sense of the world, we apply discursive skills and norms of judgment to what is going on in that stream to produce the narratives of our lives according to the framework we have made our own (on the basis of the kinds of things that normally go on around here). None of us is a "lone ranger" in this epistemological work, because we have been trained by others in the techniques of judgment and we experience many events vicariously through the stories of others.

Latching onto the ways of seeing the world that prevail around here provides one with a good idea of how the world is, what things are important in life, and how one fits in to the order of things. That learning crucially depends on being able to keep in step with others, even though, once competent, one is allowed certain idiosyncrasies. Indeed, if the intersubjective foundation is secure and a basic repertoire of cognitive skills has been mastered, we encourage individuality and creativity, recognizing (at some level) that these, too, are vital to the adaptation of the group.

We could think of the cognitive activity of integrated individuals as involving a top-down or holistic effect on the neurocognitive stream resulting from the sum total of their interactions with the environment in which language and conversation play an important role. The normally smooth coordination among discourse, perception, behavior, and the responses of others to that behavior comes apart, however, when there are deep-seated problems in the neurophysiological or neurochemical machinery or some other profound source of mismatch between these phenomena.

For the individual, autobiographical consciousness is the order that emerges out of cognitive dealings with what happens to her. Each of us is equipped with a device to track significant changes in the environment, and we have the capacity to fine-tune that device as a result of experience so as to maximize its usefulness in dealing with information from the world. The device transforms the neurocognitive stream into experiential content, and the means of transformation is structured by a set of skills of the type we convey to one another through the process called socialization.

Thus, the ordering of experience is an active cognitive skill in which we are trained through situations in which language is taught and learned. As we are trained in the requisite cognitive skills, we learn to distinguish correct from incorrect judgments about what is around us (Wittgenstein 1969) and we learn to attend to the things on which judgments of the given type criterially hinge.

Notice that, on this view, a subject's normal thinking about the world involves attention, first to the public or shared criteria underpinning judgments about the world and second to the reactions of others to those conditions. A normal subject triangulates on these and the coherence of their own narrative to form beliefs about the world and to reason about what is going on. In this task he is supported by the assurance that he is among friends who, by and large, have his best interests at heart or at least act in familiar ways. But the psychotic lacks this source of assurance because, in him or her, both access to social supports and well-practiced techniques of information gathering are defective.

Cognition is intentional (in the phenomenological sense) in that it is essentially directed toward the furniture and inhabitants of a shared world. The mind accesses that world through the conceptual techniques deployed by the subject. Thus cognition is also intertwined with action that is appropriately directed to the events, objects, and people that surround one (and is therefore intentional in the purposive sense). It follows that psychotic cognition, as Fulford (1989) has noted, is closely tied to the failure of action.

I have identified, in the cognitive task that faces each of us, the dual (and holistically connected) roles of shared discourse and individual adaptation. Our interactions with the world are shaped by techniques of information gathering and by the use of narrative techniques that integrate that information into a coherent whole. Both of these sets of skills involve others who help us carve out an autobiography on the basis of what happens to us.

PARANOID IRRATIONALITY

The subtle balance between the responses of self and the co-referential responses of others to the same conditions and events is part of what Kant calls "the *sensus communis*," or a shared and commonsense view of what the normally happens in the world. Whatever I might think in a paranoid moment, neither is there any widespread conspiracy aimed at persecuting me, nor have the people around me been replaced by replicas, nor could I be supplied with energy by a nuclear reactor within. In many and diverse ways the normative discursive context in which I operate moderates the beliefs I will accept so that they are reasonable, all things considered, and not just rationally coherent.

This task of making sense of the world results in a growing understanding of how the world works. We seem to bring to that an intuitive physics or mechanics, an interconnected web of beliefs rooted in our common practices, a fundamental conception of natural kinds, and a tendency to look to others for validation of trains of thought.

The Kantian idea of an intuitive physics or mechanics comprises a priori scientific principles that form part of the *sensus communis* (which, he notes, is not quite the same as a vulgar sense). Kant uses the colloquialism "horse sense" to indicate the pragmatic reasonableness that we all take for granted and that gives rise to full-blooded science as an intellectual discipline (1978: 24).

Campbell explores the idea of intuitive or a priori awareness of such things as objects and their causal relations and its relation to a more primitive ability to keep track of things in the world around us in his discussion of consciousness and its contents. He talks about our grasp of basic ideas such as the idea that the world comprises a number of causally active and interacting things — "the condition of a thing at any one time is causally dependent upon its condition at earlier times" (1994:

27)—or that the events around us have characteristic causes that exhibit certain regularities (66). Kant's "a priori scientific principles" are close to Campbell's "primitive" or "intuitive" physics, which we could gloss as a shared human understanding of how the world works and the kinds of things that ordinarily happen within it. These form the context of the practices and language games in which we train each other as thinkers. It is plausible that the knowledge indicated by these terms and phrases is an inclusive transformation of innate tendencies (such as the ability to track objects or presuppose their constancy) by the light that dawns gradually over the whole of our cognitive map of the world (to adapt Wittgenstein's phrase).

Wittgenstein regards the cumulative system formed by our ways of acting and interacting with the world as a means of defusing global skeptical doubts that do not make sense: "Is the hypothesis possible, that all the things around us don't exist? Would that not be like the hypothesis of our having miscalculated in all our calculations" (1969: #55). He talks of "the inherited background against which I distinguish between true and false" (#94), referring to the shared world picture within which "all testing, all confirmation and disconfirmation" occur (#105). Like Kant, he notices that this inherited background is significantly contributed to by training through which we induct our cognitive apprentices into our common techniques of judgment and forming reasonable opinions. "In order to make a mistake, a man must already judge in conformity with mankind" (#156) so that "the reasonable man does *not have* certain doubts" (#220).

It follows that we share not only conceptual techniques but also experiences, beliefs, and resulting knowledge, all of which constrain our modes of explanation and the ways that we make sense of what is going on around us. We are, according to Kant, *driven* to try and make sense of the world and to provide ourselves with a coherent narrative of the way it works as part of our cognitive inheritance. The principle of universal causality ties all this together, and it is, Kant claims, a "transcendent concept of nature" that manifests itself in our pursuit of scientific explanations. It is worth noting that in paranoia there seems to be an immoderate demand that all events be connected in a rationally explicable way, even where the resulting explanations do not comply with the informal constraints imposed by the *sensus communis*.

Understanding the pivotal defects in psychotic thinking emerges directly from an appreciation of these features of our normal epistemic techniques.

A Unifying Synthesis

Psychotic thinking is said to instance a loss of contact with reality. I have argued that this results from a loss of attunement between the cognitive skills of the psychotic person and those of others. The relevant skills are built on attentional control and selectivity that can be adjusted and refined in a social context so that the subject captures the same cues and constancies as those around them. Psychosis, it is suggested, is a state in which attention is disrupted; the mechanisms do not function smoothly and do not adjust themselves to track conditions in the world in normal ways.

The psychotic therefore finds that she is out of step with others and is driven to explain that fact in some way. However, the cognitive mechanisms undermined by the pathology of attention are also involved in constructing focused and directed trains of thought suitably sensitive to the implicit constraints (of the *sensus communis*) that others would obey in making sense of the world. Therefore, the subtle and pervasive adjustments of thought that allow us to keep track of events and to use interactions with others to update and correct our lived narratives of experience are disconnected from the guides and signposts that usually orient the mind. The psychotic is therefore alone and scared. Events happen that are alarming and make no sense, and one's fellow travelers do not seem to be on the same journey. This is an extremely unsettling state of affairs for any being whose entire cognitive system is based on principles of convergence in judgment, affirmation, and validation.

What is more, the very mechanisms that one relies on for cognitive competence are buzzing and stuttering and appear to be overloaded with data. There are several possible aberrations to which such a disorder might be plausibly expected to give rise:

1. Thought may become pressured and confused, with ideas jostling each other for conscious space and linking with one another through relatively unprincipled and haphazard sources of association. The flow of thought continues in this condition, but its coherence and reasonableness suffer so that version of events in which one seems to be caught up is chaotic and threatening and nobody else can get on to one's wavelength. *Zerfahrenheit*, as one might expect, is very scary.

2. Thought may trace a path in which the unifying skein of connectedness is bizarre. For the psychotic in the midst of this autobiographical narrative, everything connects in a narratively coherent way but in a way that nobody else believes (as if others cannot see what strikes one as glaringly obvious). This kind of *paranoid thinking* carries within it the seeds of the idea of persecution, because there could be no reason, apart from a conspiracy in which many others are involved, that something so meaningful and rationally connected with everything else that has happened could apparently escape the notice of so many. Why would so many people deny something that was so evidently true unless they themselves were subject to (or party to) a grand deception of demonic subtlety?

3. Both my place and conduct in the world and my thoughts about that world are, in the normal case, subject to implicit corrections that are smoothly integrated into a package that reveals me to myself as others see me. When I attain knowledge congruent with that ideal, I am said to have *insight* into my condition as a human being. It requires judgments that are inherently more difficult than straightforward judgments about what is going on

around me. These judgments reveal me as a narratively integrated subject and allow me to own my thoughts by placing items of experiential content accurately in relation to the operation of my mind in the world (Stephens and Graham 2000). When the thoughts in my mind are confused and clamoring for attention in a way that threatens to overwhelm me and my normal skills of ordering the neurocognitive stream are not functioning properly, the knowledge of self is likely to distintegrate and result in a *"lack of insight."* Although there is an important intersubjective foundation for this knowledge, it is not usefully collapsed into something trivial like "agreeing with your psychiatrist."

The forms of psychotic thought disorder are explicable on the basis of a subject with impaired epistemic skills trying to cope with a situation in which cognition has been seriously unsettled. This could arise from physiologically or chemically induced neurocognitive dysfunction or, conceivably, from a serious breakdown in the interpersonal pattern of exchanges that attunes and refines our cognitive adaptations to the shared world. In either case, there are likely to be stresses on the subject that worsen the suffering and loneliness of psychotic experience, and it is unlikely that in a holistic organism such as a human being, either factor operates in isolation. I have referred to this as "brain pain," because even though the brain, famously, does not feel pain, the psychotic feels the pain of a brain that has come adrift from the smooth pattern of cognitive functioning that keeps him as the person he is in tune with his context (both "physical" and "interpersonal." When that happens he begins to suffer the falling apart or terrifying distortion of his lived experience as a narrative subject that is psychosis.

REFERENCES

American Psychiatric Association (1994) *Diagnostic and Statistical Manual*, 4th ed. Washington, DC: American Psychiatric Association.

Campbell, J. (1994) *Past Space and Self*. Cambridge, MA: MIT Press.

Carter, C. S., Robertson, L. C., and Nordahl, T. E. (1992) "Abnormal Processing of Irrelevant Information in Chronic Schizophrenia: Selective Enhancement of Stroop Facilitation." *Psychiatry Research* 41: 137–46.

Fulford, W. K. M. (1990) *Moral Theory and Medical Practice*. Oxford: Oxford University Press.

Gates, R., and Hammond, R. (1993) *When the Music's Over*. Armidale, NH: University of New England Press.

Gelder, M., Gath, D., and Mayou, R. (1983) *Oxford Textbook of Psychiatry*. Oxford: Oxford University Press.

Gillett G. (1992) *Representation Meaning and Thought*. Oxford: Clarendon.

Gillett, G. (1997) "A Discursive Account of Multiple Personality Disorder." *Philosophy, Psychiatry and Psychology* 4(3): 213–22.

Gillett, G. (1999) *The Mind and Its Discontents*. Oxford: Oxford University Press.

Gillett, G. (2000) "Moral Authenticity and the Unconscious." In M. Levine (ed.), *The Analytic Freud*. London: Routledge.

Gillett, G. (2001) "Signification and the Unconscious." *Philosophical Psychology* 14(4): 477–98.

Hemsley, D. R. (1977) "What Have Cognitive Deficits to Do with Schizophrenic Symptoms?" *British Journal of Psychiatry* 130: 167–73.

Hemsley, D. R. (1992) "Cognitive Abnormalities and the Symptoms of Schizophrenia." In M. Spitzer, F. Uehlein, M. Schwartz, and C. Mundt (eds.), *Phenomenology Language and Schizophrenia*. New York: Springer Verlag.

Jaynes, J. (1990) "Verbal Hallucinations and Preconscious Mentality." In M. Spitzer, F. Uehlein, M. Schwartz, and C. Mundt (eds.), *Phenomenology Language and Schizophrenia*. New York: Springer Verlag.

Kant, I. (1789 [1929]) *The Critique of Pure Reason*. Translated by N. Kemp Smith. London: Macmillan.

Kant, I. (1798 [1978]) *Anthropology from a Pragmatic Point of View*. Translated by V. L. Dowdell. Carbondale: Southern Illinois University Press.

Laing, R. D. (1966) *The Divided Self*. London: Penguin.

Lewis, A. (1934) "The Psychopathology of Insight." *British Journal of Medical Psychology* 14: 332–48.

Luria, A. R., (1973) *The Working Brain*. Harmondsworth: Penguin.

McGhie, A. (1969) *The Pathology of Attention*. London: Penguin.

Manschrek, T. (1992) "Clinical and Experimental Analysis of Motor Phenomena in Schizophrenia." In M. Spitzer, F. Uehlein, M. Schwartz, and C. Mundt (eds.), *Phenomenology Language and Schizophrenia*. New York: Springer Verlag.

Millikan, R. (1993) *White Queen Psychology and Other Essays for Alice*. Cambridge, MA: MIT Press.

Neisser, U. (1976) *Cognition and Reality*. San Francisco: W. H. Freeman.

Perry, W., and Braff, D. L. (1994) "Information Processing Deficits and Thought Disorder in Schizophrenia." *American Journal of Psychiatry* 151(3): 363–67.

Sass, L. A. (1992) "Phenomenological Aspects of 'Zerfarenheit' and Incoherence." In M. Spitzer, F. Uehlein, M. Schwartz, and C. Mundt (eds.), *Phenomenology Language and Schizophrenia*. New York: Springer Verlag.

Spitzer, M. (1992) "Word-Associations in Experimental Psychiatry." In M. Spitzer, F. Uehlein, M. Schwartz, and C. Mundt (eds.), *Phenomenology Language and Schizophrenia*. New York: Springer Verlag.

Spitzer, M., and Maher, B. (eds.) (1990) *Philosophy and Psychopathology*. New York: Springer Verlag.

Spitzer, M., Uehlein, F., Schwartz, M., and Mundt, C. (eds.) (1992) *Phenomenology Language and Schizophrenia*. New York: Springer Verlag.

Stephens, G. Lynn, and Graham, G. (2000) *When Self-Consciousness Breaks*. Cambridge, MA: MIT Press.

Venables, P. H. (1960) "The Effect of Auditory and Visual Stimulation on the Skin: Potential Responses of Schizophrenics." *Brain* 83: 77–92.

Wittgenstein, L. (1953) *Philosophical Investigations*. Oxford: Blackwell.

Wittgenstein, L. (1969) *On Certainty*. Edited by G. E. M. Anscombe and G. H. von Wright. New York: Harper.

CHAPTER 2

....

AFFECTIVITY

Depression and Mania

....

JENNIFER HANSEN

DEPRESSION is the leading cause for disability worldwide (NIMH 2001). Researchers estimate that more than 19 million Americans suffer from depression per year (Reiger et al. 1993; Mazure et al. 2001). Its toll on human life can be measured quite concretely in dollars—$8.5 million a year are spent on antidepressant drugs; $9,265 on average for female employees of national Fortune 100 companies and $8,502 on average for male employees per year on medical, prescription drug, and disability (Birnbaum et al. 1999); and $143 million in U.S. government research funding (NARSAD 2002). More tragically, we can measure its toll in the number of lives it claims.[1] The fact that human beings are falling victim to affective disorders such as depression at catastrophic rates is a major concern for both psychiatrists and philosophers. Psychiatrists may devote more energy to searching for causes and cures, while philosophers focus more on what depression means to humanity and what it reveals about humanity.

The philosophical literature on depression proceeds along three main lines of analysis: the moral, the medical, and the social/political. Philosophers interested in moral psychology study the effect that clinical depression has on judgment, motivation, and decision making (see Caton 1986; Ardal 1993; Silberfeld and Checkland 1999; Roberts 2001). In a vein similar to that of moral psychologists, there are researchers who pursue a "melancholic epsitemology,"[2] which may shed light on one's authentic sense of self (see Graham 1991; Martin 1999). If depressed states of mind are truthful—that is, if they accurately depict or represent states of affairs in the world—then these states of mind are quite crucial for self-understanding.

Often, but not always, at odds with the moral analysis of depression are thinkers who study depression in order to clarify certain epistemological issues about psychiatric taxonomy (see Ghaemi 1999; Kramer 2000; Graham 2002). This approach, which is bound up primarily with the medical nature of depression, seeks to clarify whether depression is a natural kind, a discrete disease entity, or merely a syndrome with a multitude of irreconcilable causes (see Radden 2003).

Finally, there are philosophers who study depression as a barometer of social arrangements. This camp of thinker mines depression for what it reveals about how modernity and its political and social forces press upon humanity (e.g., Kristeva 1987; Lepenies 1992; Pensky 1993; Ferguson 1995; Rose 1996; Francassa 1999; Cheever 2000; Cheng 2000).

In this essay, I examine these three different approaches—the moral, medical, and social/political—as they apply to the study of affective disorders (mood disorders). Although affective disorders constitute a psychiatric category of illness that includes manic-depressive disorder, I focus on clinical depression because of its relation to the historical category of melancholia, which once included almost all known psychiatric categories of illness that presently exist, including cognitive disorders, volitional disorders, and psychotic disorders. Depressives sometimes alternate between the poles of sadness and mania, and much of what I outline applies equally well to manic depression. First, I point out a particularly entrenched debate between advocates of the moral and the medical perspectives regarding clinical depression, illustrating this debate by highlighting the current moral and political issues surrounding psychopharmacology ("Psychopharmacological Calvinism" versus "Pharmocentric View of the World"; see Ghaemi 1999). Second, I demonstrate how the social/political approach offers an interesting change of perspective on the significance of melancholia, by moving away from positing personhood and personal identity as the locus of philosophical analyses of psychiatric illness. Throughout this essay, I refer to the rich history of melancholia, which exists in both philosophical and medical texts, in order to emphasize the persistence and continuity of moods and their meanings to Western thinkers.

I. Depressive Realism and Psychopharmacological Calvinism

Much of the contemporary literature on clinical depression in philosophy centers on the moral and medical approaches to clinical depression. What is clear about these two different approaches is the way in which they tend to polarize any understanding of depression. Mike Martin (1999) offers a helpful way to grasp this schism between the moral and medical perspectives by representing it as the moral versus the therapeutic perspective. These clashing perspectives are best illustrated by looking more carefully at what is at stake in popular debates over whether or not Prozac and its cousins are the modern answer to the modern epidemic rates of depression.

The dilemma is as follows: given the findings of many advances in psychiatry — new research into the brain, specifically cognition and neurochemistry — should we write off depression as a mere medical problem, easily treatable and contained through the prescribing of a regimen of antidepressant pills, or is depression a more profound illness, imbuing the sufferer with truthful and important insights about his or her identity? Might there be good reasons for being depressed, or should we construe depression as pathological, mental distortion (see Graham 1991: 231)? Is there such a thing as "depressive realism" (Alloy and Abramson 1988),[3] which accurately grasps the sad and tragic features of any one person's existence (what Martin calls "feature-specific depression" [1999: 280])? Those critical of this latter stance dismiss such a perspective as "psychopharamacological Calvinism" (Klerman 1972), which clings to archaic notions of mental illness and a moralizing medical view. Peter Kramer claims that we fear the use of pharmacology because of a "cultural preference for the melancholic over the sanguine" (2000: 3). He states that "the cluster of personality traits arising from the melancholic temperament (pessimism, perfectionism, sensitivity and the rest) overlaps so strongly with our image of the intellectual that we may have difficulty crediting thinkers who are differently constituted," and this association of melancholia with intellectual prowess may in fact be an *accident* of a high historical correlation between depression and artistic genius (3). Later in this essay I consider three important problems within the moral versus therapeutic dispute: (a) the leveling of mental illness through psychiatric language, (b) the ignoring of depressed people's important insights, and (c) the issue of whether (a) and (b) are simply mistaken views drawn from bad science.

The Poetry and Prose of Depression

While modern psychiatry has become a more precise instrument, with a specialized language and better instruments for diagnosing specific and distinguishing attributes of mental illness categories, some thinkers evidence a wistfulness and nostalgia for the more subtle and profound cultural meanings historically ascribed to melancholia and mania. George Graham begins his essay "Melancholic Epistemology" with the following lines from Gerard Manley Hopkins:

> I wake and feel the fell of dark, not day.
> What hours, O what black hours we have spent
> This night! What sights you, heart, saw; ways you went!
> And more must, in yet longer light's delay. (Cited in Graham 1991: 223)

Following this epigraph, Graham asserts, "Hopkins has a knack for finding just the right descriptions—not the dulling prose of textbook clinical psychology, but the revealing metaphors of telling poetry" (223). The historical representation of melancholia and melancholy moods weave together powerful and equally horrific images of black moods, profound lassitude, and unending sadness and pain. These images still resonate with or, rather, haunt us, though we are a more rational and scientific century and these images are remnants of a more literary and mythological age. For example, the images of "black moods" metonymically refers to the diseases of black bile (*melan kole*), a humor so named because of ancient beliefs that blackness or darkness were evil, poisonous qualities. Jennifer Radden writes that "there are associations among the notions of anger, darkness, blackness surging up with anger, and blackness as poisonous (thus *cholos* [anger] and *chole* [bile] often overlap in poetic and literary usage)" (1987: 238).

The nostalgia for more literary and poetic descriptions of melancholia in the face of the "dulling prose of textbook clinical psychology" seems to come from dissatisfaction with the inability of scientific language to faithfully capture the true misery of depression. However, another, perhaps more urgent worry that motivates this dissatisfaction is that scientific language ignores centuries of passionate and poetic attempts to reckon with this disease. Connecting with this history may actually be quite cathartic for sufferers. In his "memoir of madness," William Styron tell us:

When I was first aware that I had been laid low by the disease, I felt a need, among other things, to register a strong protest against the word "depression." Depression, most people know, used to be termed "melancholia," a word which appears in English as early as the year 1303 and crops up more than once in Chaucer, who in his usage seemed to be aware of its pathological nuances. "Melancholia" would still appear to be a far more apt and evocative word for the blacker forms of the disorder, but it was usurped by a noun with bland tonality and lacking any magisterial presence, used indifferently to describe an economic decline or a rut in the ground, a true wimp of a word for such a major illness. It may be that the scientist generally held responsible for its currency in modern times, a Johns Hopkins Medical School faculty member justly venerated—the Swiss-born psychiatrist Adolf Meyer—had a tin ear for the finer rhythms of English and therefore was unaware of the semantic damage he had inflicted by offering "depression" as a descriptive noun for such a dreadful and raging disease. Nonetheless, for over seventy-five years the word has slithered innocuously through the language like a slug, leaving little trace of its intrinsic malevolence and preventing by its very insipidity, a general awareness of the horrible intensity of the disease when out of control. As one who has suffered from the malady in extremis yet returned to tell the tale, I would lobby for a truly arresting designation. "Brainstorm," for instance, has unfortunately been preempted to describe, somewhat jocularly, intellectual inspiration. But something along those lines is needed. Told that someone's mood disorder has evolved into a storm—a veritable howling tempest in the brain, which is indeed what a clinical depression resembles like nothing else—even the uniformed layman might display sympathy rather than the standard reaction that "depression" evokes, something akin to "So What?" or "You'll pull out of it" or "We all have had bad days.' " (Styron 1990: 36–38)

By stripping the larger cultural meanings from Styron's illness, modern-day psychiatrists contribute to a cultural leveling of mental illness in general. If one suffers from depression, then wellness is simply a matter of taking pills or getting involved in life rather than indulging in intellectual ruminations. Such a cultural portrait of depression is *depressing*.

"Maybe Psychiatric Well-Being Isn't Everything"

The ethicist Carl Elliott utters this thought in his mediation "Prozac and the American Dream" (2000). Elliott, among many other ethicists and philosophers, suggests another important problem with the medicalization of depression: the classic struggle between lifeworld and technology. In a spirit of scientific progress we may invent technologies that actually work against our survival and flourishing as a species. An ancient truth may manifest itself in our moods, which psychiatric pharmacology may carelessly bulldoze over in a rush to discover the "magic bullet" that will rid us of anxious, debilitating states of mind. Furthermore, as Edmund Husserl pointed out, we would be well served by distinguishing the human sciences from the theoretical sciences and not turning to a naïve positivism to understand human values and truths; psychiatry may benefit from paying more attention to the truth content of depressed moods (see Husserl 1970).

Depression may be a legitimate manifestation of truths about a sufferer's situation. Moreover, it may be an important means to self-fulfillment and self-actualization. Elliott argues that we consider some forms of depression as a form of "existential alienation," which is a "calling into question your own values, the very stuff out of which we are built" (Elliott 2000: 9). In a similar vein, Abraham Kahn highlights Soren Kierkegaard's ethico-spiritual understanding of melancholia. Psychoanalysts such as Sigmund Freud (1963 [1917]) and Melanie Klein (1975 [1955]) identify melancholia and depression as a neurotic disease, resulting from an injury to one's ego because of the loss of a loved object. Melancholia is the result of *identification* with and *introjection* of a forsaken object, wherein "the shadow of the object fell upon the ego, so that the latter could henceforth be criticized by a special mental faculty like an object, like the forsaken object" (Freud 1963 [1917]: 170). Contemporary psychiatrists, furthermore, may consider depression a case of faulty hardwiring or chemical imbalance. And, finally, evolutionary psychologists may argue "that the tendency to depression served to promote genetic survival in the environment in which it evolved" (Greenspan 2001: 329). However, all of these positions are too secular; they lack a "dimension of transcendence" (Kahn 1989: 116). Kahn, in a Kierkegaardian perspective, explains:

> On this view of the self melancholy is brought on by either neglect of refusal to free the spirit through choosing absolutely. Spirit or the ethico-spiritual element reaches a point when it is agitated, seeking to break through its mere sense-

conscious mode of existence to a higher mode. It wants to collect itself out of dispersion occasioned by the self passively cohering with the whole earthly life. (117)

Ignoring the power of the human spirit, and the subtle messages that it nudges each of us to reach beyond what is all too human, may not, in fact, lead us to greater happiness and well-being.

The *New Yorker*, in a more tongue-in-cheek spirit, began publishing a series of cartoons soon after the release of Peter Kramer's *Listening to Prozac*. One of the more memorable cartoons, entitled "If They Had Prozac in the Nineteenth Century," featured Karl Marx saying, "Sure! Capitalism can work out its kinks!" and Friedrich Nietzsche saying to his mother after church, "Me, too, Mom. I really liked what the priest said about all the little people" (Martel 1993). The implication is clear: what might we have lost as a culture if psychopharmacology had prevailed in earlier times?

Modern psychiatry, particularly psychopharmacology, may deprive us of the *Homo melancholis*, whose pained, yet imaginative insights push human knowledge beyond itself. The association between cultural genius and melancholia extends back to ancient medicine. Aristotle's writings on melancholia, for example, left an indelible mark on the cultural imagination regarding the connection of this infliction with philosophic and literary genius. In the *Problemata*, he asks, "Why is it that all men who have become outstanding in philosophy, statesmanship, poetry or the arts are melancholic, and some to such an extent that they are infected by the diseases arising from black bile?" (quoted in Radden 2000: 57). Marsilio Ficino's Platonism led him to associate melancholia with the divine mania of poets that Plato discusses in the *Ion, Republic*, and *Phaedrus*. Melancholics are inspired by God and given prophetic sight, though this gift carries with it a horrible burden. Ficino exalts the mad philosopher above all, writing: "But of all learned people, those especially are oppressed by black bile, who, being sedulously devoted to the study of philosophy" (quoted in Radden 2000: 90).

Immanuel Kant argues that melancholia is a result of the mind's imagination run riot, thereby the overstepping of the boundaries of reason. Nonetheless, Kant claims that the melancholy man

> has above all a *feeling for the sublime*. Even beauty, for which he also has a perception, must not only delight him but move him, since it also stirs admiration in him. The enjoyment of pleasures is more earnest with him, but is none the smaller on that account. All emotions of the sublime have more fascination for him than the deceiving charms of the beautiful. His well-being will rather be satisfaction than pleasure. He is resolute. On that account he orders his sensations under principles. They are much less subject to inconstancy and change, the more universal this principle is to which they are subordinated. (Kant 1960: 64–65)

Kant's melancholic may settle for satisfaction rather than pleasure—a state of achievement that Kramer's beloved Prozac might perhaps offer us all—but his satisfaction restrains a mind capable of sublime insights. Likewise, for David Hume, melancholia was a state indigenous to the true philosopher, who must be skeptical of all philosophical positions and arguments. This skepticism was sure to bring about a melancholic attitude, which would dissipate once the philosopher earned a deeper and more profound insight into the working of the world (see Livingston 1998). Pall Ardal argues that "philosophy has some therapeutic value to those who enjoy it. There were no pills available that helped cure depression. But, since reason is incapable of effecting a cure, Hume is driven to philosophizing" (1993: 542). While philosophical analysis cures Hume's depression, it is precisely the activity that led John Stuart Mill into a profound depression (see Anderson 1991; Graham 1991; Nelson 1985; Martin 1999). Graham reports that "Mill surmised that his depression was caused in part by his being overanalytical, too detached and intellectual, and that his life lacked sufficient aesthetic pleasure" (1991: 241). Yet, in Mill's case, depression is a *pharmakon*, a poison and a gift, for his descent into depression leads him to reformulate his father's and Jeremy Bentham's utilitarianism. Because reading Wordsworth's poetry began to lift Mill out of his depression, he came to realize that poetry and other aesthetic endeavors were of the utmost importance to the development of character and moral beneficence.

Because of this long and profitable connection between depression and philosophical greatness, some ethicists worry that the recent turn to psychopharmacology is the worst kind of reductionism. A. M. Weisberger accuses Peter Kramer, for example, of the genetic fallacy that "the claim that to know the causes is to know the whole story" (1995: 70). Weisberger continues:

> For perhaps we may one day know the exact cause of Michelangelo's creative abilities and visions, but this will not provide a blueprint for producing a Michelangelo over a Velvet Elvis painter. Even if we could neurochemically deduce the exact cause of the "aesthetic response" to great art, or being "head over heels in love" none of this will help us to understand the felt quality of these experiences. In other words, what is produced in us by listening to Mozart or by creating poetry can never be reduced to talk of brain firing or optimal neurotransmitter blends. This distinction should serve to prevent us from drifting too far in the direction of the disintegration of the unique characteristics of persons. (70)

By searching for the common denominator for human beings in the minutiae of brain chemistry or in the depleted resources of serotonin, we are robbing ourselves of our humanity.

The highly regulated, organized, sanguine, and mass-medicated utopias depicted in the science fiction novels *Brave New World* and *The Giver* may now be more truth than fiction. Instead of soma we are handed Prozac to deal with a world increasingly cruel to human life. Recently, for example, a free month of Prozac Weekly was directly mailed to potential consumers of this drug. The accompanying letter read, "Congratulations on being one step to full recovery" (*New York Times* July 6, 2002). Somehow Eli Lilly, the manufacturer of Prozac, got access to private medical records in order to send free samples of their drug. While this action may seem simply pharmaceutical marketing gone awry, it also echoes the societies depicted in science fiction in which technology has made illnesses and weaknesses a thing of the past partially through coercing those who are less than well to medicate themselves. This mass prescribing, and now aggressive marketing of antidepressants, may be another casualty in the reign of terror of scientific, positivistic thinking in the twentieth century.

Pharmacological Calvinism

While a belief in the moral significance of depression steers the philosophical criticism of contemporary research and treatment of depression, a countervailing philosophical position asserts these arguments are specters, haunting us from the grave of old, outdated, outmoded scientific theories. A moral approach to treatment is a throwback to an archaic understanding of medicine as a form of moral education. Recent developments in neuroscience, psychiatry, and psychopharmacology have revolutionized the medical approach to mental illness. We need to purge modern medicine of theological concerns.

Gerard Klerman argues that criticisms of psychopharmacology on the grounds that it hinders personal growth are "basically a secular variant of the theological view of salvation through good works" (1972: 3). Many historians of melancholia trace this theological view of melancholia to ancient and medieval conceptions of mental illness, which view medicine as a tool of moral education. To clarify the humoral model of Galenic medicine, Jean Starobinski explains that

> the patient must be willing to receive instructions; he must learn to recognize the moral necessity for numerical proportion, and be prepared to make the effort to improve his behaviour. He must see the error of his ways, must learn to be more sensible about his choice of food and divide his time better between exertion and repose. . . . Greek medicine was a process of education (*paideia*) in which men learned to treat their bodies on rational principles. (1962: 15)

In the period between antiquity and the Renaissance, the church held sway over all intellectual pursuits, and therefore physicians from this period considered melancholia to be a specific sin: *acedia* or *tristitia*. Both of these concepts persisted in later writings on melancholia under the heading "religious melancholia." Those diagnosed with *acedia* were neglecting their spiritual duties and feigning illness in order to avoid the difficult labor of monastic life. Melancholia and its alternate pole, mania, were diseases brought about by indulging in sins such as lust or greed. Medieval romances modified the earlier iconography of melancholia by portraying the characters *Tristesse* and *Merencolyie* as "threatening female figures wreaking allegorical havoc on poor young knights and lovers" (Schiesari 1992: 98). Furthermore, the figure of Dame Melancholy symbolized the danger and destruction that melancholia waged on pious men (99). Finally, Melancholia was also known as the Noon-Day Demon, tempting many from living a humble and moral existence (see Starobinski 1962: 32). In sum, iconography and medical treatises during the Middle Ages viewed melancholia through the lens of moral and spiritual weakness.

Given the incredible advances of medical science, moral and theological condemnations of depressed persons are bad science. Psychiatrists who refrain from treating patients suffering from sleeplessness, anxiety, or suicidal thoughts are perhaps more to blame than those critical of new psychopharmacological treatments. While these critics also worry that treatment of depression through pills reflects an overly reductionistic and abstract view of human beings, Ghaemi points out that those who deny patients the relief that comes from these medicines may be guilty of the same abstractions and reductionism. Ghaemi reports:

> A common argument before the 1970s was that biological treatments might reduce anxiety, depression, and psychosis, thereby removing the kind of painful impetus that alone could push patients to discover the "true" underlying causes of their misfortunes. A kernel of truth notwithstanding, such a perspective reeks of the sacrifice of human beings to abstractions. Contemporary objections to the "medicalization" of depression share a similar fault. (1999: 292)

If both psychopharmacological hedonists and psychopharmacological Calvinists commit the sins of reductionism, then, perhaps, to clarify which reductionism is more harmful, we should determine which theoretical model is more accurate or more representative of current scientific advances.

Graham points out that concepts of mental illness or disorder are semantic norms that "determine the class of individuals to whom the concept applies" (2002: 113). Furthermore, these concepts compare this class of individuals to a standard of proper function. How we determine what a proper function is for a human being ought to reflect in part what we now know about the physiological and psychological functioning of human beings. That is, philosophers who fail to heed or work with theorists in evolutionary biology, cognitive neuropsychology, neurobiology, and similar fields will perhaps proceed from assumptions or norms that have been disproved through new scientific evidence. For example, to claim that depressed persons are simply avoiding their spiritual work or responsibilities is to ignore epidemiological evidence of disfunction. If anxious moods can be traced to neurochemical imbalances, then it seems quite inappropriate to berate a sufferer for failing to struggle toward salvation. To make a medical analogy, if depression is more akin to diabetes, then to suggest that a sufferer chooses his or her misery in failing to work toward salvation makes no sense. Disfunction, in this scenario, is not a product of human will or choice. To allow such presuppositions or assumptions to guide one's moral judgments is a failure of scientific and philosophical thinking. It is simply bad science to persist in viewing depression as an expression of personal moral struggle.

II. AN AGE OF MELANCHOLY

The moral versus medical debate over the significance and meaning of depression takes as its focus the rational, autonomous individual and considers whether this individual gains truthful, justified wisdom from his or her depression or is simply ill and in need of proper medical attention. However, Continental philosophers tend to take a slightly different approach, using melancholia as an analytical category of social and political *systems*, rather than individuals. Though the social/political analysis of depression (melancholia) acknowledges the health concerns of individual sufferers, it begins with different metaphysical assumptions of identity and selfhood.

Following Freud, many social theorists such as Herbert Marcuse (1955), Louis Althusser (1970), Jacques Lacan (1977), and Julia Kristeva (1989) argue that identity formation is a complex process of negotiation. While Freud focuses largely on the metapsychology of the self, and the conflict between the id, ego, and superego, social theorists after Freud extrapolate from his metapsychology to think about social systems. In any given social system, there are forces that are (a) normalizing, like Freud's superego, (b) dissident, such as the id, and finally, (c) a compromise between (a) and (b), much like Freud's notion of the ego. Human beings become who they are, then, in the midst of countervailing, conflicting forces that push and pull them toward becoming one sort of person over another. The struggle to become an individual who is essentially "normal" may involve complex processes of self-denial and self-abnegation.

When Freud analyzed melancholia, he asserted that it was the result of the ego's failure to grieve or mourn the loss of someone, something, or some idea. In melancholic patients, he said, we see a "devotion to its mourning, which leaves nothing over for other purposes or other interests" (1963 [1917]: 165). The melancholic identifies with the lost object, introjects this loss into him- or herself, and then fails to compensate for it. What may have been a struggle with an object external to the self becomes an internal struggle of identity and loss.

Transferring this metapsychological explanation of melancholia to social systems, many theorists diagnose elements of modernity and identity formation that mimic the melancholic ego. In Freud's interpretation, one becomes melancholy generally because of the loss of a loved object. What a new generation of theorists offer is an analysis of the conditions of modernity and the norms of identity specific to Western culture that incorporate a loss of self that is not recoverable through healthy mourning or grieving. Instead, those who are forced to renounce parts of themselves or parts of their traditions become profoundly melancholic. On these terms, then, melancholia is not only individual pathology but also the pathology of modernity. In the next sections I consider two examples of social analyses of melancholia.

Melancholic Modernity

Social theorists who labor to understand what modernity means after the Holocaust, the dropping of the bomb on Hiroshima, and other modern warfare deem modernity as the age of melancholia. Julia Kristeva writes:

A tremendous crisis of thought and speech, a crisis of representation, has indeed emerged; one may look for analogues in past centuries (the fall of the Roman empire and the dawning of Christianity, the years of devastating medieval plagues and wars) or for its causes in economic, political, and juridical bankruptcies. Nonetheless, never has the power of destructive forces appeared as unquestionable and unavoidable as now, within and without society and the individual. The despoliation of nature, lives, and property is accompanied by an upsurge, or simply a more obvious display of disorders whose diagnoses are being refined by psychiatry — psychosis, depression, manic-depressive states, borderline states, false selves, etc. (1987: 221–22)

For Kristeva, the horrors of modernity and industrialization cost us our mental health. A rise in the population of the clinically depressed, for example, may in fact speak to the sickness of our culture. In a similar vein, Socrates claims in the *Apology* that to corrupt others ineluctably leads to the corruption of the state. If the state is unhealthy, then the individuals will be unhealthy. In fact, after the attacks on the World Trade Center and the Pentagon on September 11, 2001, various journalists began reporting on the high rates of depression, suicide, and substance abuse that followed. A new epidemic of depression and anxiety plagues the American landscape as many of us begin to feel that our lives are far more vulnerable than we had allowed ourselves to imagine.

In the midst of this wound, this failure of our best political and economic systems to foster human flourishing, we may find ourselves nostalgic for a lost social order, a past that — in fact — never was. Naomi Schor writes, "After the alleged affectlessness of postmodernism . . . a pervasive depression or, as some might have it, a 'melancholic mourning' hovers like some nasty hangover over legions of consumers of antidepressants" (1996: 1). Gillian Rose suggests that this melancholic age or this impossible grieving is for the very belief in utopia. Postmodern analyses, mindful of the failure of communism, offer little suggestion that a world of social harmony is possible. Perhaps we are more depressed now because we are more than ever aware of the fact that our political states and our ethical systems nonetheless lead to murder and violence. We are mourning the loss of a belief that global politics is indeed working toward a more perfect future. Gillian Rose writes:

This is no work of mourning: it remains baroque melancholia immersed in the world of soulless and unredeemed bodies, which affords a vision that is far more disturbing than the salvific distillation of disembodied spirit. . . . For if all human law is sheer violence, if there is no positive or symbolic law to be acknowledged — the law that decrees the absence of the other, the relinquishing of the dead one, returning from devastating inner grief to the law of the everyday and of relationships, old and new, with those who live — then there can be no *work*, no exploring of the legacy of ambivalence, working through the contradictory emotions aroused by bereavement. Instead, the remains of the dead one will be incorporated into the soul of the one who cannot mourn and will manifest themselves in some all too physical symptom. (1996: 69–70)

In this postmodern age, we may be depressed because we no longer believe in redemption. We are all too secular, and hence souless. We are without hope. Rose is not arguing that depression is a symptom of an individual's loss of faith; she is not simply reverting to a tradition of acedia or religious melancholia. Rather, she is characterizing a culture, a political and ethical order, as increasingly nihilistic. Along with Kristeva, she argues that this era of nihilism manufactures psychic disorders.

Melancholic Gender

Among the hostilities of modernity is homophobia and sexism. Judith Butler (1997) analyzes cultural hostility to gays and lesbians and shows how norms of sexuality actually produce melancholic subjects. In fact, Butler makes the bold claim that gender is essentially melancholic. The process of developing a gendered identity requires renouncing other crucial parts of oneself that cannot be replaced or easily mourned. For Butler, part of becoming a "normal" subject in Western culture involves renouncing any desire for same-sex love. Heterosexual love is the norm of our culture, and our notions of gender follow from a basic assumption that we are essentially heterosexual. "Male" and "female" make sense only with reference to a heterosexual matrix. Homosexual subjects, for Butler, cannot properly be male or female, since such identities follow from heterosexual practices. The cultural norms that pressure us into either a male or a female identity create a loss within us for same-sex love. Our culture struggles to come to grips with what sort of sexual identity same-sex love encompasses, if it is not male or female. Butler writes:

> To the extent that homosexual attachments remain unacknowledged within normative heterosexuality, they are not merely constituted as desires which emerge and subsequently become prohibited; rather, these desires are proscribed from the start. And when they do emerge on the far side of the censor, they may well carry the mark of impossibility with them. . . . As such, they will not be attachments that can be openly grieved. This is, then, less a refusal to grieve . . . than a preemption of grief performed by the absence of cultural conventions for avowing the less of homosexual love. (147)

Butler extends Freud's theoretical apparatus to show that heterosexuals become so identified through cultural prohibitions or proscriptions of nonheterosexual desire. This prohibition becomes a loss that is impossible to mourn. Differing from Freud, Butler clarifies that it is not a "devotion to mourning" but rather an inability to grieve. We simply do not have the language, the cultural conventions, to work through this loss.

Butler also clarifies how homosexual melancholy works. While homosexuality may be culturally prohibited, subjects who desire same-sex subjects nevertheless come to be. While our norms are impressive, they are not total. Those whose identity struggles against normative pressures to assimilate to heterosexuality suffer a distinct form of melancholia. Butler writes:

> Gay melancholia . . . contains anger that can be translated into political expression. It is precisely to counter this pervasive cultural risk of gay melancholia (what the

newspapers generalize as "depression") that there has been an insistent publiciza-
tion and politicization of grief over those who have died of AIDS. The Names
Project Quilt is exemplary, ritualizing and repeating the name itself as a way of
publicly avowing limitless loss. Insofar as grief remains unspeakable, the rage over
loss can redouble by virtue of remaining unavowed. And if that rage is publicly
proscribed, the melancholic effects of such a proscription can achieve suicidal proportions. (147–48)

In this passage, Butler clearly demonstrates how her analysis acknowledges the real
suffering of the gay community—that is, how this community becomes a victim of
depression and suicide. However, she clearly chooses against analyzing epidemic
suicide rates and depression in the gay community within a medical paradigm.
Such a paradigm, in her estimation, takes individual suffering out of a larger social
context. Moreover, the medical paradigm understands identity and traumas of self,
perhaps, too far outside a social context. Those who are gay and depressed cannot
be properly attended to if one does not understand the dynamics of identity formation.

Butler interprets this epidemic in political terms, and likewise she foresees its
solution in political protest. The health of the gay community depends not on psychotherapy or psychopharmacology, claims Butler, but in opening up spaces for political protest as, for example, the Names Project Quilt does. She further writes: "The
emergence of collective institutions for grieving are thus crucial to survival, to reas-
sembling community, to rearticulating kinship, to reweaving sustaining relations"
(148). The danger of a medical approach and medical intervention is that it may miss
the forest for the trees. While individual gays may be relieved of their suffering with
antidepressants, for example, the opportunity to understand the political circumstances of this epidemic will be lost. To resort to a medical metaphor, we will treat
the symptom and ignore the disease.

In similar fashion, a great deal of feminist research is appearing that ties the high
rates of depression in women to gender oppression (see Schiesari 1992; Zita 1998;
Hansen 1999; Restuccia 2000). Women are depressed because they are oppressed.
Repeatedly, psychiatric epidemiology reports show that women fall into depression
twice as often as men, "regardless of racial and ethnic background or economic
status," and this "same ratio has been reported in eleven countries all over the world"
(U.S. Department of Health and Human Services 1994; Wilhelm et al. 1997). Women
are also prescribed antidepressants at higher rates than men (Ashton 1991; Silverstone
1998). While many theorists study female biology and its unique proclivities toward
depression in the wake of this data, other feminists follow the lead of Continental
social theorists by attending to the hostility of Western culture toward femininity and
how this affects female identity development.

What is important to clarify about much of this feminist research is that it does
not ignore female biology as an aspect of female depression, nor does it wholeheartedly eschew psychopharmacological intervention. What these feminist analyses do is
change the focus from individual biology or pathology to social context. Because
some psychiatrists achieve a great deal of success by prescribing new, powerful anti-

depressants for their female patients, we take a chance when we ask important questions about how oppressive political forces affect female mental health.

For example, some of the criteria for the diagnosis of depression overlap with cultural patterns of female identity. The DSM-IV claims that depressed persons have "feelings of worthlessness or excessive or inappropriate guilt" and that depressed persons have "diminshed ability to think or concentrate" (American Psychiatric Association 1994: 327). Morever, because pervasive stereotypes portray women as indecisive, fickle, insecure, and passive, ad nauseum, physicians and psychiatrists might too quickly make judgments that women are suffering a major mood disorder and therefore are in need of antidepressants. Once the female patient's complaints become heard within a medical, psychiatric framework, the health provider may in fact stop listening to the patient's history. In this scenario, the medical community becomes increasingly complicit in shifting political questions concerning the conditions of women in Western culture away from political analyses.

It may be that women do largely suffer from mood disorders that leave them feeling worthless, guilt-ridden, inefficacious, or listless. Many of the symptoms of this suffering may indeed be alleviated by medical intervention. However, what many contemporary feminist theorists are pointing out is that we may very well be able to understand this suffering, this mood disorder among women, as a reasonable response to a culture that devalues and disrespects women. Plenty of psychologists and psychiatrists are well aware of this particular interpretation of women's depression (see, for example, Nolen-Hoeksema 1990; McGrath 1990; Mazure et al. 2002). However, as psychiatry becomes increasingly dominated by psychopharmacology, which proceeds by abstracting the human person from a social context in order to study internal neurochemical functioning, the fear is that the culture will continue to oppress women. We may make women better able to function in that culture by administering pills, and we may make them suffer less, but we will have done little to attack the problem at its roots.

CONCLUSION

The field of philosophical literature on depression and melancholia is bountiful. Although this essay demonstrates the variety of perspectives, and how these perspectives often clash with one another, we are richer for it. Philosophical research on mood disorders repeatedly demonstrates that the field is essentially interdisciplinary. The strength of interdisciplinary work is that many important minds are coming together to think through the crucial questions that depression poses for humanity. Whether these thinkers challenge each other to change the focus of their conceptual lenses, or to reformulate the essential nature of the meaning of depression, the psychiatric and philosophical communities can only benefit.

In this brief survey, I have only scratched the surface of research and writings on mood. As one digs deeper into the literature on depression, it becomes clear that as long as humans have asked questions and written down their observations and insights, depression has been a central domain of study. Depression and mania also have a special relationship to the philosopher; such human ailments both inspire and horrify the curious mind. In her work highlighting the high correlation between manic-depressive illness and artistic temperament, Kay Jamison remarks that Lord Byron "represents the fine edge of the fine madness — the often imperceptible line between poetic temperament and psychiatric illness" (1993: 7). Perhaps philosophers and other creative people are doomed to muse about depression as long as they muse about anything. And if I am right, then the debates concerning what depression means and how to cope with it will not cease but only multiply as we encounter new problems of communal living and self-identity.

NOTES

1. According to the *National Vital Statistics Report* for 1999, suicide was the eleventh ranking cause for death in the United States. Suicide claims more deaths in the United States than homicide (29,199 deaths compared to 16,889) (Hoyert et al. 2001). It is estimated that 90 percent of those who killed themselves were either depressed or had a substance abuse disorder (NIMH 2001).

2. In "Melancholic Epistemology," George Graham considers depression from an "epistemic point of view" (1991: 399). "Melancholic epistemology" searches for criteria with which to evaluate the truthful beliefs of depressed persons. Graham argues that depressed persons may be justified or warranted in their depressed states of mind and suggests that those states of mind may in fact offer truthful information. Graham's interest in this paper is in part to challenge Aaron Beck's view that depressed thinking is largely illogical inferences and hence without any truthful content.

3. Lauren Alloy and Lyn Abramson (1988) developed their notion of "depressive realism" as an alternate view to the popular view held by Aaron Beck (1967) that most depressed people's negative views are a result of logical errors in interpreting reality.

REFERENCES

Alloy, Lauren B., and Abramson, Lyn Y. (1988) "Depressive Realism: Four Theoretical Perspectives." In L. B. Alloy (ed.), *Cognitive Processes in Depression*. New York: Guilford Press.

Althusser, Louis, and Balibar, Etienne (1970) *Reading Capital*. Translated by Ben Brewster. New York: Pantheon Books.

American Psychiatric Association (1994) *Diagnostic and Statistical Manual of Mental Disorders*, 4th ed. Washington, DC: American Psychiatric Association.

Anderson, Elizabeth S. (1991) "John Stuart Mill and Experiments in Living." *Ethics* 102 (October): 4–26.

Ardal, Pall S. (1993) "Depression and Reason." *Ethics* 103 (April): 540–50.

Ashton, Heather (1991) "Psychotropic-Drug Prescribing for Women." *Bristish Journal of Psychiatry* 158 (suppl. 10): 30–35.

Beck, Aaron T. (1967) *Depression: Clinical, Experimental, and Theoretical Aspects.* New York: Harper and Row.

Birnbaum, H. G. et al. (1999) "Work-place Burden of Depression: A Case Study in Social Functioning using Employer Claims Data." *Drug Benefit Trends* 11(8).

Butler, J. (1997) *The Psychic Life of Power: Theories in Subjection.* Stanford, CA: Stanford University Press.

Caton, Hiram (1986) "Pascal's Syndrome: Positivism as a Symptom of Depression and Mania." *Zygon* 21(3): 319–51.

Cheever, Abigail (2000) "Prozac Americans: Depression, Identity, and Selfhood." *Twentieth Century Literature* 46(3): 346–68.

Cheng, Anne Anlin (2000) *The Melancholy of Race.* New York: Oxford University Press.

Elliott, Carl (2000) "Pursued by Happiness and Beaten Senseless: Prozac and the American Dream." *Hastings Center Report* 30(2): 7–12.

Ferguson, Harvie (1995) *Melancholy and the Critique of Modernity: Søren Kierkegaard's Religious Psychology.* New York: Routledge.

Francassa, Moira (1999) "Medicating the Self: The Roles of Science and Culture in the Construction of Prozac." *Journal of Popular Culture* 32(4): 23–28.

Freud, Sigmund (1963 [1917]) "Mourning and Melancholia." *General Psychological Theory.* Edited by Philip Rieff. New York: Collier Books.

Ghaemi, S. Nassir (1999) "Depression: Insight, Illusion, and Psychopharmacological Calvinism." *Philosophy, Psychiatry and Psychology* 6(4): 287–94.

Graham, George (1991) "Melancholic Epistemology." In James H. Fetzer (ed.), *Epistemology and Cognition.* Boston: Kluwer Academic.

Graham, George (2002) "Recent Work in Philosophical Psychopathology." *American Philosophical Quarterly* 39(2): 109–34.

Greenspan, Patricia (2001) "Good Evolutionary Reasons: Darwinian Psychiatry and Women's Depression." *Philosophical Psychiatry* 14(3): 327–38.

Hansen, Jennifer (1999) "Re-membering the Self: Gender, Melancholia, and Philosophical Method." Ph.D. dissertation, State University of New York, Stony Brook.

Hoyert, D. L., Arias, E., Smith, B. L., Murphy, S. L., and Kochanek, K. D. (2001) "Deaths: Final Data for 1999." *National Vital Statistics Report,* 49 (8). DHHS Publication No. (PHS) 2001-1120. Hyattsville, MD: National Center for Health Statistics. Available at http://www.cdc.gov/nchs/data/nvs47_19.pdf

Husserl, Edmund (1970) "The Vienna Lecture." In *The Crisis of European Sciences and Transcendental Philosophy: An Introduction to Phenomenological Philosophy.* Evanston: Northwestern University Press.

Jamison, Kay Redfield (1993) *Touched with Fire: Manic-Depressive Illness and the Artistic Temperament.* New York: Free Press Paperbacks.

Kahn, Abraham H. (1994) "Melancholy: An Elusive Dimension of Depression?" *Journal of Medical Humanities* 15(2): 113–22.

Klein, Melanie (1975 [1955]) "On Identification." In *Envy and Gratitude and Other Works 1946–1963.* New York: Free Press.

Klerman, Gerald (1972) "Psychotropic Hedonism vs. Pharmacological Calvinism." *Hastings Center Report* 2: 1–3.

Kramer, Peter D. (2000) "The Valorization of Sadness: Alienation and the Melancholic Temperament." *Hastings Center Report* 30(2): 13–18.

Kristeva, Julia (1987) *Black Sun: Depression and Melancholia.* Translated by Leon S. Roudiez. New York: Columbia University Press.

Lacan, Jacques (1977) *Ecrits: A Selection.* Translated by Alan Sheridan. New York: Norton.

Lepenies, Wolf (1992) *Melancholy and Society.* Cambridge, MA: Harvard University Press.

Marcuse, Herbert (1955) "Eros and Civilization: A Philosophical Inquiry into Freud." Boston: Beacon Press.

Martel, Huguette (1993) "If They Had Prozac in the Nineteenth Century (Political Cartoon)." *New Yorker,* Vol. 69, Issue 37, No. 8.

Martin, Mike (1999) "Depression: Illness, Insight, and Identity." *Philosophy, Psychiatry and Psychology* 6(4): 271–86.

Mazure, C. M., Keita, G. P., and Blehar, M. C. (2002) *Summit on Women and Depression: Proceedings and Recommendations.* Washington, DC: American Psychological Association.

McGrath, E., et al. (1990) *Final Report of the American Psychological Association's National Task Force on Women and Depression.* Washington, DC: American Psychological Association.

NARSAD (National Alliance for Research on Schizophrenia and Depression) (2002) "Quick Facts." Available at http://www.mhsource.com/narsad/help/numbers.html

Nelson, Alan (1985) "John Stuart Mill: The Reformer Reformed." *Interpretation* 13: 359–401.

NIMH (National Institutes of Mental Health) (2001) *In Harm's Way: Suicide in America.* NIH Publication No. 01-4594. Washington, DC: NIMH. Available at http://www.nimh.nih.gov/publicat/harmaway.cfm

Nolen-Hoeksema, Susan (1990) *Sex Differences in Depression.* Stanford: Stanford University Press.

Pensky, Max (1993) *Melancholy Dialectics: Walter Benjamin and the Play of Mourning.* Amherst: University of Massachusetts Press.

Radden, Jennifer (1987) "Melancholy and Melancholia." In David Michael Levin (ed.), *Pathologies of the Modern Self: Postmodern Studies on Narcissism, Schizophrenia, and Depression.* New York: New York University Press.

Radden, Jennifer (2000) *The Nature of Melancholy: From Aristotle to Kristeva.* New York: Oxford University Press.

Radden, Jennifer (2003) "Is This Dame Melancholy?: Equating Today's Depression and Past Melancholia." *Philosophy, Psychiatry and Psychology* 10(1): 37–52.

Reiger, D. A. et al. (1993) "The De Facto U.S. Mental Addictive Disorders Service System." *Archives of General Psychiatry* 50: 85–94.

Restuccia, Frances (2000) *Melancholics in Love: Representing Women's Depression and Domestic Abuse.* Lanham, MD: Rowman and Littlefield.

Roberts, John Russell (2001) "Mental Illness, Motivation and Moral Commitment." *Philosophical Quarterly* 51(202): 1–59.

Rose, Gillian (1996) *Mourning Becomes the Law: Philosophy and Representation.* New York: Cambridge University Press.

Schiesari, Juliana (1992) *The Gendering of Melancholia: Feminism, Psychoanalysis, and the Symbolics of Loss in Renaissance Literature.* Ithaca, NY: Cornell University Press.

Schor, Naomi (1996) *One Hundred Years of Melancholy: The Zaharoff Lecture.* Oxford: Clarendon Press.

Silberfeld, Michel, and Checkland, David (1999) "Faulty Judgement, Expert Opinion, and Decision-Making Capacity." *Theoretical Medicine and Bioethics* 20: 377–93.

Silverstone, Trevor (1998) "Women and Pharmacological Therapies." In Sarah E. Romans (ed.), *Folding Back the Shadows: A Perspective on Women's Mental Health*. Dunedin, New Zealand: University of Otago Press.

Starobinski, Jean (1962) *History of the Treatment of Melancholy from the Earliest Times to 1900*. Basel: J. R. Geigy.

U.S. Department of Health and Human Services, National Institutes of Health, National Institutes of Mental Health (1994) *Depression: What Every Woman Should Know*. NIH Publication 95-3871. Washington, DC: U.S. Government Printing Office.

Weisberger, A. M. (1995) "The Ethics of Broader Usage of Prozac: Social Choice or Social Bias?" *International Journal of Applied Philosophy* 10: 69–74.

Wilhelm, K., Parker, G., and Hadzi-Pavlovic, D. (1997) "Fifteen Years On: Evolving Ideas in Researching Sex Differences in Depression." *Psychological Medicine* 27: 875–83.

Zita, Jacqueline (1998) *Body Talk: Philosophical Reflections on Sex and Gender*. New York: Columbia University Press.

CHAPTER 3

DESIRE

Paraphilia and Distress in DSM-IV

ALAN G. SOBLE

IN 1940, psychologist Clifford Allen called sexualities that depart from ordinary heterosexuality (e.g., fetishism, homosexual activity) "perversions" and "paraphilias"—that is, "diseases" of sexuality.[1] Even though the most recent version of the handbook of the American Psychiatric Association—the *Diagnostic and Statistical Manual of Mental Disorders*, 4th edition—excludes homosexual orientation from the sexual mental disorders, and even though it eschews the pejorative "perversion" in favor of the clinical "paraphilia" in naming other sexualities, one might still ask whether American psychiatry, 60 years after Clifford, offers just another nod to premodern, traditional, or theological notions of sexual perversion. The answer, I think, is that DSM-IV embodies cultural biases "masquerading"[2] as scientific medical truth but also expresses a more liberal view of human sexuality. Philosophers have subjected earlier incarnations of DSM to critical scrutiny.[3] Some of these investigations have been fruitful; by intention or fortuitously, DSM-IV has incorporated proposals made in the critical literature. But DSM-IV has also been the target of attack—often incredulous and virulent.[4]

The revolutionary change in the earlier DSM-III was its not including homosexuality per se as a mental disorder,[5] despite homosexuality's different desire structure and gay promiscuity, some of it anonymous. DSM-IV retains this change. But psychically distressing ("ego-dystonic") homosexuality was included in DSM-III and appears in DSM-IV. Under "Sexual Disorder Not Otherwise Specified," there is the diagnosis "Persistent and marked distress about sexual orientation" (538). This category includes distressing homosexuality *and* distressing heterosexuality.[6] Unlike DSM-III, DSM-IV doesn't use "ego-dystonic" to name distressing homosexuality; indeed, it doesn't even use "homosexuality" to name it. DSM-III's discussion of ego-dystonic homosexuality (281–82) is longer and more nuanced than this single sentence DSM-IV devotes to it.

In response to this change in the pathological status of homosexuality, it has been argued that the reasons for excluding homosexuality also apply to some paraphilias: homosexuality and some paraphilias do not involve conduct harmful to others; the illegality of these behaviors does not warrant in itself a sexual mental disorder judgment; paraphiliac desire deviates no more radically from heterosexuality than does homosexuality; and paraphiliacs lead lives no more functionally impaired than those of homosexuals.[7] So, if homosexuality is replaced by the less populous category of distressing homosexuality, only distressing paraphilia should be a mental disorder.[8] DSM-IV largely conceded this point by adding "distress" to the diagnostic criteria of paraphilia.

Problems remain even after distress is added as a diagnostic criterion. First, once distress is a diagnostic criterion, the *sexual* nature of the acts becomes irrelevant: distressing fetishism and distressing psoriasis, for example, belong in their own category of "ego-dystonic" disorders.[9] Similarly, some cases of paraphilia might be better classified as volitional disabilities or disorders of impulse control, rather than as sexual disorders.[10] Second, DSM-IV claims that for the diagnosis of mental disorder, distress must be endogenous, due to something "in the individual," and not exogenous, not "primarily" caused by conflicts between the "deviant" person and society (xxi–xxii).[11] As DSM-III says about ego-dystonic homosexuality, "distress resulting from a conflict between a homosexual and society should not be classified here" (282). Yet, whether paraphiliac distress, when it exists, is mostly endogenous is not clear.[12] Third, perhaps there is still pathology, or more pathology, if paraphilias such as voyeurism and pedophilia are "ego-syntonic," if the person is *not* distressed by his behavior. DSM-IV-TR (the "text revision" of DSM-IV) partly agrees, since it demotes distress as a diagnostic criterion of paraphilia when the behavior involves nonconsenting victims (566, 840). DSM-IV-TR, however, seems not to demote distress *because* absence of distress in such cases is a stronger sign of pathology than its presence.[13]

The diagnostic mission of psychic distress is specified in DSM-IV's definition of "paraphilia":

> The *Paraphilias* are characterized by recurrent, intense sexual urges, fantasies, or behaviors that involve unusual objects, activities, or situations and cause clinically significant distress or impairment in social, occupational, or other important areas of functioning. (493)

Note three things: the objects or activities are "unusual"; distress, even without impaired functioning, constitutes sexual mental disorder (psychic pain is a noxious condition to be remedied); and the fantasies, urges, or behaviors—not something else—*cause* the distress. DSM-IV lists eight numerically coded paraphilias: exhibitionism, fetishism, frotteurism, pedophilia, sexual masochism, sexual sadism, transvestic fetishism, and voyeurism. DSM-IV expands its list of paraphilias in its diagnostic category "Paraphilia Not Otherwise Specified" (532), adding telephone scatologia, necrophilia, partialism, zoophilia, coprophilia, urophilia, and klismaphilia.[14]

DSM-IV asserts that being unusual (deviant) is necessary for sexual fantasies, urges, or behaviors to be paraphiliac, but not sufficient: "Neither deviant behavior (e.g., political, religious, or sexual) nor conflicts that are primarily between the individual and society are mental disorders" (xxii). There must also be distress or impairment in functioning (xxi). But if it is unlikely that there could be sexual deviance but *no* conflict with society's sexual norms, it is also unlikely that there could be sexual deviance but *no* distress. To the extent that this distress is exogenous, no one qualifies as a paraphiliac. This is paradoxical. Paraphilias are sexual mental disorders for DSM-IV in part because they are unusual, but in virtue of being unusual, their associated distress might be exogenous, which blocks the diagnosis.

DSM-IV cannot get far with "unusual," anyway. Consider a two-hour marathon of heterosexual fellatio. Alan Goldman (2002) asserts about such an act that its being unusual per se does not make it "abnormal." Something else is required; he proposes that the unusual component must be "the *form of the desire* itself in order to constitute sexual perversion" (53). This is incompatible with DSM-IV. DSM-IV does not fault homosexual desire, even though it is unusual and defies sexuality's reproductive function, and once heterosexual desire is no longer privileged, to claim that the unusual, nonreproductive desires of klismaphilia and partialism are disordered is unsupportable. DSM-III had explained its choice of the term "paraphilia" by saying that it "is preferable [to "sexual deviation"] because it correctly emphasizes that the deviation (para) is in that to which the individual is attracted (philia)" (266–67). This rationale is odd (and missing from DSM-IV); homosexuality, which DSM-III does not label a paraphilia, involves a deviation, in a descriptive sense, "in that to which the individual is attracted." DSM-IV is explicit in not faulting paraphiliac desire per se: unusual desires are disordered only if they cause distress or impairment. Yet, DSM-IV tries to distinguish nondisordered desire from paraphiliac desire by claiming that paraphilia often involves an impaired capacity for "reciprocal, affectionate sexual activity" (524). Both editions of DSM (III, 267; IV, 524) regard this as an "associated feature" of paraphilia, but this indicator of impairment is incautious and perniciously value-laden.[15] Further, even if straight and gay sexuality do not often involve such impairment (which is dubious, not only for bathhouse gays but also for "sexually addicted" straights),[16] there *are* couples who engage in affectionate sadomasochism, urophilia, and klismaphilia. The class of the sexually mentally disordered becomes smaller, perhaps restricted to those who are not lucky enough to find a sexual soul mate. Even in these cases, distress might be more exogenous than endogenous.

DSM-IV maintains that being unusual is only necessary and adds, instead of a criterion based on the form of desire, that the fantasies, urges, or behaviors cause distress or impairment. But if distress and impairment are *that* important, more important than the form of desire, it seems that whether fantasies, urges, and behaviors are unusual is irrelevant. Even common activities, say, masturbation, if distressing or impairing, should be a matter of psychiatric concern.[17] Indeed, DSM-IV grants that being unusual is irrelevant: distress over having a heterosexual orientation is a sexual mental disorder, even though being heterosexual (like masturbating) is hardly unusual.

DSM-IV also claims that unusual sexuality is not paraphiliac if it "is not the individual's preferred or obligatory pattern" (525). A fantasy, urge, or behavior's being obligatory is therefore a necessary condition of paraphilia.[18] A connection between obligatoriness and impairment seems in part why paraphilia is disordered. For example, "Usually the fetish is required or strongly preferred for sexual excitement, and in its absence there may be erectile dysfunction" (DSM-IV, 526; DSM-III, 268). However, even though erectile dysfunction is an impairment, it is not the fetish condition that causes this impairment but the absence of the stimulus. The stubbornly flaccid husband who no longer finds his wife arousing is not necessarily impaired. The stimulus is inadequate, or a stimulus that would work for him—another woman—is missing. What DSM-IV might be driving at is that the exclusivity of a paraphiliac stimulus causes impairment through a decrease in overall sexual satisfaction. If the paraphiliac does not have access to his stimulus, he has (unlike the bored husband) no other way of achieving satisfaction and is significantly deprived and hence impaired. Yet, that satisfaction is decreased because the stimulus is obligatory is a social contingency—what other people like and dislike—and not inherent to the condition. Were other people, the "normals," themselves less sexually exclusive, more would enjoy sexual enemas and the klismaphiliac's suffering would be attenuated. DSM-IV also points out that "in some instances, the unusual behavior . . . may become the major sexual activity in the individual's life" (523). DSM-IV would be on firmer ground reserving mental disorder for cases in which the activity is the person's major activity *simpliciter*, with implications for impairment in other areas of life (see DSM-III, 267–68).[19]

Suppose we focus on the distress a paraphiliac might have over the fact that his sexual stimulus is obligatory.[20] It seems that there should not be much distress over exclusivity itself, especially if the preferred act is sufficient for sexual pleasure. (If a person *were* distressed merely over the exclusivity of his sexual interest, perhaps that *would* be a disorder.) A belief held by the individual that the desire or act is in some way wrong seems required. Heterosexuals are not distressed over the exclusivity of their sexual interest because straight exclusivity is not accompanied by judgments condemning heterosexual desire. Paraphiliac distress, then, results from the tension between the person's sexuality and his beliefs. If so, it matters little that the desires are narrow or the acts obligatory: what matters is that distress results from tension between desires and beliefs, and this can occur more generally, for any type of sexuality and any type of desire.

Under what conditions should distress count as, or be symptomatic of, mental disorder? The formula provided by DSM-IV for distinguishing mental-disorder (endogenous) distress from nonmental-disorder (exogenous) distress—that, to be endogenous, distress must be caused by the sexual fantasies, urges, or behavior (493, 523) or must result from something "in the individual" (a psychological, behavioral, or biological dysfunction [xxi]) and must not be "primarily" the result of a conflict between the person and society (xxii) — is not always easy to apply. What situations are "conflicts" between a person and society? How are the "psychological" dysfunctions that underlie mental disorder to be identified? Sometimes the formula permits us to sort out disordered from nondisordered states. But not always.

DSM-IV mentions that "social and sexual relationships may suffer if others find the unusual sexual behavior shameful or repugnant or if the individual's sexual partner refuses to cooperate in the unusual sexual preferences" (523). To me, such distress seems exogenous and hence not indicative of mental disorder.[21] Being reactively distressed that one's mate sneeringly rejects one's sexual requests is different from being endogenously distressed at one's sexual urge itself. Now consider a description of "ego-dystonic homosexuality" from DSM-III:

> Generally individuals with this disorder have had homosexual relationships, but often the physical satisfaction is accompanied by emotional upset because of strong negative feelings regarding homosexuality. In some cases the negative feelings are so strong that the homosexual arousal has been confined to fantasy. (281)

For DSM-III, this distress is both endogenous and due to tension between a person's sexual desires and his beliefs or attitudes ("negative feelings") about those desires. Thus, DSM-IV's claim that sexual fantasies, urges, or behaviors *cause* distress is inaccurate. They do not cause distress on their own; the beliefs or attitudes with which they don't fit are also causally relevant.

The endogenous distress in the described case is brought about by desires and attitudes that are *the individual's*. The desire, no matter where it comes from, is the person's desire, part of *his* psychological makeup; even if the "negative attitudes" come from society, broadly construed (from where else could they come?), that they are held by the individual makes them *his*. As DSM-III says, "The factors that predispose to Ego-dystonic Homosexuality are those negative societal attitudes toward homosexuality that have been internalized" (282). The resulting distress, arising from tension between desire and belief, is endogenous, even if much of a person's psychology is social in origin. The ontological point is that some mental disorders *in* a person are caused by external entities: parents, trauma, "society." That a belief is socially imposed and causes psychic distress neither entails nor is equivalent to the distress's being the result of a "conflict" between the person and society. When DSM-III says that "distress resulting from a conflict between a homosexual and society should not be classified here" (282), it doesn't mean that if the distress-causing belief comes from society, a mental disorder diagnosis cannot be sustained.

While discussing paraphilia, DSM-IV describes a state similar to DSM-III's ego-dystonic homosexuality: some paraphiliacs "report extreme guilt, shame, and depression at having to engage in an unusual sexual activity that is socially unacceptable or that they regard as immoral" (524).[22] DSM-IV's reference to a person's own morality (absent from DSM-III [267]) implies that there can be mental disorder with respect to behaviors society condones or tolerates, as long as the person believes they are wrong; distressing heterosexuality and distressing promiscuity thus become candidate mental disorders. In this situation, therapy may accept the belief and pinpoint the desire as the main culprit in causing the distress. Further, DSM-IV's reference to a person's own morality carves out space for mental disorder to result primarily from mistaken belief: the desires might be innocuous and the behavior might not be demonstrably immoral (masturbation), yet the person believes that it is. In this situation, therapy may accept the desire and pinpoint the false or unsupported belief as the main culprit in causing the distress. Again, it doesn't matter that the beliefs come from society; if society instills the "bad" beliefs, nonetheless the person ends up disordered.[23]

Let us return to the idea that "the factors that predispose to Ego-dystonic Homosexuality are those negative societal attitudes toward homosexuality that have been internalized" (DSM-III, 282). Note "predispose": DSM-III implies that not everyone who internalizes these attitudes experiences distress. Some people are endogenously more sensitive or overreact to tension between their desires and internalized attitudes. It might be possible to conceive of distressing homosexuality and paraphilia as an endogenous disproportionate reaction to lack of fit between belief and desire. Recall another thing DSM-III said about ego-dystonic homosexuality: "In some cases the negative feelings are so strong that the homosexual arousal has been confined to fantasy" (281). Distress that is "so strong" as to kill behavior altogether is a disproportionate response to tension between desire and belief. Here distress is not *reducible* to tension between desire and belief; it cannot be altogether explained by lack of fit between desire and belief, but is in part the result of a dysfunction "in the individual." Alexander Portnoy might be the paraphiliac equivalent.

Culver and Gert (1982) propose that if suffering "persist[s] much longer than is normal for the species, for example, if the grief period is significantly prolonged, then one does begin to explain the suffering as due to something wrong with the person" (98).[24] But what period or intensity of distress is psychologically "normal for the species"? If that cannot be answered, then even if prolonged or intense distress is "due to something" about the person, we cannot assert that it is due to something *wrong* with the person. Under "Adjustment Disorders," DSM-IV says that "the diagnosis of Adjustment Disorder may be appropriate [for bereavement] when the reaction is in excess of, or more prolonged than, what would be expected" (626; see xxi). Neither "longer than is normal for the species" nor "in excess of . . . what would be expected" is satisfactory. Whether distress is excessive, then, probably rests on whether it is impairing. In this way, impairment is a more important diagnostic criterion than distress. How else is an Adjustment Disorder going to be a disorder unless impairment is caused by its associated distress? How else can we tell that distress is excessive, or make sense of the claim, if not through its effects on functioning?[25]

DSM-III eliminated homosexuality as a mental disorder, retaining only distressing homosexuality; DSM-IV continues this trend, diagnosing paraphiliac disorder only when the sexuality is distressing or impairing. But if paraphilia should be handled the same way as homosexuality, why does DSM-IV devote ten pages to paraphilia and only seven words to homosexuality? Perhaps DSM-IV assumes that paraphilia is frequently impairing, even though paraphiliacs do not often present themselves clinically (DSM-IV, 523, 524). It is not empirically clear that paraphiliacs are in any worse position than homosexuals. DSM-IV acknowledges, "Many individuals with these disorders assert that the behavior causes them no distress and that their only problem is social dysfunction as a result of the reaction of others to their behaviors" (524), but it doesn't comment on the veracity of the defense. If there is little distress and the functional problems are "primarily" the result of conflicts with society, it is wrong, by its own criteria, for DSM-IV to speak about "individuals *with these disorders.*" By including that phrase, DSM-IV rejects their defense: the "many individuals" are in denial. DSM-IV refuses to give paraphiliacs the benefit of the doubt, the way it gives the benefit of the doubt to homosexuals.[26]

NOTES

1. See his book's title and, for example, 57.

2. Suppe [1987], 112.

3. Culver and Gert; Gert; Margolis; Suppe.

4. Davis; National Organization of Women; "Psychiatric Diagnosis: Manufacturing Madness." I discussed DSM-IV briefly in my [1996], 160–63, 173.

5. The change had already been made in 1973–74 as a revision to DSM-II (Conrad and Schneider, 208–9).

6. DSM-IV thereby conceded a point made by Conrad and Schneider (209), Margolis (292), and Suppe ([1987], 118). For DSM-IV-TR, distress at one's sexual orientation explicitly includes distressing bisexuality (535).

7. See Suppe [1984], 21; [1987], 130–31.

8. See Silverstein, 34–35. Suppe claimed that the "decision [of DSM-III] to include just one ego-dystonic condition [homosexuality] as a mental disorder seems highly arbitrary" ([1984], 14; [1987], 118). This is not quite true: see obsession-compulsion (III, 359; IV, 418). Further, if "ego-dystonic" in part means "distressing," DSM-III describes sexual disorders other than homosexuality as distressing (e.g., 278, 283).

9. Culver and Gert, 107; Suppe [1984], 13–14, 21–23; [1987], 119–20, 130–32.

10. Culver and Gert, 103; Suppe [1984], 23, 26; [1987], 129, 131.

11. Culver and Gert offer another version: "the suffering is explained primarily as due to something wrong with the person rather than something abnormal about his environment" (97).

12. For Culver and Gert, "the primary reason why certain recurring sexual behaviors are maladies is that they are ego-dystonic. The person engaging in the behavior is distressed by it" (104). Hence, voyeurs "have a sexual malady to the extent that their peeping is ego-dystonic" (106). This might be right, and it is (absent impairment) DSM-IV's view, but it is misleading. Only endogenous distress makes the voyeur's condition a mental disorder (as Gert [167] acknowledges).

13. I discuss DSM-IV-TR at length in my "Alternative Desires, Arousals, and Satisfactions: The Paraphilias in DSM-IV" (in preparation). Write to the author at asoble@uno.edu for a typescript.

14. DSM-IV might have included others; see Katharine Gates's profusely illustrated book and web site, and chapter 1 of my [2002]. Deserving mention are an attraction to smoking women (see Allen, 174); sexual desire for obese or anorexic women, or for ampu-

tees; sexual interest in women with hairy armpits, legs, or forearms or those dressed in jeans and heavily cosmeticized; and sexual arousal from spit, snot, vomit, or the ejaculate of women or men (DSM-III [275] included "Mysophilia (filth)," which is missing from DSM-IV). Several of these might be subsumed, with some stretching, under fetishism or partialism.

15. See Davis and Herdt, 953; Primoratz, 181–28; Suppe [1987], 124–26. An associated feature is not a diagnostic criterion, because it is "insufficiently sensitive or specific" (DSM-IV, 8).

16. "DSM-III cannot view impaired capacity for reciprocal affectionate *sexual* activity as a disability in the case of the [paraphilias] while denying that it is for homosexuality" (Suppe [1984], 21). Some gays (like some straights) know well the life of nonaffectionate sexuality, about which DSM-IV never raises a diagnostic or therapeutic eyebrow.

17. Carnes, 39–40; Culver and Gert, 104, 107; Suppe [1984], 13, [1987], 118.

18. But DSM-IV claims that "Not uncommonly, individuals have more than one Paraphilia" (523). So, if "paraphilia" is defined in terms of the obligatory quality of a stimulus, there are not many (genuine) paraphiliacs.

19. Further, as Neu argues, exclusivity "cannot be used to mark off homosexuality as perverse without marking off (excessively strong) commitments to heterosexuality as equally perverse" (92). The same seems to apply to paraphilia.

20. DSM-IV does not require that distress be at, about, or over something; that is, the diagnostic criteria of paraphilia do not require that the distress have an intentional object. DSM-IV says that the fantasies, urges, or behavior *cause* distress; this can happen with or without an intentional object. But DSM-IV does allow that the distress is intentional, both in general (524) and in the definition of particular sexual disorders (e.g., 538).

21. Culver and Gert apparently agree: distress that results from "the consequences that are contingent on" the behavior is not diagnostic of mental disorder (107).

22. Several decades before DSM-IV, Philip Roth (in his mock epigraph) described something like distressing paraphilia caused by one's moral beliefs. He defined "Portnoy's Complaint" as

> A disorder in which strongly felt ethical and altruistic impulses are perpetually warring with extreme sexual longings, often of a perverse nature. Spielvogel says: "Acts of exhibitionism, voyeurism, fetishism, auto-eroticism and oral coitus are plentiful; as a consequence of the patient's 'morality,' however, neither fantasy nor act issues in genuine sexual gratification, but rather in overriding feelings of shame and the dread of retribution, particularly in the form of castration."

23. Distress might occur because a person "has internalized mistaken standards." So "an individual can suffer from an unjustified (but perhaps socially encouraged) self-loathing" (Neu, 102n13).

24. See Gert, 159.

25. DSM-IV apparently agrees: "distress or impairment in functioning . . . is frequently manifested as decreased performance at work or school" (624; see 626).

26. For their help, I thank W. Scott Griffies, Edward Johnson, John Kleinig, Jerome Neu, Igor Primoratz, Jennifer Radden, Kristin von Ranson, Alan Wertheimer, and students in my fall 2002 Philosophy of Sex seminar. Please browse my web site (http://www.uno.edu/~asoble) for essays and other material that relate to this chapter.

REFERENCES

Allen, Clifford (1979 [orig. 1940, 1949]) *The Sexual Perversions and Abnormalities: A Study in the Psychology of Paraphilia*. Westport, CT: Greenwood Press.

American Psychiatric Association (1980) *Diagnostic and Statistical Manual of Mental Disorders*, 3rd ed. [DSM-III]. Washington, DC: American Psychiatric Association.

American Psychiatric Association (1994) *Diagnostic and Statistical Manual of Mental Disorders*, 4th ed. [DSM-IV]. Washington, DC: American Psychiatric Association.

American Psychiatric Association (2000) *Diagnostic and Statistical Manual of Mental Disorders*, 4th ed., Text Revision. [DSM-IV-TR]. Washington, DC: American Psychiatric Association.

Carnes, Patrick (2001) *Out of the Shadows: Understanding Sexual Addiction*, 3rd ed. Center City, MN: Hazelden.

Citizens Commission on Human Rights (1997) "Psychiatric Diagnosis: Manufacturing Madness." In *Psychiatry: Destroying Religion*. Los Angeles, CA: Citizens Commission on Human Rights, pp. 44–47.

Conrad, Peter, and Schneider, Joseph W. (1980) *Deviance and Medicalization: From Badness to Sickness*. St. Louis, MO: C. V. Mosby.

Culver, Charles M., and Gert, Bernard (1982) *Philosophy in Medicine: Conceptual and Ethical Issues in Medicine and Psychiatry*. New York: Oxford University Press.

Davis, Dona, and Herdt, Gilbert (1997) "Cultural Issues and Sexual Disorders." In Thomas A. Widiger, Allen J. Francis, Harold Alan Pincus, Ruth Ross, Michael B. First, and Wendy Davis (eds.), *DSM-IV Sourcebook*, vol. 3. Washington, DC: American Psychiatric Association, pp. 951–57.

Davis, L. J. (1997) "The Encyclopedia of Insanity." *Harper's* (February 1997), pp. 61–66; see also "Letters," *Harper's* (May 1997), pp. 4–7.

Gates, Katharine (2000) *Deviant Desires: Incredibly Strange Sex*. New York: Juno Books. See her web site <www.deviantdesires.com> and "fetish roadmap" <www.deviantdesires.com/map/mappics/map81002.gif>.

Gert, Bernard (1992) "A Sex Caused Inconsistency in DSM-III-R: The Definition of Mental Disorder and the Definition of Paraphilias." *Journal of Medicine and Philosophy* 17: 155–71.

Goldman, Alan (2002) "Plain Sex." In Alan Soble (ed.), *The Philosophy of Sex: Contemporary Readings*, 4th ed. Lanham, MD: Rowman and Littlefield, pp. 39–55.

Margolis, Joseph (1975) "The Question of Homosexuality." In Robert Baker and Frederick Elliston (eds.), *Philosophy and Sex*, 1st ed. Buffalo, NY: Prometheus Books, pp. 288–302.

National Organization of Women (1997) "Testimony from Physicians and Psychiatrists for the S/M Policy Reform Statement," 3/22/97. Available at <members.aol.com/NOWSM/Psychiatrists.html>.

Neu, Jerome (1995) "Freud and Perversion." In Robert Stewart (ed.), *Philosophical Perspectives on Sex and Love*. New York: Oxford University Press, pp. 87–104.

Primoratz, Igor (1999) *Ethics and Sex*. London: Routledge.

Roth, Philip (1969) *Portnoy's Complaint*. New York: Random House.

Silverstein, Charles (1984) "The Ethical and Moral Implications of Sexual Classification: A Commentary." *Journal of Homosexuality* 9(4): 29–38.

Soble, Alan (1996) *Sexual Investigations*. New York: New York University Press.

Soble, Alan (2002) *Pornography, Sex, and Feminism*. Amherst, NY: Prometheus.

Suppe, Frederick (1984) "Classifying Sexual Disorders: The *Diagnostic and Statistical Manual* of the American Psychiatric Association." *Journal of Homosexuality* 9(4): 9–28.

Suppe, Frederick (1987) "The Diagnostic and Statistical Manual of the American Psychiatric Association: Classifying Sexual Disorders." In Earl E. Shelp (ed.), *Sexuality and Medicine*, Vol. 2: *Ethical Viewpoints in Transition*. Dordrecht: D. Reidel, pp. 111–35.

CHAPTER 4

....

CHARACTER

Moral Treatment and the Personality Disorders

....

LOUIS C. CHARLAND

ONE interesting philosophical question about personality disorders is whether people diagnosed with such conditions should be held morally responsible for their actions (Elliott 1996). Another philosophical point of interest lies in the fact that these disorders usually involve deviations from social rather than physiological norms, meaning that they are evaluative and not simply descriptive diagnostic categories (Agich 1994). But what really *are* personality disorders? There are standard clinical answers to this question, of course, but philosophically the answer is far from obvious.

The argument advanced here is that the conditions we now call "personality disorders" actually constitute two very different kinds of theoretical entities. In particular, several core personality disorders are actually really moral, and not medical, conditions. Accordingly, the categories that are held to represent them are really moral, and not medical, theoretical kinds. Strategically, the idea is to work back from the possibility of treatment to the nature of the kinds that are allegedly treated. Along the way, we will revisit the eighteenth-century idea of moral treatment. The discussion closes with a reflection on how the ambiguous medical status of personality disorders and their treatment today is reminiscent of the ideological tug of war that pits alienist "mad doctors" like Pinel against their lay counterparts such as Tuke as they battled over who should be in charge of treating the mad.

BRIEF HISTORY OF THE PERSONALITY DISORDERS

Personality disorders have proven to be rather transient theoretical kinds. To understand this aspect of their nature and the argument to come, it is important to appreciate their history. For our purposes, that history starts with publication of the third edition of the *Diagnostic and Statistical Manual of Mental Disorders* (APA 1980). Loosely understood, personality disorders have a history that arguably predates the publication of DSM-III by hundreds of years (Millon and Davis 1995). Some prefer to trace their origins to the late nineteenth century, when the modern concept of personality first appeared (Healy 2002: 14). But it is only with the publication of DSM-III that the personality disorders achieved widespread official recognition as a separate clinical diagnostic class of their own. Indeed, some researchers even distinguish between a "pre-" and "post"-DSM-III era in the study of personality disorders (Livesely 2000).

The publication of DSM-III marked a turning point in the evolution of personality disorders and, indeed, the DSM itself. The chief factor responsible for this change was the introduction of a multiaxial system of classification. Prior to DSM-III, by default all mental disorders were located on a single diagnostic axis. The move to a multiaxial system of classification has been compared by some to a Kuhnian "paradigm shift" (Millon and Davis 1995: 17). In that shift, personality disorders were placed on a separate axis, namely, Axis II. Axis I was reserved for the more serious clinical "mental" disorders such as schizophrenia and depression. Axis II was the domain of "personality" disorders and mental retardation, both enduring conditions with a relatively early onset. Finally, Axes III, IV, and V were left for more general medical and psychosocial factors relevant to treatment and diagnosis (APA 1994: 25–31).

Scientific experts in the area of personality disorders do not hesitate to say that the classification of personality disorders proposed in DSM-III was just as much a political compromise as was their classification in DSM-I (APA 1952) and DSM-II (APA 1968). In all cases, the guiding methodological principle has been to systematize and codify trends in current diagnostic practice using surveys and special committees and workgroups. As might be expected, this has meant that DSM classifications are highly vulnerable to political and economic influences and interests, a fact that even sympathetic insiders freely admit. Personality disorders have proven especially vulnerable to these forces. As Lee Ann Clark states, "it is no secret that the official classification of personality disorders . . . embodied in the DSMs represents a compromise among the often competing interests of clinicians, researchers, educators, and statisticians with various training backgrounds and orientations (1995: 482). Others are even more critical, stating that "in many ways, the DSM-IV classification of personality disorders is more like a political or philosophical statement than a scientific classification" (Livesely 1995: 500). These criticisms by sympathetic "insiders" are significant and not very far removed from the more polemical criticisms by "outsiders" (Caplan 1995; Kirk and Kutchins 1992).

In DSM-IV, a personality disorder is defined as "an enduring pattern of inner experience and behavior that departs markedly from the individual's culture, is pervasive and inflexible, has an onset in adolescence or early adulthood, is stable over time, and leads to distress and impairment" (APA 1994: 629). Personality disorders are defined as collections of personality traits that have passed a certain "threshold" and "cause significant functional impairment or subjective distress" (633). More specifically, "only when personality traits are inflexible and maladaptive and cause significant distress do they constitute Personality Disorders" (630). Table 4.1 contains a list of the DSM-IV personality disorders and their predecessors. It nicely illustrates the transient nature of these peculiar theoretical kinds.

The placement of personality disorders on a separate axis represented a statement of faith in their empirical validity as important clinical conditions in their own right (Livesely 1995a: iv; Tyrer 1995: 29). It encouraged and eventually led to a large quantity of research devoted to the DSM personality disorders and their criteria sets (Livesely 1995: v; Shea 1995: 397). Recently, however, research in the area has been dwindling. Critics, even sympathetic insiders, are calling for change. The problem is that too many efforts have gone into measuring and defining the DSM criteria sets. Some have gone as far as calling this "an indictment of academia" (Tyrer 1995: 30). The present categorical system itself has come under heavy fire. A categorical approach works best when "all the members of diagnostic class are homogenous, when there are clear boundaries between classes, and when the different classes are mutually exclusive" (APA 1994: xxii). Unfortunately, many mental disorders do not satisfy those conditions, and therefore categorization has to be more flexible. The solution has been to retain the categorical approach but with "poltythetic" criteria sets (xxii). According to that method, one need not satisfy all the criteria for a disorder in order to have it. One need only satisfy "a subset of items from a longer list" (xxii).

DSM-IV contains a brief mention of the fact there is a dimensional alternative to the present categorical system (APA 1994: 633–34). There are now many commentators who believe that more efforts need to be put into developing a dimensional approach to classification (Blashfield and McElroy 1995; Clark 1995; Shea 1995; Widiger and Sanderson 1995). It is probably not an exaggeration to say that the adoption of a dimensional model of classification for personality disorders would signify a scientific revolution in the area. But why reject the categorical model? According to many experts, it poses vexing problems, particularly in the case of personality disorders. First, its adoption was based on committee consensus and not scientific merit. Second, according to many, it simply does not accord with the facts. In summarizing a large amount of research in the area, John Livesley flatly states that "the simple categorical model adopted by the DSM-IV is not supported by the facts" (Livesley 1995: 499). He argues that "the results of all relevant studies consistently support a dimensional model of phenotypic traits of personality disorders (Livesely 1995: 499).

Table 4.1. DSM Personality Disorder Classifications

DSM-I	Inadequate, schizoid, cyclothymic, paranoid, emotionally unstable, passive-aggressive, compulsive, antisocial, dysocial (APA 1952: 7).
DSM-II	Paranoid, cyclothymic, schizoid, explosive, obsessive-compulsive, hysterical, asthenic, antisocial, passive-aggressive, inadequate (APA 1968: 9).
DSM-III	Dependent, histrionic, narcissistic, antisocial, compulsive, passive-aggressive, schizoid, avoidant, borderline, paranoid, schizotypal (APA 1980: 19).
DSM-IV	Paranoid, schizoid, schizotypal, antisocial, borderline, histrionic, narcissistic, avoidant, dependent, obsessive-compulsive (APA 1994: 23).

This of course makes the transient character of our current personality disorders even more shaky than it already is.

PERSONALITY DISORDERS AS INTERACTIVE MORAL KINDS

The preceding historical sketch is very hard to reconcile with the idea that personality disorders might be naturally occurring disease entities. In the language of philosophers, it makes it doubtful they are "natural kinds." The reason is that they are very transient and rest on a very weak empirical base. How then are we to understand their nature? This is an area where psychiatry can benefit from contemporary discussions in the philosophy of science.

Personality disorders may not be what philosophers call natural kinds. But they do appear to be distinct theoretical kinds nonetheless. In Ian Hacking's terms, they are *interactive* kinds. The distinction between natural and interactive kinds is particularly helpful in trying to make sense of the transient character of personality disorders. Indeed, it helps explain why they are so transient. Hacking's doctrine of interactive kinds provides a helpful way for understanding the ontology of personality disorders that at the same time acknowledges their transient character. Exploring this thesis will set the stage for the central argument of this essay, which is that several of the core personality disorders are really moral, and not medical, theoretical kinds.

According to Hacking, natural kinds are "a kind of event found in nature and hooked up to other events by laws of nature" (1995: 59). Typical examples include "water, sulphur, horse, tiger, lemon, multiple sclerosis, heat and the color yellow"

(Hacking 1999: 107). Natural kinds are *indifferent*: they are simply there, unaware of being classified by the terms used to classify them. In that respect they are different from interactive kinds. Those are kinds "that, when known, by people or those around them, and put to work in institutions, change the ways in which individuals experience themselves—and may even lead people to evolve their feelings and behavior in part because they are so classified" (104). Thus, interactive kinds interact with what they classify. For example, consider plutonium: it is a natural, or indifferent, kind; it "does not interact with the idea of plutonium, in virtue of being aware that it is plutonium, or experiencing existence in plutonium institutions like reactors, bombs, and storage tanks" (105). In contrast, hyperactivity is an interactive kind: a hyperactive child can be aware of the fact that he is classified as such and this can shape his future behavior. In general, "terms for interactive kinds apply to human beings and their behavior" (123). What makes them interactive as opposed to indifferent is that "they interact with the people classified by them" (123). Interactive kinds thus have a characteristic *looping effect* that connects what is classified with what does the classifying (105, 121).

Asking the question what personality disorders are using Hacking's distinction between natural and interactive kinds has interesting consequences for the debate whether the current categorical system should be retained or replaced with a dimensional alternative. On the one hand, the notion of an interactive kind fits nicely with the transient character of some of the personality disorders generated by the current categorical approach. On the other hand, speaking of personality disorders as natural kinds seems to make more sense in the context of a dimensional approach, particularly where the suggested dimensions are held to be measurable biological variables. On a biological dimensional approach, the idea is to work "bottom-up" from biological mechanisms to disorders, rather than "top-down" from folk psychological descriptions determined by clinical practice. Cloninger's (1986, 1987) hypothesis that personality disorders are heritable dispositions that derive from malfunctions in monoaminergic pathways is a good example of a "bottom-up" biological dimensional approach. If that hypothesis is sound, there is an important sense in which personality disorder categories might turn out to be genuine disease conditions, or natural kinds.

On Hacking's view, some mental disorders look very much like genuine natural kinds; schizophrenia and mental retardation are the examples he cites. Alternatively, he says, anorexia and hyperactivity look more like interactive kinds (Hacking 1999: 101–2). Note that it is also possible for a kind to be both natural *and* interactive. Schizophrenia and depression are probably like this. But before we try to sort personality disorders into their respective kind status, we need to look at another element in how this talk of "kinds" relates to them. The connection lies in the fact that natural kinds can be of different sorts. They can be geological, chemical—or medical. Diseases like multiple sclerosis and tuberculosis are examples of medical conditions that are natural kinds. Is the same true of personality disorders?

On his side, Carl Elliott is skeptical about construing personality disorders as medical kinds, noting that "the idea that personality disorders are illnesses should give us pause" (1996: 62). However, unlike Thomas Szasz, who argues that mental illness is a myth, Elliott does not say that the DSM personality disorders are mythical. Nor is what he says consistent with this. He appears to take their existence seriously; at least enough to inquire into their implications for questions of moral responsibility. His view appears to be that, despite their ambiguous nature, we can and do generalize about the different "kinds" of personality disorders nonetheless. In other words, there is something to the general category and its putative individual kinds. In sum, personality disorders may not be medical kinds, but they are "kinds" of some sort. They do exhibit some theoretical uniformity, provide some explanatory and predictive power, and enable us to capture a modest amount of generalizations.

PROBLEMS WITH TREATMENT

Treatment plays a central role in Elliott's argument that the medical status of personality disorders is doubtful. In that argument, he asserts that "for personality disorders there is often no effective treatment" (Elliott 1996: 62). However, if we are to believe the most recent edition of *Treatments of Psychiatric Disorders*, this situation is changing. In the introduction to that volume, the claim is made that "advances in the diagnostic understanding and treatment of the personality disorders have been substantial" (APA 2001: 2223). Indeed, some personality disorders are now held to be "eminently treatable with psychotherapy" (2223). This suggests that at least some personality disorders may be illnesses after all. In turn, that suggests that they may, in fact, be medical conditions. The controversial premise here is nicely captured by Bill Fulford's claim that "*medical* interventions require *medical* grounds" (Fulford 1999: 164, 182). If a condition is a medical condition, then it is no surprise that it requires medical intervention. In the case of personality disorders, successful medical treatment would then be confirmation of the fact that these constitute conditions of a medical sort; that they are *medical* kinds.

The treatments for personality disorders referred to in *Treatments of Psychiatric Disorders* include both pharmacological and psychological therapies. Sometimes pharmacological therapies are recommended because of concurrent Axis I comorbid conditions. In practice, pharmacological treatments might also be administered even though they are not therapeutically specific to the conditions they are applied to (APA 2001: 2225). For example, antidepressants and neuroleptics might form part of the recommended treatment for some personality disorders even though there is no full-fledged Axis I indication for them (Healy 2002: 346). In that respect, such treatments resemble and function like the pharmacological tonics of earlier eras (Healy 1997: 257; 2002: 65–67). On the psychotherapeutic side, a variety of approaches are possible. Virtually all them are said to require the establishment of a "therapeutic alliance" and "empathy." Pharmacological and psychotherapeutic treatment recommendations are not divided equally across the different personality disorders. As might be expected, pharmacotherapies tend to be favored in the case of disorders that are suspected to have strong biological determinants; for example, the schizotypal and avoidant types (APA 2001: 2223). In other cases, pharmacological interventions are prescribed on a "creative" basis, depending on the individual details of the case (2223).

Let us grant there now exists a widespread variety of therapies that are more or less effective in treating some of the personality disorders. Let us also grant that the pharmacological therapies involved sometimes target genuine Axis I conditions and so are clearly medically indicated. What I want to suggest is that this leaves an important subset of personality disorders out of the medical loop, beyond the boundaries of medical intervention, strictly speaking. The disorders I have in mind are the antisocial, borderline, histrionic, and narcissistic types. These, I suggest, are not genuine medical kinds; they are really moral kinds. As we shall see, this goes beyond merely suggesting that they are evaluative in nature (Agich 1994).

The central thesis of this discussion is that historically the DSM personality disorders tend to fall into two groups: a moral group and a nonmoral group. Part of the inspiration for this distinction is the division of personality disorders into clusters found in DSM-IV (APA 1994: 629–30). There personality disorders are divided into three classes. Cluster A consists of paranoid, schizoid, and schizotypal; this is referred to as the "eccentric" group of personality disorders. Cluster B consists of antisocial, borderline, histrionic, and narcissistic; this is referred to as the "dramatic" or "theatrical" group. Finally, Cluster C consists of avoidant, dependent, and obsessive-compulsive; this is the "anxious" or "fearful" group. This division of personality disorders into clusters is based on "descriptive similarities" (629). We are also told it has not yet been "consistently validated" (630).

In fact, the division of personality disorders into clusters is on the right track but does not go far enough. It *cannot* go far enough because the criteria for clustering are supposed to be limited to purely descriptive, factual terms. This is understandable, since the DSM professes to be a descriptive, objective scientific text. Terms with strong or even weak moral or evaluative connotations are to be avoided as much as possible. Psychiatry is part of medicine, and medicine is supposed to be based on science. And science, of course, is supposed to be based on fact, not value. The point is to identify and describe mental categories and conditions that are of "clinical" relevance, not to morally evaluate those conditions and the persons who suffer from them.

However laudable this might be as a general statement of ideological commitment and priority, the DSM fails to live up to its pledge to fact and objectivity. The general point that many of the DSM categories and criteria are heavily evaluative is well known and has been ably defended from a variety of different points of view (Agich 1994; Fulford 1999; Szasz 1961). The evaluative nature of the personality disorders is particularly transparent (Elliott 1996: 57–67). Even the notion of a mental "disorder" is evaluative. As Hacking notes, "disorder' often suggests something bad, unhealthy, and undesirable" (Hacking 1995: 17). On the other hand, "order" typically means something good—what is healthy and desirable. This precisely is how the concept of a personality disorder appears to function in psychiatric diagnosis and treatment. Personality disorders are undesirable and unhealthy traits of character that medical specialists hope to alleviate or cure through treatment. Therefore, the concept of a personality disorder is inherently evaluative. It is based largely on value and not simply on fact.

TREATMENT AS MORAL CONVERSION

To say that personality disorders are evaluative and not simply descriptive categories is not the same as stating they are specifically *moral* categories; the moral is only one subdomain of the evaluative. Thus the thesis that some of the central personality disorders are really moral categories requires a separate argument. The disorders in question are those in Cluster B: antisocial, borderline, histrionic, and narcissistic. Those Cluster B conditions are fundamentally moral in nature, while Cluster A and C conditions are not. The thesis that the Cluster B disorders are moral and not medical can be defended on the basis of the *kind* of treatment required for their "cure." Call this the "Argument from Treatment."

It is impossible to imagine a successful "treatment" for the Cluster B disorders that does not involve a *moral commitment* to therapy. The central issue is whether there exists a *moral willingness* to change together with a sustained readiness to make the *moral effort* to make and sustain that change. Thus it is impossible to imagine a successful "treatment" or "cure" for those conditions that does not involve some sort of conversion or change in *moral character*. On this basis, it can be argued that these are fundamentally moral conditions and, consequently, that their treatment requires a sort of *moral treatment*. None of this should be taken to imply that Cluster B disorders cannot or do not admit of treatment using other means. Rather, the point is simply that those other treatment interventions can never be sufficient for complete treatment or recovery. A full cure requires moral willingness, moral change, and moral effort. Of course, these moral desiderata are not mentioned in most standard psychotherapeutic interventions recommended for the treatment of personality disorders. Scientific objectivity does not permit it. But the point is that those desiderata are ultimately required for successful treatment and cure.

To see why, consider very briefly the nature of the individual Cluster B disorders. Antisocial personality disorder is said to involve a "pervasive pattern of disregard for and violation of the rights of others" (APA 1994: 649). Narcissistic personality disorder is said to involve a "lack of empathy" (661). The moral nature of histrionic personality disorder is more implied than explicit but is clear nonetheless. Here the "excessive attention seeking" and "inappropriate sexually seductive and provocative behavior" referred to is flatly inconsistent with a pattern of empathy and regard for others (657–58). Finally, the "inappropriate, intense anger" and "instability in interpersonal relationships" cited in the diagnostic criteria for borderline personality disorder again imply clear moral deficits in empathy and regard for others. There is therefore no escaping the conclusion that, either by explicit mention or by implication, persons diagnosed with Cluster B personality disorders exhibit morally objectionable and reprehensible behavior toward others.

Clearly, moral shortcomings of some sort appear to be necessary conditions of the DSM Cluster B personality disorders. It follows that unless those moral problems can be overcome or eliminated, successful treatment and cure are impossible. Someone who is empathic and caring of others cannot logically be said to suffer from antisocial or narcissistic personality disorder in the way these are presently characterized in the DSM. Likewise, someone who has reached the point of being morally committed to being more respectful and considerate of others can plausibly be said to be improving and recovering from histrionic personality disorder. The case of borderline disorder is more difficult, but here as well it is plausible to imagine that a moral commitment to being patient and loving with both others and oneself is an essential ingredient of any serious treatment and cure. Note that the same cannot be said of psychotherapeutic interventions for many other sorts of conditions. There are no such moral presuppositions for desensitization behavioral therapy for phobias or even cognitive therapy for depression. Willingness, commitment, and effort are of course required for therapy to succeed in these and many other cases. But *moral* willingness, commitment, and effort of the sort we have been discussing are not required. In addition, successful pharmacological interventions to reduce conditions like depression and anxiety for the Cluster B disorders may well help foster positive growth and development, but without a *moral* commitment to change, those interventions are doomed to remain insufficient and will elude any thorough cure.

WHAT PERSONALITY DISORDERS ARE

We are now in a position to answer our opening question about what personality disorders are. Keeping in mind the distinction between the Cluster B personality disorders and their moral presuppositions, which are absent from the Cluster A and C disorders, the answer is this.

First, Cluster B disorders are not natural kinds in any plausible sense. They are a species of interactive kinds that are simply too transient to count as genuine natural disease entities. In fact, precisely because they are interactive, their transient character should be no surprise. It is a predictable consequence of the fact that as social and political conditions change, so do the boundaries of deviant moral behavioral syndromes that are thought to require special social attention and behavioral control. Nonetheless, despite their transient interactive character, Cluster B disorders still stand for genuine theoretical kinds. They represent behavioral syndromes that are nomologically uniform and distinct enough to permit various limited explanatory projects and activities.

Second, Cluster B disorders are moral and not medical kinds. Both their identification and treatment rest on and require articulation in moral terms and concepts. In particular, treatment requires a sort of moral willingness and commitment to change that is typically absent in consent to therapy for other sorts of mental and behavioral disorders. Willingness and commitment to developing the capacity for empathy is an important milestone in psychotherapeutic treatment for Cluster B disorders. So is the willingness and commitment to relate honestly in the therapeutic alliance. Any psychotherapeutic intervention directed at Cluster B disorders must pass these two milestones if it is to be successful. Moreover, this remains true even if the theoretical vocabulary in which that therapeutic theory is couched makes little or no explicit mention of any such notions. Two interesting contemporary therapeutic initiatives to consider here are Moral Reconation Therapy for antisocial personality disorder (Little and Robinson 1988) and Dialectical Behavioral Therapy for borderline individuals (Linehan 1993).

Third, turning to Cluster A and C disorders, we can say that these appear to be very different in kind from their Cluster B counterparts. Whether they constitute natural and independent disease entities is doubtful but remains to be seen. However, that they are not moral kinds seems much clearer. Consider the fact that the definition of the Cluster A and C disorders does not appear to employ or imply moral terms and notions, while the definition of Cluster B disorders does. In effect, most of the behaviors captured by the Cluster A and C groupings are morally neutral. Thus, the avoidant person simply avoids others but does not necessarily dislike or hate them. In other words, dislike and hate are not logically presupposed or implied by the diagnosis. Likewise, the dependent individual may annoy others but does not necessarily intend to annoy them for the sake of it. Again, the intention to annoy is not logically presupposed or implied by the diagnosis. Finally, the obsessive-compulsive individual may embarrass or ignore others as a result of that condition, but typically this is not because he intends to do so. Here again, there is nothing in the diagnosis that logically presupposes or implies the intention to embarrass or ignore others. Of course, cure and treatment for these three conditions do require willingness and effort—but not the sort of *moral* willingness and effort required by the Cluster B disorders. You can be fully cured of obsessive-compulsive, avoidant, or schizoid personality disorder but still have an evil character and intend to perform immoral actions. However, you cannot be fully "cured" of antisocial, borderline, histrionic, or narcissistic personality disorder and regularly intend to be systematically cruel, dishonest, and indifferent to the feelings of others. Successful treatment here requires a moral commitment and character change of a significant sort. This invites the question why treatment should be administered by medical professionals. The issues go to the heart of the professional status of psychiatry as a medical discipline and the conditions it claims to treat. The situation is also reminiscent of the ideological and professional disputes associated with the eighteenth-century practice of moral treatment.

REVISITING MORAL TREATMENT

In its widest sense, moral treatment had to do with restoring inmates to orderly and socially appropriate conduct. For example, William Tuke's York Retreat was run according to a strict code of "moral management" defined by basic rules of house-keeping and personal conduct that included everything from regular dining and bed-time hours to leisure activities like gardening, games, and strolls in the countryside. Every effort was made to inspire and instill a family atmosphere, and intimacy with patients was paramount. The idea was to manage all aspects of inmates' lives in order to restore them to reason and emotional equilibrium. These general presuppositions of moral treatment were accompanied by moral interventions of a narrower sort. Intimacy with inmates was thought necessary to address these narrower, more im-mediate moral concerns (Scull 1993: 148). Therapy consisted of efforts to rouse and nurture inmates' moral feelings, as well as their sense of moral discipline. Appeal to the desire for self-esteem was held to be a central component of this task (Scull 1993: 101). Overall, this was a system supposed to be governed by "kindness" (Scull 1993: 102; Porter 2001: 291). Tuke repeatedly insisted on the nonmedical character of moral treatment and refused even to say that it was based on any theory. According to him, this was clearly not a professional intervention requiring special theoretical skills. And yet it proved surprisingly successful, if recent historical assessments of the official records are to be believed (Scull 1993: 102, 148–55; Porter 2002: 105–15; Whitaker 2002: 19–38).

The nonmedical character of moral treatment posed no problem for Tuke and his lay followers, but it did pose a problem of allegiance for medical proponents like Pinel. Why were medical professionals needed to administer nonmedical moral treat-ments? The same question is pertinent today. If the Cluster B disorders are funda-mentally moral in nature, then it is unclear why their treatment should fall in the province of medicine or any other "scientific" form of treatment, including various psychotherapies. Strictly speaking, the moral treatment of the Cluster B disorders falls in the province of what psychiatrist David Healy calls the quest for *authenticity* (1990: 28–33, 200–204, 214–15). Standard psychotherapy may help and sometimes even be required for moral recovery, but it can never be sufficient on its own. It should be clear that, for the Cluster B disorders at least, moral treatment must form the core of any successful treatment and recovery (Borthick et al. 2001; Deniker and Sempé, 2001). The fact that this recommendation might seem naïve and utopian just shows how far we have strayed from the ideals of hope and humanity that drove Tuke and Pinel to undertake their reforms.

REFERENCES

Agich, George J. (1994) "Evaluative Judgment and Personality Disorder." In John Z. Sadler, Osborne P. Wiggins, and Michael A. Shwartz (eds.), *Philosophical Perspectives on Psychiatric Classification.* Baltimore, MD: John Hopkins University Press, pp. 233–45.

American Psychiatric Association (1952) *Diagnostic and Statistical Manual of Mental Disorders,* 1st ed. [DSM-I]. Washington DC: American Psychiatric Association.

American Psychiatric Association (1968) *Diagnostic and Statistical Manual of Mental Disorders,* 2nd ed. [DSM-II]. Washington, DC: American Psychiatric Association.

American Psychiatric Association (1980) *Diagnostic and Statistical Manual of Mental Disorders,* 3rd ed. [DSM-III]. Washington, DC: American Psychiatric Association.

American Psychiatric Association (1994) *Diagnostic and Statistical Manual of Mental Disorders,* 4th ed. [DSM-IV]. Washington, DC: American Psychiatric Association.

American Psychiatric Association (1995) *DSM-IV Casebook.* Washington, DC: American Psychiatric Association.

American Psychiatric Association (2001) *Treatments for Psychiatric Disorders,* 3rd ed. Washington DC: American Psychiatric Association.

Blashfield, Roger K., and McElroy, Ross A. (1995) "Confusions in the Terminology Used for Classificatory Models." In John W. Livesley (ed.), *The DSM-IV Personality Disorders.* New York: Guilford Press, pp. 407–16.

Bloch, Sidney, Chodoff, Paul, and Green, Stephen A. (1999) *Psychiatric Ethics,* 3rd ed. Oxford: Oxford University Press.

Borthick, Annie, Holman, Chris, Kennard, David, McFetridge, Mark, Messruther, Karen, and Wilkins, Jenny (2001) "The Relevance of Moral Treatment to Contemporary Mental Health Care." *Journal of Mental Health* 10(4): 427–39.

Caplan, Paula (1995) *They Say You're Crazy.* Reading, MA: Perseus Books.

Clark, Lee Anna (1995) "The Challenge of Alternating Perspectives in Classification: A Discussion of Basic Issues." In John W. Livesley (ed.), *The DSM-IV Personality Disorders.* New York: Guilford Press, pp. 482–97.

Cloninger, C. R. (1986) "A Unified Biosocial Theory of Personality and Its Role in the Development of Anxiety States." *Psychiatric Developments* 3: 167–220.

Cloninger, C. R. (1987) "A Systematic Method for Clinical Description and Classification of Personality Variants." *Archives of General Psychiatry* 44: 573–88.

Deniker, Pierre, and Sempé, Jean-Claude (2001) "Les personnalités psychopathiques: essai de définition structurale." *L'Encéphale* 27(1): 136–56. Originally published in 1967.

Elliott, Carl (1996) *The Rules of Insanity: Moral Responsibility and the Mentally Ill Offender.* Albany: State University Press of New York.

Foucault, Michael (1965) *Madness and Civilization.* New York: Vintage Books.

Fulford, William (1999) "Analytic Philosophy, Brain Science, and the Concept of a Disorder." In Sidney Bloch, Paul Chodoff, and Stephen A. Green (eds.), *Psychiatric Ethics,* 3rd ed. Oxford: Oxford University Press, pp. 161–93.

Hacking, Ian (1995) *Rewriting the Soul: Multiple Personality and the Sciences of Memory.* Cambridge, MA: Harvard University Press.

Hacking, Ian (1998) *Mad Travelers: Reflections on the Reality of Transient Mental Illness.* Charlottesville: University of Virginia Press.

Hacking, Ian (1999) *The Social Construction of What?* Cambridge, MA: Harvard University Press.

Healy, David (1997) *The Antidepressant Era*. Cambridge, MA: Harvard University Press.

Healy, David (1990) *The Suspended Revolution: Psychiatry and Psychotherapy Re-examined*. London: Faber and Faber.

Healy, David (2002) *The Creation of Psychopharmacology*. Cambridge, MA: Harvard University Press.

Kirk, Stuart A., and Kutchins, Herb (1992) *The Selling of DSM: The Rhetoric of Science in Psychiatry*. New York: Aldine de Gruyter.

Linehan, Marsha (1993) *Cognitive-Behavioral Treatment of Borderline Personality Disorder*. New York: Guilford Press.

Little, Gregory L., and Robinson, K. D. (1988) "Moral Reconation: A Step-by-Step Treatment System for Treatment Resistant Clients." *Psychological Reports* 62: 135–51.

Livesley, John W. (ed.) (1995) *The DSM-IV Personality Disorders*. New York: Guilford Press.

Livesley, John W. (2000) Introduction. *Journal of Personality Disorders* 14(1): 97–99.

Livesley, John W., and Jang, Kerry L. (2000) "Toward an Empirically Based Classification of Personality Disorder." *Journal of Personality Disorders* 14(2): 137–52.

Millon, Theodore (2000) Reflections on the Future of DSM Axis II. *Journal of Personality Disorders* 14(2): 30–42.

Millon, Theodore, and Davis, Roger (1995) "Conditions of Personality Disorders: Historical Perspectives, the DSM, and Future Directions." In John W. Livesley (ed.), *The DSM-IV Personality Disorders*. New York: Guilford Press, pp. 3–29.

Paris, Joel (1995) "Commentary on Narcissistic Personality Disorder." In John W. Livesley (ed.), *The DSM-IV Personality Disorders*. New York: Guilford Press, pp. 213–17.

Porter, Roy (1998) *The Greatest Benefit to Mankind: A Medical History of Humanity*. New York: Norton.

Porter, Roy (2001) "Mental Illness." In Roy Porter (ed), *The Cambridge Illustrated History of Medicine*. Cambridge: Cambridge University Press.

Porter, Roy (2002) *Madness: A Brief History*. Oxford: Oxford University Press.

Reznek, Laurie (1987) *The Nature of Disease*. London: Routledge.

Sadler, John Z., Wiggins, Osborne P., and Schwartz, Michael A. (1994) *Philosophical Perspectives on Psychiatric Classification*. Baltimore, MD: Johns Hopkins University Press.

Scull, Andrew (1993) *The Most Solitary of Afflictions*. New Haven: Yale University Press.

Shea, Tracie (1995) "Interrelationships among Categories of Personality Disorders." In John W. Livesley (ed.), *The DSM-IV Personality Disorders*. New York: Guilford Press, pp. 397–407.

Siever, Larry J., Bernstein, David P., and Silverman, Jeremy M. (1995) "Schizotypal Personality Disorder." In John W. Livesley (ed.), *The DSM-IV Personality Disorders*. New York: Guilford Press, pp. 71–90.

Szasz, Thomas (1961) *The Myth of Mental Illness: Foundations of a Theory of Personal Conduct*, rev. ed. New York: Harper and Row.

Tryer, Peter (1995) "Are Personality Disorders Well Classified in DSM-IV?" In John W. Livesley (ed.), *The DSM-IV Personality Disorders*. New York: Guilford Press, pp. 29–42.

Western, Drew, and Shedler, Jonathan (2000) "A Prototype Matching Approach to Diagnosing Personality Disorders: Toward DSM-V." *Journal of Personality Disorders* 14(2): 109–27.

Widiger, Thomas A. (1999) "Depressive Personality Traits and Dysthimia: A Commentary on Ryder and Bagby. *Journal of Personality Disorders* 13(2): 135–42.

Widiger, Thomas A. (2000) "Personality Disorders in the 21st Century." *Journal of Personality Disorders* 14(2): 3–17.

Widiger, Thomas A., and Sanderson, Cynthia J. (1995) "Toward a Dimensional Model of Personality Disorders." In John. W. Livesley (ed.), *The DSM-IV Personality Disorders.* New York: Guilford Press, pp. 433–59.

Whitaker, Robert (2002) *Mad in America: Bad Science, Bad Medicine, and the Enduring Mistreatment of the Mentally Ill.* Cambridge, MA: Perseus.

World Health Organization (1992) *The ICD-10 Classification of Mental and Behavioral Disorders.* Geneva: World Health Organization.

....

CHAPTER 5

ACTION

Volitional Disorder and Addiction

....

ALFRED R. MELE

THE expression "volitional disorder" lacks a standard meaning. According to one way of understanding it, a volitional disorder is a motivational or executive analogue of a cognitive disorder that excuses a person from moral and legal responsibility for certain actions. In an instructive book on conditions under which mentally disordered people should and should not be held morally responsible for their actions, Carl Elliott distinguishes between "volitional disorders" (1996: 40) and cognitive disorders.[1] His examples of the former include pyromania, kleptomania, pathological gambling, obsessive-compulsive disorder, exhibitionism, pedophilia, voyeurism, frotteurism, necrophilia, and some fetishes (pp. 3–5, ch. 3). Very powerful phobias also seem to be likely candidates for inclusion on the list. Elliott writes: "Cognitive tests [for insanity] generally ask whether a person's mental illness prevented her from knowing what she was doing, and volitional tests ask whether her mental illness prevented her from being able to control what she was doing" (2). One can say that such volitional tests test for volitional disorders. Insofar as being "prevented . . . from being able to control" what one is doing is central to volitional disorders, people who believe that a defining characteristic of addiction is the person's inability to control pertinent actions of hers may say that addictions are volitional disorders.

In this essay, I place some of the literature on volitional disorders and addictions in a philosophical context that dates back to Plato and Aristotle in an attempt to shed light on issues that a theorist who wishes to analyze the idea of a volitional disorder will face.

1. Weakness of Will and Irresistible Desires

"Weakness of will" has perplexed philosophers since Plato's time. In Plato's *Protagoras*, Socrates examines the common idea that "many people who know what it is best to do are not willing to do it, though it is in their power, but do something else" (352d). His statement of the common idea marks a central question in ancient and contemporary philosophical discussions of *akrasia* (want of self-control, weakness of will). Is it possible for sane people to perform uncompelled, intentional actions that, as they recognize at the time, are contrary to what they judge best, the judgment being made from the perspective of their own values, principles, desires, and beliefs? More briefly, is *strict* akratic action possible (cf. Mele 1987: 7)? Agents of strict akratic actions are commonly distinguished from agents who are *unable*, at the time of action, to control what they are doing. If this inability is a defining feature of volitional disorders, *akrasia* is not such a disorder.

One way to try to draw the line between the "weak-willed" person and the volitionally disordered one is in terms of resistibility of pertinent desires. It may be said that the difference is that akratic agents, when they act akratically, are motivated by resistible desires, whereas the pertinent desires of the volitionally disordered are irresistible. This naturally raises the question what it is for a desire to be irresistible, and there is an interesting body of philosophical literature on that topic (Elliott 1996: ch. 3; Feinberg 1970: ch. 11; Glover 1970: 97–107; Mele 1992: ch. 5; Neely 1974; Watson 1999). There are also philosophers who argue that strict akratic action is impossible and that we sometimes mistakenly identify cases in which an agent is moved by an irresistible desire as cases of strict akratic action (see Socrates in Plato's *Protagoras*; Hare 1963: ch. 5; Pugmire 1982; Watson 1977).[2]

Some philosophers doubt the existence of irresistible desires. Joel Feinberg, for example, writes: "strictly speaking, no impulse is 'irresistible.' For every case of giving in to a desire, . . . if the person had tried harder, he would have resisted it successfully" (1970: 282). Is it a necessary condition of a desire's being irresistible that the agent would not resist it successfully no matter how hard he were to try? A relatively obvious point is that an agent who would successfully have resisted a desire if he had tried harder to resist might not have been able to try any harder than he did. Perhaps such an agent's desire should count as irresistible even though Feinberg's condition is true of him.

Is a desire that an agent would be able to resist under some external conditions ipso facto a resistible desire independently of the agent's actual external condition? Suppose that a certain heroin addict with a craving for the drug is able to resist his impulse to use it now, while a policeman is present. Does it follow that he would also be able to resist it if no worrisome authorities were present? Wright Neely's account of irresistibility is relevant in this connection: "A desire is irresistible if and only if it is the case that if the agent had been presented with what he took to be good and sufficient reason for not acting on it, he would still have acted on it" (1974: 47; cf. Glover 1970: 97–107, 173). Elsewhere, I raised several objections to this proposal (Mele 1992: 87–88). Here I mention just one.

Even in extreme cases of phobia or addiction, we can usually imagine *some* reason such that if the agent had had that reason for not acting as he did, he would not have so acted. This seemingly does not entail that the desires on which the agent acted were resistible by him at the time of action. Consider the following scenario. Fred has agoraphobia. His fear is so strong that he has not left his house in ten years, despite our many attempts to persuade him to do so. We decide finally that we just have not been presenting Fred with the right reasons, and we threaten to burn his house to the ground if he does not open his door today. When it becomes evident that the threat will not work, we start throwing flaming brands through his windows. Fred is even more afraid of raging fires than of leaving his house. He judges that he has a good reason to leave his house, and he acts accordingly.

Fred's situation is comparable to that of the woman who, under ordinary circumstances, cannot even budge a 300-pound weight but who, upon finding her child pinned under a 400-pound timber, manages, because of a sudden burst of adrenalin, to raise it. Surely, it would be misleading to say that she can lift 400 pounds, if we leave it at that. Rather, we should say that in ordinary circumstances she cannot do this (no matter how hard she tries), although in a certain kind of exceptional circumstance she can. Similarly, it seems conceivable that under ordinary circumstances Fred cannot successfully resist his desire to remain in his house, no matter how hard he tries, even though a raging fire would drive him out. Arguably, the topic of basic concern should be the irresistibility of a desire under the circumstances that obtain at the time of action, whether those circumstances are ordinary or exceptional.

The problem I have raised for Neely's account of irresistible desire is also a problem for an account of moral responsibility developed by John Fischer and Mark Ravizza (1998) and for an associated way of distinguishing between akratic and compelled action. Fischer and Ravizza defend the thesis that "an agent is morally responsible for an action insofar as it issues from his own, moderately reasons-responsive mechanism" (1998: 86). The same can be said of an agent's performing an action freely. On their view, an agent makes a mechanism his own by "taking responsibility" for it. "Moderate reasons-responsiveness consists in *regular reasons-receptivity*, and at least *weak reasons-reactivity*, of the actual-sequence mechanism that leads to the action" (89; italics added). Reasons-receptivity is "the capacity to recognize the reasons that exist," and reasons-reactivity is "the capacity to translate reasons into choices (and then subsequent behavior)" (69). "It is a defining characteristic of *regular* reasons-receptivity that it involves an understandable pattern of (actual and hypothetical) reasons-receptivity" (71; italics added). A mechanism of an agent that issues in the agent's A-ing in the actual world is at least *weakly* reasons-reactive provided that there is some possible world with the same laws in which a mechanism of this kind is operative in this agent, "there is a sufficient reason to do otherwise, the agent recognizes this reason, and the agent does otherwise" (63) for this reason.

It may be suggested that strict akratic action differs from compelled action contrary to the agent's better judgment in that whereas the akratic agent's action "issues from his own, moderately reasons-responsive mechanism," the compelled agent's action does not. Although both agents may satisfy the conditions for regular reasons-receptivity, the akratic agent's "mechanism . . . is at least weakly reasons-reactive" and the compelled agent's mechanism is not. In the case of the latter agent, there is no world of the specified sort in which he "does otherwise." It may be said that this, indeed, is precisely what it is for a desire to be irresistible and, hence, to have compelling force.

In Mele 2000—using a variant of a story like Fred's in which he judges it best to leave his house for his daughter's wedding next door but remains at home—I argued that weak reasons-reactivity is too weak to do the work that Fischer and Ravizza want it to do for moral responsibility.[3] The objection advanced there bears on the present issue, as well. Fred's relevant mechanism is weakly reasons-reactive. We can suppose that it is also regularly reasons-receptive and that it is Fred's own mechanism. (Nothing in Fred's story precludes this.) Thus, on Fischer and Ravizza's view, Fred is morally responsible for staying at home on his daughter's wedding day (in the actual world), and on the view at issue about akratic action, Fred *akratically* stays home. However, this is implausible. Other things being equal (e.g., Fred is not morally responsible for his agoraphobia), if Fred's fear is so debilitating that it would take something as frightening as a raging fire to move him to decide to leave his house or to leave it intentionally, then he seems *not* to be morally responsible for staying home. Similarly, the problem he manifests in staying home on his daughter's wedding day seems much more severe than *akrasia*.

Even if an acceptable analysis of irresistible desire is offered, it is an open question whether volitional disorder should be defined in terms of irresistible desire. Might some volitionally disordered people have relevant desires that are resistible but extremely hard to resist? Should we say that the volitional problem from which people like this suffer is not weakness of will but something more severe? Elliott defends the idea that what is characteristic of volitionally disordered persons is acting under *duress*, rather than being moved by irresistible desires.[4] Often, a person suffering from a volitional disorder "is faced with the choice between (1) acting on desires that he finds morally repellent and shameful, and (2) refraining, which causes him considerable distress" (1996: 48).

2. ADDICTION AND SELF-CONTROL

Although it is common to believe that addicts are victims of irresistible desires, this idea has encountered significant opposition in several fields of study (Bakalar and Grinspoon 1984; Becker and Murphy 1988; Heyman 1996; Peele 1985, 1989; Szasz 1974). My concern in this section is some theoretical issues surrounding a strategy for self-control of potential use to addicts on the assumption that their pertinent desires *fall short* of irresistibility.[5] I offer no defense of this assumption; rather, I treat it as a point of departure for one approach to understanding addiction in action. If volitional disorders may involve desires that are extremely hard to resist but resistible, addictions may be or encompass volitional disorders even if relevant desires of addicts fall short of irresistibility.[6]

Most desires have more than a momentary existence. If there are irresistible desires, desires that are irresistible at some times may be resistible at others. What I identified as the guiding assumption of this section has at least two distinct interpretations. In articulating them, some shorthand will prove useful: I use "*a*-desires" as shorthand for "desires characteristic of addicts." On a strong reading, the assumption is that no *a*-desire is irresistible at any time. On a weaker reading, it is assumed that every *a*-desire is resistible at some time or other. Imagine a crack cocaine addict who has exhausted his supply and desires to use more crack as soon as he can. Suppose that, owing partly to this desire, he drives to an acquaintance's house and steals some crack. His driving where he does is motivated by this desire, and the desire in still in place when he acquires the drug. On the strong reading of the assumption, this desire is not irresistible even when he gains possession of the drug. On the weak reading, it might be. If the desire is irresistible now, then even though the addict might have been able successfully to exercise self-control in resisting it earlier, there is no longer any chance of that. I leave both readings of the assumption open here.[7]

Work by George Ainslie on self-control and its contrary sheds light on the behavior of addicts and their prospects for self-control, on the assumption just discussed. In early work, Ainslie marshals weighty evidence for a view that I summarized in Mele 1987 (85) as follows:

1. "The curve describing the effectiveness of reward as a function of delay is markedly concave upwards" (Ainslie 1982: 740). That is, a desire for a "reward" of a prospective action, other things being equal, acquires greater motivational force as the time for the reward's achievement approaches and after a certain point motivation increases sharply.
2. Human beings are not at the mercy of the effects of the proximity of rewards. They can bring it about that they act for a larger, later reward in preference to a smaller, earlier one by using "pre-committing devices," a form of self-control (Ainslie 1975, 1982).[8]

These ideas in Ainslie 1975 and 1982 are developed more fully in Ainslie 1992 and 2001. Later, I will apply them specifically to addiction. A broader focus is useful for introductory purposes.

In Ainslie's view, "personal rules are the most flexible and acceptable precommitting device" (1992: 154). He opens a discussion of hyperbolic discount functions and personal rules with the following claim:

It is possible to deduce a mechanism for willpower from the existence of deeply concave discount curves . . . if we assume only that curves from multiple rewards combine in an additive fashion. In brief, choosing rewards in aggregates rather than individually gives later, larger rewards a major advantage over smaller, earlier ones; and the perception of one's current choice as a precedent predicting a whole series of choices leads to just such aggregations. (144–45)

Consider Sally. She judges it best to adopt a certain exercise routine as a means of losing weight, but, as she knows, she has a record of violating her exercise resolutions. If Sally has come to believe the following assertion, *P*, about herself, she might enjoy more success in the future: (*P*) Whatever choice I make and execute the first time I am tempted to violate my new exercise routine is the choice I will uniformly make and execute on subsequent occasions of temptation. This assertion is not absurd: after all, given that the temptations are similar, how she chooses and acts on the first occasion is evidence about how she will choose and act on relevant subsequent occasions. Believing *P*, Sally should regard herself now, at time *t*, as faced with a choice between the following two items: (1) the series of "rewards" to be obtained should she *not* abide by the exercise plan, both on the first occasion of temptation and on all subsequent occasions, and (2) the series of "rewards" to be obtained by *abiding by* this plan on the first and all subsequent occasions of temptation. If, at *t*, Sally deems the latter series of rewards better, on the whole, than the former, she should choose 2 over 1 (if she can).

Regarding temptation, Ainslie writes: "The crucial time at which preference between . . . two whole series of rewards changes [is the time, t_i] at which the value *V'* of the series of larger rewards equals the value V of the series of smaller ones," the time of "indifference" (1992: 145). "If the choice is made before $\lfloor t_i \rfloor$, it will favor the series of larger, later rewards, and if it is made after $[t_i]$, it will favor the series of smaller, earlier rewards" (145).

If, at *t*, Sally chooses the series of "larger, later rewards" to be obtained by abiding by her plan, she thereby adopts a *personal rule* about exercise. "The force of a personal rule," Ainslie writes, "is proportional to the number of delayed rewards that are perceived to be part of the series at risk" (1992: 174): "In principle, personal rules make it possible for a person never to prefer small, early alternatives at the expense of the series of larger, later ones. He may be able to keep temptations close at hand without succumbing to them" (193).

On Ainslie's view, some personal rules are, as I wish to put it, more *self-protective* than others, in virtue of certain properties of the rules themselves. The term "self-protective" should be understood in a double sense: protective of the *rule*, including both its persistence or survival and its not being violated, and protective of the person whose rule it is, or, more precisely, of the person's prospects for maximizing reward. Ainslie summarizes the major self-protective features of rules as follows:

> To be cost-effective, a personal rule must be drawn with three characteristics: (1) The series of rewards to be waited for must be long enough and valuable enough so that it will be preferred over each impulsive alternative. (2) Each member of the series and its impulsive alternatives must be readily identifiable, without ambiguity. (3) The features that exclude a choice from the series must either occur independently of the person's behavior or have such a high intrinsic cost that he will

not be motivated to bring them about just for the sake of evading the rule. (1992: 162)

Relatively precise rules — rules with "bright lines" — that one has explicitly endorsed (163–73) are harder to ignore than vague impressions about how one ought to conduct oneself. Rules that one views as serving the maximization of reward, that are precise enough to leave little room for doubt about their application to particular cases, and that are explicitly formulated with a view to excluding the voluntary production of conditions that satisfy the rules' escape clauses, are — in virtue of these very properties — less likely to be violated, other things being equal, than rules that lack one or more of these features.[9] If Ainslie is right, Sally may benefit from adopting an exercise rule with these features.[10]

On Ainslie's view, like Plato's (*Protagoras* 355e–357e), the perceived *proximity* of a reward tends to exert a powerful positive influence on the strength of an agent's motivation to pursue it, an effect that precommitment strategies of self-control, including the tactic of personal rules, are designed to counter.[11] He contends that "it is in the *addictive* behaviors that the influence of proximity on the temporary preferences is especially evident: For instance, an alcoholic may plan not to drink, succeed if he keeps sufficiently distant from the opportunities, become overwhelmingly tempted when faced with an imminent chance to drink, but later wholeheartedly regret this lapse" (1992: 98; italics added). He says, in the same vein, that "the behaviors that seem best to fit the description 'temporarily preferred' are often called addictions. They have a clear phase of conscious though temporary preference, followed by an equally clear period of regret" (97). On Ainslie's view, "Acts governed by willpower evidently are both diagnostic and causal. Drinking too much is diagnostic of a condition, alcoholism out of control, but it causes further uncontrolled drinking when the subject, using it to diagnose himself as out of control, is discouraged from trying to will sobriety" (203).

Merely choosing (or deciding, or intending) to refrain from a certain kind of tempting activity indefinitely (e.g., cocaine use) is not sufficient for using the tactic of personal rules. To use the tactic, one must view what is to be gained by resisting as a series of rewards stretching out over a considerable time. Ainslie contends that people who take this long view of things will tend to do better at resisting relevant temptations than people who do not; for, other things being equal, the longer the series of similar rewards one has in view, the more strongly motivated one will be to actualize the series.[12] The point about motivation is plausible; how often the resultant motivation will be enough to sustain resistance is an empirical matter.

The success of the tactic of personal rules also depends on how well tailored one's rules are to oneself. A sedentary, middle-aged man concerned about his deteriorating physical condition might envision a lengthy series of rewards associated with daily exercise. But if he deems it highly unlikely that he would abide by a daily exercise routine, a rule requiring exercise three days a week may prove more beneficial. Given that one's motivation to follow a rule is partly a function of one's subjective probability that one will succeed in following it and achieve the associated rewards, the man may be more motivated to pursue the less demanding routine, even though he believes that the daily routine would yield greater rewards were he to follow it faithfully. Some failures by agents who employ the tactic of personal rules may be attributable not to any flaw in the tactic itself but to their setting their sights unrealistically high.

Whether the tactic of personal rules works and how reliably it works are empirical matters, of course. If we can satisfy ourselves, independently of their succeeding in resisting temptation, that a group of people are employing the tactic, we can wait and see how well they fare in resisting temptation. And we can see how well they fare relative to people who judge it best to resist but do not employ this tactic.

Whatever the facts about personal rules and about addiction may be, what view of addiction would be most usefully held by the general public? A popular view treats addictions as incurable diseases (that might be manageable with considerable expert assistance). It is not difficult to locate apparent pragmatic grounds for promulgating such a view: acceptance of it by those who have not yet experimented with addictive substances, for example, might seem, intuitively, to tend to steer them away from such substances.[13] Setting aside the question of the actual preventive effects of acceptance of this popular view of addiction, consider its likely effect on many addicts, given a position like Ainslie's. If a particular addict's motivation to resist a relevant temptation on any given occasion is partly determined by her estimation of the chance that she will uniformly or normally successfully resist in the future, her accepting the popular view would be a considerable obstacle to successful resistance. This is not a criticism of Ainslie's position, of course. The popular view may be evidentially unwarranted. Whether widespread acceptance of that view is unwarranted from a *pragmatic* perspective is a complicated and interesting question. If we could successfully promulgate two distinct views of addiction, one for nonaddicts and one for addicts, matters might be easier. But, of course, that is not feasible. One hopes that a sustained search for the truth about addiction will yield a theory that is both well supported by the evidence and well suited (at some level of description) for salutary public consumption.

3. CONCLUSION

Theoretical notions are invented for theoretical uses. One use for the notion of volitional disorder is to help us make judgments about the moral or legal responsibility of an agent for an action. A theorist with this interest may understand volitional disorders by analogy with insanity-level cognitive disorders, cognitive disorders that absolve agents of moral and legal responsibility for certain actions, provided that the agents are not themselves morally or legally responsible for the disorders. Whether various addictions properly count as volitional disorders, so understood, depends on whether they provide legitimate, relevant excuses for actions to which they lead. The same is true of any candidate for a volitional disorder.

It is an interesting question whether someone sufficiently self-possessed successfully to use personal rules in resisting temptations associated with addictions or other problems can count as volitionally disordered. Again, Elliott counts such things as the following as volitional disorders: pyromania, kleptomania, pathological gambling, obsessive-compulsive disorder, exhibitionism, pedophilia, voyeurism, frotteurism, necrophilia. How well may the tactic of personal rules be expected to work with each of these disorders? Are those people in whom it would work properly regarded as volitionally disordered? Perhaps whether or not a person can master a problem simply through the use of the technique of personal rules can be used as one rough mark of distinction between volitional problems that do not qualify as volitional disorders and those that do.[14]

NOTES

1. Also see Ferrell et al. 1984 on "volitional disability." Ronald Zec (1995: 216) reports that Emil Kraepelin maintained that "the 'dementia' of dementia praecox was primarily a disorder of volition, rather than one of intellect."

2. For recent worries about whether akratic agents are distinguishable from addicts and others who supposedly are compelled to act as they do, see Buss 1997, Tenenbaum 1999, and Wallace 1999. For a response, see Mele 2002.

3. For a reply, see Fischer and Ravizza 2000: 470–72.

4. For an instructive discussion of a duress model of *addiction*, see Watson 1999.

5. For detailed accounts of self-control, see Logue 1995 and Mele 1995: chs. 1–7.

6. For discussion of four distinct interpretations of addiction, see Herrnstein and Prelec 1992.

7. Notice that even the weaker reading is quite strong. Consider a crack addict's desire to use some crack *now*, a desire he just acquired. If that desire is resistible at some time, the relevant time is now. Incidentally, even the much less demanding assumption that *some* desires characteristic of addicts are resistible will suffice for present purposes.

8. For further discussion, see Mele 1987: 84–86, 90–93 and Mele 1992: ch. 4. Also see Elster 1985 on imperfect rationality and precommitment.

9. I set aside the technical question what, exactly, would count as violating (or not violating) a vague or ambiguous rule.

10. An additional alleged feature of personal rules is that behavior guided by them tends to increase the probability that the agent's relevant subsequent behavior will also be guided by them. In Mele 1996, I defend Ainslie's position on this feature of personal rules against criticisms advanced in Bratman 1996.

11. On motivational strength and our prospects for control in this sphere, see Mele 2003: chs. 7 and 8.

12. Among the relevant "other things" are subjective probabilities. In some cases, a lengthening of a series might include a significant decrease in one's subjective probability of achieving its rewards and a net decrease in motivation. For some people, a New Year's resolution (personal rule) like "Don't eat between meals this month" might be more effective in

the long run than a resolution *never* again to eat between meals. A person who succeeds for a whole month in this endeavor might then be in a much better position consistently to abide by the latter personal rule.

13. For criticism of this intuitive idea, see Peele 1985 and 1989.

14. Parts of this article derive from Mele 1992, 1996, and 2002.

REFERENCES

Ainslie, G. (1975) "Specious Reward: A Behavioral Theory of Impulsiveness and Impulse Control." *Psychological Bulletin* 82: 463–96.

Ainslie, G. (1982) "A Behavioral Economic Approach to the Defense Mechanisms: Freud's Energy Theory Revisited." *Social Science Information* 21: 735–80.

Ainslie, G. (1992) *Picoeconomics.* Cambridge: Cambridge University Press.

Ainslie, G. (2001) *Breakdown of Will.* New York: Cambridge University Press.

Bakalar, J., and Grinspoon, L. (1984) *Drug Control in a Free Society.* Cambridge: Cambridge University Press.

Becker, G., and Murphy, K. (1988) "A Theory of Rational Addiction." *Journal of Political Economy* 96: 675–700.

Bratman, M. (1996) "Planning and Temptation." In L. May, M. Friedman, and A. Clark (eds.), *Mind and Morals.* Cambridge, MA: MIT Press.

Buss, S. (1997) "Weakness of Will." *Pacific Philosophical Quarterly* 78: 13–44.

Elliot, C. (1996) *The Rules of Insanity: Moral Responsibility and the Mentally Ill Offender.* Albany, NY: SUNY Press.

Elster, Jon (1985) *Ulysses and the Sirens.* Cambridge: Cambridge University Press.

Feinberg, J. (1970) *Doing and Deserving: Essays in the Theory of Responsibility.* Princeton, NJ: Princeton University Press.

Ferrell, R., Price, T., Gert, B., and Bergen, B. (1984) "Volitional Disability and Physician Attitudes toward Noncompliance." *Journal of Medicine and Philosophy* 9: 333–51.

Fischer, J., and Ravizza, M. (1998) *Responsibility and Control: A Theory of Moral Responsibility.* New York: Cambridge University Press.

Fischer, J., and Ravizza, M. (2000) "Replies." *Philosophy and Phenomenological Research* 61: 467–80.

Glover, J. (1970) *Responsibility.* London: Routledge and Kegan Paul.

Hare, R. M. (1963) *Freedom and Reason.* Oxford: Oxford University Press.

Herrnstein, R., and Prelec, D. (1992) "A Theory of Addiction." In G. Loewenstein and J. Elster (eds.), *Choice over Time.* New York: Russell Sage Foundation.

Heyman, G. (1996) "Resolving the Contradictions of Addiction." *Behavioral and Brain Sciences* 19: 561–610.

Logue, A. (1995) *Self-Control.* Englewood Cliffs: Prentice Hall.

Mele, A. (1987) *Irrationality.* New York: Oxford University Press.

Mele, A. (1992) *Springs of Action.* New York: Oxford University Press.

Mele, A. (1995) *Autonomous Agents.* New York: Oxford University Press.

Mele, A. (1996) "Addiction and Self-Control." *Behavior and Philosophy* 24: 99–117.

Mele, A. (2000) "Reactive Attitudes, Reactivity, and Omissions." *Philosophy and Phenomenological Research* 61: 447–52.

Mele, A. (2002) "Akratics and Addicts." *American Philosophical Quarterly* 39: 153–67.

Mele, A. (2003) *Motivation and Agency.* New York: Oxford University Press.

Neely, W. (1974) "Freedom and Desire." *Philosophical Review* 83: 32–54.

Peele, S. (1985) *The Meaning of Addiction*. Lexington, MA: Lexington Books.

Peele, S. (1989) *Diseasing of America: Addiction Treatment out of Control*. Lexington, MA: Lexington Books.

Plato (1953) Protagoras. In *The Dialogues of Plato*. Translated by B. Jowett. Oxford: Clarendon Press.

Pugmire, D. (1982) "Motivated Irrationality." *Proceedings of the Aristotelian Society* 56: 179–96.

Rachlin, H. (1995) "Self-Control: Beyond Commitment." *Behavioral and Brain Sciences* 18: 109–59.

Szasz, T. (1974) *Ceremonial Chemistry*. Garden City, NY: Anchor Press.

Tenenbaum, S. (1999) "The Judgment of a Weak Will." *Philosophy and Phenomenological Research* 59: 875–911.

Wallace, R. J. (1999) "Three Conceptions of Rational Agency." *Ethical Theory and Moral Practice* 2: 217–42.

Watson, G. (1977) "Skepticism about Weakness of Will." *Philosophical Review* 86: 319–39.

Watson, G. (1999) "Excusing Addiction." *Law and Philosophy* 18: 589–619.

Zec, R. (1995) "Neuropsychology of Schizophrenia According to Kraeplin: Disorders of Volition and Executive Functioning." *European Archive of Psychiatry and Clinical Neuroscience* 245: 216–23.

....

CHAPTER 6

SELF-ASCRIPTION

Thought Insertion

....

GEORGE GRAHAM

IMAGINE. You're in New York. It's spring. You are an urbane world traveler. Your thoughts turn to Paris. You love Paris in the springtime.

You walk into a travel agency, spot a Parisian tour that you wish to take, ask an agent what it costs, make a reservation, write a deposit check, hand it to the agent, and leave. In the course of this activity you undergo a variety of conscious thoughts, feelings, and actions, which, in their very occurrence, you experience as your own. You self-ascribe them, so that if asked to report what is going on, you remark: "I am thinking of Paris." "I must ask what it costs." "I am writing a deposit check." Now substitute the following twist. Imagine that instead of experiencing these occurrences as *your* thoughts, feelings, and actions, you experience them as if somehow made for or done to you by an external agent or individual: a person or intelligent force other than yourself. You think about Paris but report: "He treats my mind like a screen and flashes his thoughts onto it like you flash a picture" (Mellor 1970: 17). You inquire about costs but exclaim: "The force moved my lips. I began to speak. The words were made for me." You sign a check but announce: "My fingers pick up the pen, but I don't control them. What they do is nothing to do with me" (18).

The human capacity for experiencing one's own conscious activity in a self-ascribed manner, for undergoing conscious thoughts, feelings, and actions as one's own, can break down and become disordered or distorted. One startling manner in which the capacity for self-ascription breaks down is in a phenomenon known as *thought insertion*. Thought insertion is a disorder of self-ascription that takes place in people diagnosed with schizophrenia and related forms of mental illness. An instance of thought insertion is reported in the first quote from Mellor. Indeed, it is one of schizophrenia's defining symptoms (Fulford 1989: 220; see also Gelder et al. 1983). Thought insertion typically coexists with disorders such as alien voices, thought withdrawal, and other so-called passivity experiences (Schneider 1959; Sartorius et al. 1977). Thought insertion is a delusion, which means, in part, that its victim represents the experience to himself, although objectively, of course, it is grossly misleading, as something of whose inserted nature he is absolutely convinced and from which he cannot be dissuaded. The level or sincerity of conviction may be sustained with a bizarre or confabulatory explanation (Stephens and Graham 2004). When asked how thoughts can be inserted into you, you might reply with an outlandish remark like: "He treats my mind like a screen and flashes thoughts onto it like you flash a picture."

In this chapter I offer a brief philosophical perspective on thought insertion as a disorder or breakdown in the human capacity for self-ascription of one's own conscious activity. I begin by defining thought insertion. I end with speculation about how best to link the phenomenology or experience of thought insertion with neuropsychological research. In the middle sections of the chapter, I consider an epistemological or identification puzzle about thought insertion that has bothered philosophers of psychiatry and others. I show how the puzzle may be resolved.

WHAT IS THOUGHT INSERTION?

Thought insertion consists, in part, in undergoing conscious thoughts and directly knowing what they are of or about (their content) but failing, in some sense, to experience them as one's own. One fails to self-ascribe. A patient of Frith (1992: 66) reports: "Thoughts come into my head like 'Kill God.' It's just like my mind working, but it isn't." Persons who experience inserted thoughts also—and here is *the* critical feature—believe that *another* person's or agent's thoughts somehow have been inserted or engendered into their mind or stream of consciousness. One's thoughts are experienced as if they belong to another. Frith's patient continues: "They come from this chap, Chris. They're his thoughts" (66). As Cahill and Frith (1996: 278) describe the phenomenon: "Patients report that . . . the thoughts which occur in their heads (are) not actually their own. It is as if another's thoughts have been . . . inserted in them. One of our patients reported physically feeling the alien thoughts as they entered his head and claimed that he could pin-point the point of entry!"

Marked clinical similarities exist in patient presentation between thought insertion and various other disorders of self-ascription or self-consciousness. To mention just two examples: (1) So-called made feelings, a disorder in the self-attribution of feelings and emotions, are described by patients similarly to inserted thoughts. One patient says: "They project upon me laughter, for no reason, and you have no idea how terrible it is to laugh and look happy and know it is not you, but their emotions" (Mellor 1970: 17). (2) Inner or subvocal speech may be experienced as the voices of external agents, even in cases in which there is no distinguishable auditory or acoustic phenomenology. This phenomenon, which Stephens and I call "alien voices," and which is classified as verbal auditory hallucination (although not always accurately since there may be no auditory phenomenology), is a type of disorder of self-ascription (Stephens and Graham 2000).

Clinical similarities among thought insertion, other-ascribed feelings, alien voices, and certain other disorders of self-ascription that could be mentioned may mean that such disorders are species or instances of the same general internal dysfunction or deficit that achieves different forms in individuals on different occasions. If so, then such clinically similar disorders should be explained in a similar manner at some level or levels, perhaps by reference to similar neuropsychological structures or subpersonal information processing activities. I speak about subpersonal processes later in the chapter, when I discuss how to construct a subpersonal model of thought insertion.

Thought insertion should not be confused with experiences of thought influence or control. Fulford (1989: 221) states that in believing that an external agent influences or controls one's thinking, one does not believe that the other actually is *doing* the thinking, "whereas in the case of thought insertion it is (bizarrely) the thinking itself" that the patient believes is done by another. Wing (1978: 105) remarks: "The symptom is not that [the patient] has been caused to have unusual thoughts . . . but [that] the thoughts *themselves* are not his."

THOUGHT INSERTION'S MISIDENTIFICATION PUZZLE

Consider the kinds of evidence to which I may appeal in establishing the truth of the following statements. [Relevant circumstances of utterance are specified in brackets.]

(1) This [said when pointing] hair is graying.
(2) This [said when pointing] is my graying hair.
(3) [Said when introspectively reporting] I am thinking about Paris.

The evidence that would support the truth of (1) might include the following: how the hair looks in a mirror, what the barber says about the hair, time-delayed photographs of the top of a head, and so on. The evidence that would support the truth of (2) might include the following: how my hair looks in a mirror, what the barber says about my hair, time-delayed photographs of the top of my head, and so on.

Let's call the evidence just cited for (1) and (2), "indirect" evidence. We are calling this evidence "indirect" because I must *infer* from the evidence to something about the hair: that it is graying and that it is my graying hair, respectively. In both cases the evidence may mislead. I am not impervious to being misled. Mirrors, barbers, and photographs lie. Indirect evidence leaves room for drawing incorrect inferences.

We should distinguish between indirect evidence for (1) and for (2). When I say that *this* hair is graying, I am not self-ascribing the hair. When I say that this is *my* graying hair, I am self-attributing the hair. I am saying something that requires additional and different evidence from evidence merely for referring to graying hair.

Let's compare with (3). What about (3)? The evidence that supports the truth of (3) is not indirect. It is direct, self-evident, or noninferential. Another word that is sometimes used for evidence of this sort is "immediate." My thought about Paris, self-evidently, is a Paris-thought and it would appear equally to be, self-evidently or immediately, my thought. After all, to know that a thought is of Paris one has merely to think of Paris. One doesn't have to look in mirrors, talk to barbers, or examine photographs. Someone asks, "What's going through your mind right now?" I reply, "Thought of Paris." My direct or immediate appeal for this claim is the experience of thinking. There is no room for inference. Direct evidence precludes being misled. We know, writes Heil (1992: 182), "immediately and with certainty what we are thinking." Likewise, direct evidence of thinking of Paris is or appears at the same time to be direct or immediate evidence of self-ascription—that is to say, of *my* thinking of Paris. It seems that there cannot be an error of (what may be called) "thinker-identification" or "self-identification" in this case. If I say, "I am thinking of Paris," I cannot be right that someone is thinking of Paris but wrong about who this person is. I cannot misidentify the thinker (see esp. Shoemaker 1968 and 1986 for discussion). By comparison, in the case of graying hair, if I say "My hair is graying," I can be right that someone's hair is graying but mistaken about whose hair it is. Perhaps I am looking in a mirror and misidentify the top of someone else's head as my own. Therein I get the person with the graying hair wrong. I misidentify myself as the person with the hair.

So much seems noncontentious, if a bit esoteric. Such points about direct evidence and self-ascription are points that only a philosopher may care to make. Now, however, a perplexing puzzle about thought insertion arises that is worrisome to philosophers of psychiatry and others. It's a worry about misidentification of the thinker. It can be expressed as follows.

Thought insertion appears to violate a principle suggested by the example of my thinking of Paris. I refer to it as the *principle of present-tense ascription immunity* (or simply the *principle of ascription immunity*). The principle may be expressed as the follows: *It is impossible for anyone to have or entertain thoughts without being aware—immediately or self-evidently—that he is thinking those thoughts.* My thoughts (the thoughts that I myself have) are experienced as mine. Your thoughts are experienced as yours. However, it seems, contrary to the principle, thought insertion reveals that a person can be in ascription error. I can have or entertain thoughts of Paris but attribute these to another person or thinker. Suppose as a victim of thought insertion I say: "Thoughts come into my head like 'Go to Paris.' It's just like my mind working, but it isn't. They come from this chap, Pierre. They're his thoughts." I am directly aware of certain thoughts but ascribe them to another. Although their content or occurrence is self-evident, their self-ascription to me apparently is not self-evident. Campbell (1999: 609–10) remarks, "what is so striking about the phenomenon . . . is that it seems to involve an error of identification. Thought insertion seems to be a counterexample to the thesis that present-tense introspectively based reports of [thoughts] cannot involve errors of identification." Can this really be so? Can I fail to be correct in identifying the "thinker" of my thoughts?

Let us make sure that we understand what is puzzling about thought insertion before we try to tackle or resolve the puzzle. The identification puzzle posed by thought insertion is not a worry over *past* thoughts about whose ownership I am mistaken. Perhaps last year I had thought of Paris and now remember that someone thought of Paris but misremember the identity of that person. Likewise, the puzzle is not about entertaining thought contents of whose reliability or veridicality I am ignorant. I may think of Paris, and report this, but hold mistaken or unreliable beliefs about Paris. Furthermore, the puzzle is not a worry about my being able to identify the type of attitude of which my Paris thought is a part. I may interpret my thought as a mere wish to go to Paris, when it is hardly just a wish as I saunter into a travel agency to buy tickets. My thought of Paris is, in such an instance, an intention or part of an intention. The range of errors that I can make about my own thoughts and conscious attitudes is widely discussed in the philosophical literature (see Heil 1992: 151–83). There is much about my conscious life, including past conscious life, about which I am not infallible or even privileged and can be wrong or mistaken. However, it seems that there are at least two things—two self-evident facts—about my thoughts about which I cannot be mistaken. Having or entertaining thoughts is inseparable from immediately grasping their content. And—were it not for a puzzle like that posed by thought insertion—entertaining thoughts seems inseparable from experiencing them as my own: that is, as belonging to me.

So, the question is, is thought insertion a counterexample to the principle of ascription immunity? Therein sits the puzzle.

A handful of theorists, this author included, have argued, independently, that thought insertion is compatible with the principle of ascription immunity and does not constitute a counterexample to the principle (Campbell 1989; Gallagher 2000; Graham 2002; Stephens and Graham 1994, 2000). The heart of the argument (which I recast later in terms that I have helped to develop with Stephens) goes like this.

First-person reports of inserted thoughts are equivocal. In reports, as well as in experiencing inserted thoughts, victims experience thoughts as belonging to themselves, in one sense, but also as belonging, in another sense, to another person or thinker. So, victims actually do experience thoughts as their own (in the first sense, to be described momentarily), and thought insertion does not violate the ascription immunity principle. The principle says only that my thoughts are experienced as mine. It does not say that I must or do experience them as mine in each of the two relevant senses.

The next two sections of the chapter detail the argument.

COMPATIBILITY OF THOUGHT INSERTION WITH ASCRIPTION IMMUNITY

Suppose that lightening strikes a man in a parking lot. After his neurons settle, he says:

4. I am short. I am tall.

The man contradicts himself, does he not? He seems to violate a principle that philosophers call the *principle of noncontradiction*. Lightning can wreak terrible havoc. However, suppose that common-sense observation reveals two important facts about the circumstances of the man. To his left is a large professional basketball player. To his right is a small young child. Thus, we may presume, charitably, that the man is not contradicting himself. We may presume that what he means goes something like this: "With respect to the basketball player, I am short, although with respect to the child, I am tall." The actual statements of the man are incomplete. Moreover, when properly recast, they do not violate the noncontradiction principle.

Suppose that lightening strikes me on a campus walkway. After my neurons settle, I say:

5. Thoughts of Paris are occurring in me. However these are not my Paris thoughts. They have been inserted into me by this chap, Pierre. They're Pierre's thoughts.

I seem to be violating the ascription immunity principle, do I not? I seem to be ascribing present-tense thoughts of whose content I am directly aware, and, of course, which are mine, to an external individual. Once again, lightning can wreak terrible havoc. However, recall the case of the apparent self-contradictor in the parking lot. Arguably, something similar is taking place on the campus walkway. My report of thought insertion is equivocal or misleading. When the statements are properly recast, I do not violate the ascription immunity principle.

Reports or experiences of thought insertion exhibit two distinct ways or senses in which a thought can be (said to be) mine. In one sense, I am the subject in which thought occurs. In another or second sense, I am the active thinker or agent of the thought. Arguably, as a victim of thought insertion, I recognize that thoughts of

Paris—episodes of thought with content—are occurring in me as subject. (Recall that Frith's patient says that thoughts are being put into his head.) I experience myself as the subject in whom Paris thoughts occur. However, what I fail to experience or recognize is my own involvement in the *activity* of thinking of Paris. I fail to grasp my own personal agency in thinking of Paris. I attribute the activity—the thinking as *doing* (to use Fulford's term)—to another agent or person, specifically to Pierre.

I try to explain what this means in a moment (in the next section of the chapter), when I consider what it is like to experience inserted thoughts. My present point is this: if we can distinguish within thought insertion between the experience of being subject and agent of thinking, thought insertion can be interpreted in a manner that is not inimical or antithetical to the principle of ascription immunity. Thought insertion is bizarre, of course, but it does not violate the principle. We can protect the principle by recognizing that it is best conceived as a principle about immunity from misidentifying oneself as the subject ("thinker" in the subjectivity sense) in whom thoughts occur and not as immunity from misidentifying oneself as the agent behind the thinking ("thinker" in the agency sense). As Gallagher (2000: 205) puts it, "we are always correct on this score." The principle is not about immunity with respect to identifying oneself as the individual *doing* thinking.

So, ultimately, the immunity principle is no more violated by thought insertion than, analogously, the noncontradiction principle is violated by the utterance of the man in the parking lot. Tall basketball player to the left, short child to the right, and there is no violation of the principle of noncontradiction. Thoughts are said to be in me, but are represented or experienced as Pierre's activity, and there is no violation of the principle of ascription immunity. Ascription immunity is not violated because ascription immunity is about thoughts being experienced as mine subjectively. It is not about experiencing them as my deeds or activities.

The solution sketched above to the puzzle posed by thought insertion shows that thought insertion is compatible, conceptually, with the principle of ascription immunity. One can appreciate the unusual character of thought insertion without abandoning the principle. However, is the solution factually accurate? Do victims actually experience thoughts as the solution requires?

PHENOMENOLOGY OF THOUGHT INSERTION

"Activity verbs," Place notes, "refer to an ongoing activity in which an individual can be engaged and on which he or she can spend time" (1999: 381). I claim that prototypically "thinking" is an activity verb. Forms of thinking are multitudinous and include activities such as studying, theorizing, scrutinizing, pondering, planning, relishing, wondering, concentrating, and so on.

In a prototypical case, there is a distinctive *phenomenology*—a what-it's-like aspect—to thinking. Taking myself as a representative example, this what-it's-like aspect includes both (a) a generic phenomenology of thinking and (b) a more specific phenomenology of being engaged in specific thoughts in a manner that I self-attribute or experience as my own. Thinking self-attributively means taking my thoughts to be part of or to stem from me, perhaps from my beliefs, attitudes, or features of my current task or situation. For example, I may experience *myself thinking* of Paris because I know that I want to go to Paris and that I am in a travel agency making a reservation. The generic phenomenology of thinking includes operative knowledge of how to think: that is, how to focus thoughts; control, terminate, redirect them; and so on. There is a what-it's-like aspect to each of these bits of know-how: a what-it's-likeness to focusing, to redirecting, and so on. If, for example, I am trying to write a professional philosophy paper, with an agonizingly difficult central argument, the generic phenomenology appears when I process and act responsively to the construction of the argument. "I am articulating the conclusion clearly, but I cannot seem to keep the number of premises under control," I mutter to myself. "The argument is becoming too complicated. My thought processes are contorted. Simplify. Simplify." I repeat this methodological mantra to myself.

In referring to what it is like to think I don't mean to refer to a sensory phenomenon. Thinking needs not consist of mental images of a sensory or qualitative sort (visual, acoustic, or tactile). Sometimes thinking occurs in image-like form (e.g., as sentences spoken silently in the imagination). Other times, however, it does not. Sometimes, that is, thoughts occur that are "wholly determinate in their content yet quite diaphanous, lacking any experiential character other than the meaning [content] they carry" (Dainton 2000: 13). In referring to the phenomenology of thinking, I mean to refer to the manner in which thinking immediately or self-evidently appears in the first person (i.e., to the person thinking), generically and with respect to specific thoughts on which the person is spending time. It is this first-person appearance to which I am referring as the what-it's-likeness or phenomenology of thinking.

Not every episode of thinking is experienced as something that one does. Thoughts sometimes occur unbidden, willy-nilly or otherwise so as not to reflect being mine in any sense but as episodes in my stream of consciousness. I may think willy-nilly of a jingle from a TV commercial, for example. This jingle has meaning to me, but I do not experience the jingle as something that I actively think. The what-it's-likeness of thoughts appearing as mere episodes and not as activity occurs if (a) and (b) are truncated or lacking altogether. I don't experience myself directing or focusing thoughts. I don't attribute their specific content to details of my self or situation.

Now what about thought insertion? What is the phenomenology of thought insertion? In thought insertion, thinking is experienced as an activity. However, although episodes of thinking are experienced as occurring in oneself (as subject), the activity itself is experienced as if conducted or engaged in by *someone else* (as the agent). An analogous phenomenon occurs in silent inner speech in schizophrenia in which I (as victim) seem to hear another person's voice. I experience the voice not as a random bit of doggerel but as the intelligent speech act of another. No other is speaking to me, but I believe that another is speaking. "Mother Teresa is urging me to attend not to philosophical arguments but to the poor," I report. So, perhaps the phenomenology of alien voices is similar to that of inserted thoughts (Stephens and Graham 2000). In any case, in thought insertion, the structure or process of the phenomenological displacement of the self by attribution to the other proceeds, roughly, as in the following example.

I think of Paris. Paris-thoughts occur to me. However, I experience my thinking of Paris as the activity of another person. There is a distinctive phenomenology—a what-it's-like aspect—in experiencing thinking as the activity of another person or agent. It consists of two main elements. One is a generic phenomenology of episodes occurring in me—that is, in my stream of consciousness, but in which operative knowledge of how to think (e.g., of how to control or focus these episodes) is attributed to another person or agent. The second element is a phenomenology as if specific thoughts (say, about Paris) that occur to me match or express not me or my situation but the self or situation of another person or agent. Somehow—perhaps quite spontaneously—I assume that the contents of my stream of consciousness express the beliefs, attitudes, or situation of someone else. The assumption of another as *doing* the thinking may be voiced in a silent, perhaps normally absent, narrative wherein I provide running introspective commentary on my thinking. "These thoughts belong to Pierre, not me. He loves Paris. I don't. I am strictly a New Yorker. I want never to leave Manhattan."

UNITY AND FRAGILITY OF SELF-ASCRIPTION

Brook (2001) remarks that, normally, when engaged in thinking, a person is directly aware of herself not just as someone in whom thoughts or mental activities occur but as the single common agent of various mental acts. The experiences of being subject and agent are phenomenologically intertwined. If this is true, and I assume that, in some manner, normally it is, it follows that thought insertion is a disorder or deficit in a person's capacity to distinguish her agency from nonagency, her mental deeds from her nonactivities or from another's mental acts. Thought insertion represents a disturbance in the normal subjective and agentic unity of the activity of thinking.

Certain other and more profound disorders of self-ascription, as Radden (1999) cautions, are more dramatically personally distorting than thought insertion. Some disturbances actually rob a person of the capacity for self-ascription and unity of conscious activity altogether—"along with robbing them of a self" (354).

TOWARD A COMPLETE THEORY OF
THOUGHT INSERTION

An advertisement for the phenomenology of thought insertion might read "Where thought insertion occurs" or "When and why it occurs." Thought insertion occurs in experience (it is a disorder in the phenomenology). It occurs when the phenomenology of experiencing oneself as *thinker* is displaced. It occurs because the seeming "personal" intelligence or direction of thinking appears as alien to one's self or situation and as suited to an external agent. However, as critically important and fascinating as it is to describe matters at a phenomenological level, an exclusive single-level phenomenological analysis of thought insertion is, by its nature, partial or incomplete. The incompleteness of phenomenology is something that Stephens and I (2000) mentioned in our book-length treatment of thought insertion and alien voices. However, given the phenomenological focus of that book, we did not pursue the theme of incompleteness. Now I wish to say something about it, although since the incompleteness of phenomenological description and explanation is a huge topic, I explore it here only briefly.

I plan to offer no grand lesson about incomplete and complete theories—phenomenological or otherwise—here. However, it is useful to distinguish between two ways in which an exclusively phenomenological analysis of thought insertion is incomplete. It is incomplete *horizontally* (neglecting the cultural and social situation of the victim of thought insertion, as well as facts about the victim's attentional set, motivation, and learning history) and *vertically* (making no contact with levels of aggregation and analysis discussed in neuropsychology and cognitive neuroscience).

Horizontal analyses, including phenomenological analysis, take place at the level of the whole person and her perceived situation. Vertical analyses, unlike phenomenological analysis, take place at the level of information processing parts or subsystems of the person.

Much of the credit for interest in describing linkages between thought insertion and subpersonal systems and, ultimately, brain regions must be given to a neuropsychological model of thought insertion offered by Christopher Frith (1992; Frith et al. 2000: 1783). Frith's model, offered prominently in 1992 and currently undergoing refinement, interprets thinking as a kind of motor activity and thought insertion as a failure in subpersonal or subconscious monitoring of motor/thinking activity (see Feinberg 1978).

The notion that thinking is a motor activity is far from intuitively obvious, although Frith does try to intuitively lubricate the notion. Frith's motive for focusing on motor activity as a model for thought insertion is, in part, as follows. If thought insertion is a deficiency in the sense of agency, which Frith assumes that it is, then the best picture of how to understand the phenomenon may be drawn from investigation of the subpersonal monitoring and control of action (Campbell 1999). Motor processes are "actions" in a motion or movement sense. Various abnormalities associated with schizophrenia and related delusional illnesses such as supernumerary limbs, alien or anarchic hands, passivity experiences, and so on stem or arise, in part, from subpersonal motor control and monitoring failures. That is Frith's surmise. Then Frith proposes that we extend the surmise *all the way in*. Picture thinking as a motor process. Picture thought insertion as a subpersonal monitoring failure of thinking as a motor process.

It is too soon (given its ongoing refinement and potential for connecting with other models) to summarily evaluate the success of Frith's motor control and monitoring failure model of thought insertion, although there is reason for skepticism. The counterintuition resists lubrication. Thinking is a different kind of action, a different sort of "motion," than bodily movement. "Thinking," Frith writes, "like all our actions, is normally accompanied by a sense of effort and deliberate choice as we move from one thought to the next" (1992: 81). I am not sure what Frith intends to be saying by this claim. Certainly individual thoughts are not deliberately produced. Certainly we do not choose to think specific thoughts (contents) and could not on pain of regress. (See Stephens and Graham 2000 for discussion.)

In certain tasks, of course, such as trying to construct a philosophical argument or negotiating a difficult career decision, thinking can be effortful and infused with choice if not, as already noted, of specific thoughts, then of themes or desired general lines or directions of content. However, such overt direction and detailed vigilance is absent in most day-to-day experiences of thinking.

If thinking is not a subpersonal motor control monitoring failure, then what type of subpersonal model applies to thought insertion? It may help to step back and decide what a subpersonal model of thought insertion should accomplish. In the narrow sense, it should link the phenomenology of thought insertion with neural structures or correlates. It may be presumed that neural correlates are internal loci of control—full or partial—for elements in thought insertion: that is, that the correlates, in some sense, produce and regulate, or help to produce and regulate, phenomenological features of thought insertion. One way in which to discover or build such a model is to seek direct neural instantiations of the phenomenology. This manner of proceeding, which sometimes is referred to as the development of modular models, is common in cognitive neuroscience. It lies behind Frith's motor control monitoring failure model of thought insertion. According to Frith's model, for instance, the thoughts (contents) one ends up thinking are compared, in some manner subpersonally, with thoughts that the brain "commands" or "intends." If commanded and then activated or conscious thoughts fail to mesh or match, the conscious thoughts become candidates for being experienced as inserted thoughts. They are experienced as inserted given relevant activity in other parts of the model or its modules. This means that Frith's model includes a comparator apparatus or a comparator subsystem and other relevant subsystems (such as a system that commands thought) for the experience of thought insertion.

In my opinion, the brain's massively parallel processing implies that the existence of comparators between thinking and the brain's alleged commands to think is unlikely. The problem, crudely put, with assuming a role for comparators in the production and execution of thinking is that a comparator system must compare thoughts with something that, although preconscious, is thoughtlike in its content. However nothing thoughtlike in content seems to be localized in the brain. There is no place in the brain (unlike, for contrasting example, the role which the cerebellum plays as a location for comparing premotor commands and their actual implementation [Brooks 1986]) where commands with thoughtlike contents such as "Think 'Paris' " occur. Absent some sort of preconscious content with which thought content is compared, thought content is incomparable by a subpersonal apparatus. To make the same point in slightly different terms, instead of deploying modules that are specialized with comparators for examining one-to-one correlations between preconscious and conscious content, the brain somehow produces thinking through parallel activity in many different and distributed brain structures. No one of these structures compares preconscious content with conscious content, although just how conscious and specific thought is produced is not (on my reading of the scientific literature) currently known.

If I were a subpersonal modeler, I would take a different course than Frith's in developing models of linkages between neural structures and the experiences of thinking and thought insertion. I would not appeal to motor control or motor acts as a model for understanding thought. I would appeal to what we know of perception and perceptual processing.

One major lesson of the recent history of cognitive neuroscientific modeling of conscious perceptual processes and activities is that information drawn from subpersonal modeling can play a role in developing a proper understanding of salient features of the phenomenology of perceptual experience. The experience of building subpersonal models of conscious visual perception and evidence from a variety of sources associated with describing the visual system (such as lesion studies and brain imaging techniques) have revealed that perceiving, while certainly not the same sort of action as movement, is a kind of act. It is an act in the following sense: in order for subjects to perceive, they must make various kinds of subpersonal decisions (or, perhaps better expressed, such decisions must occur in them), and these decisions imply that perceptual experience has an active or agentlike component. Let me explain.

Perceiving an object, visually, consciously, does not consist in the passive occurrence of visual awareness of an object. It consists, instead, in controlling the visual search for objects and fixing perception on an object in the teeth of distractions or conflicting demands on the visual system. Visual perception is selective attention. It enables a creature to notice or heed some objects rather than others. It enables a creature not merely to refer to objects and to extract information about them (which, as studies of the phenomenon of blindsight reveal, can be done nonconsciously, although in extremely informationally impoverished terms) but to track and categorize them in an informationally enriched manner.[1] (See Place 2000.)

I like to put this by saying that conscious visual perception is active contrastive perception rather than passive categorical awareness. Philosophers of perception often assume that visual perception is an epistemically more or less passive two-place categorical relation: I perceive P (e.g., the bear in the woods, the bird in the tree). Recent subpersonal models suggest that visual perception is a three-place subpersonal, decision-driven contrastive relation: I perceive P rather than P* (e.g., the bear rather than the bird). I visually track the bear, not the bird, which may recede or remain in the preconscious or preattentive background. There is no such thing as visually perceiving an object, unless one does this as opposed to perceiving another object. Perception thus reflects a decision within the visual system about which object in the environment on which to visually attend, while leaving other objects (remaining much more ill defined in received character) to visually nonconscious information extraction.

Visual perception sometimes has, on occasion, a phenomenologically or consciously explicit selective-attention or active-heeding component. A person explicitly heeds or attends to an object or stimulus in cases in which visual stimuli (e.g., bright lights) suddenly enter consciousness, as if demanding attention or in which behavioral demands (e.g., I am a hunter tracking a bear) require perceptual focusing and behavioral regimentation. However, a selective attention component is at work — subpersonally — even in cases in which heeding is not part of the phenomenology. Visual perception is allocated, subpersonally, contrastively, to an object. It is always selective attention.

What about thinking and the phenomenology of thought insertion? Does the subpersonal modeling of perception contain a lesson for modeling thinking and, in particular, the phenomenology of thought insertion?

I assume that the subpersonal correlates of thinking currently are unknown. However, perhaps we can speculate that the task of fully or partially controlling the experience of self-ascription — or helping to regulate attributively attending, as it were, to the self as *thinker* or agent — is a major subpersonal component of thinking. Just as subpersonal control of perceptual attention is essential to conscious visual perception, so subpersonal regulation of self-ascription is empirically essential for being a thinker and, most important, for the experience mentioned by Brook of being the single common subject and agent of various mental acts. To borrow a metaphor from Braff (1999: 259), we may assume that the mind/brain has one or more spatially distributed bins or pools that are devoted to the experience of self-ascription of thinking. Just when and how such resources are actively deployed is a matter of subpersonal decision, as it were, if the contrastive picture of visual perception is, at least in part, properly suggestive of what happens in thinking.

Suppose I think:

"It's springtime. Paris is wonderful in the spring."

Suppose in thinking of Paris in this manner I come to the completion of the thought, the fulfillment of its line of content. Suppose I experience as the completed activity:

"So, I had better get myself to a travel agent and buy a ticket to Paris."

Now I might experience myself as the single common agent behind the completed line of thought. However, suppose I do not experience myself as completing the thought. The content doesn't seem to me to come from or represent me or to arise from my situation or circumstance, although, because of its apparent direction and intelligence, it may seem to have been engendered in me by another person or agent. I say to myself: "I have no desire to go to Paris. The desire for Paris is Pierre's. These are his thoughts." As one schizophrenic patient puts it, "I am picking up thoughts from other people. It's like being a receiving station" (quoted in Fulford 1992: 11).

My hypothesis is that one function of subpersonal activity in helping to produce the experience of thinking is, in part, to produce or support the sense at the phenomenological level of thinking as my activity (when it is genuinely my activity and not something random or willy-nilly). Even though (I assume contrary to Frith) my brain does not, in motor fashion, command specific thoughts, the subpersonal level does allocate resources for "tracking" or experiencing one's thinking as one's own. Its pools and bins regulate or help to regulate self-ascription. Thought insertion represents, in part, a breakdown or mismanagement at the level of those resources. This is at least somewhat akin to the subpersonal selective allocation of perceptual resources. In the normal case of perceiving, I don't perceive the bear. I perceive the bear *rather than* the bird. In the prototypical case of thinking, I don't just entertain a Paris-thought. I take *myself* to be *thinking* of Paris. When I think of Paris, I experience this as my activity. However, in an abnormal case like that of thought insertion, self-attributive phenomenology is displaced.

A critical scientific question is how subpersonal information processes and the neural correlates of thinking allocate resources for the experience of self-attribution (for being the thinker in the sense of agent). One also may wonder where in the brain these resources are located or may be found. The prefrontal cortex, which is an area consistently identified as abnormal in various symptoms of schizophrenia, should be among the candidates. Abnormalities in the prefrontal cortex are particularly robust when victims have been asked to engage in cognitive activity commonly affected by the illness, such as working-memory tasks. Are working-memory tasks more generally implicated in thought insertion? Is memory partly at fault? Is thought insertion brought about, in some measure, because victims fail to retain or actually forget what they believe, intend, or currently are doing?

I offer the hypothesis that it is by controlling or regulating memory and attention to one's self and situation that subpersonal information processing serves as a locus of control for the self-attribution of thinking. In general, one's grasp of oneself as thinker or agent goes substantially beyond what is experienced in the immediate moment. It reflects a conception of oneself and one's situation and of what one is doing. Memory of who one is and recognition of what one is doing is necessary for self-ascription of ongoing thinking activity. Self-ascription is influenced by subpersonal systems, which have access to or process information about the memory and attentional resources of a person. Only when subpersonal activity gives rise to conscious experience of thinking, and does so in a manner that a person believes expresses herself or her situation, does the phenomenology of thinking as a self-ascribed activity take place.

Researchers into thought insertion also need to look at time-linked variability in reports of thought insertion. Schizophrenic patients' performances notoriously exhibit complex dynamical properties in which, among other things, patterns of highly organized, stereotypical behavior fluctuate with periods of disorganization and disturbance. Concordant with this temporal pattern, victims don't experience thought insertion all the time. Why? Does temporal variability somehow mean that the hypothesis of subpersonal resource allocation for the experience of self-ascription is on the right track? Just as the visual system must operate attentively in the teeth of distractions and conflicting demands, so "self-ascription" of conscious activity must navigate through stresses and strains on the activity of thinking. These stresses and strains do not always occur, but when they do they are dealt with, in some sense, in the form of allocations at the subpersonal level for the phenomenological ingredients of self-ascription. When distractions cannot be resisted—perhaps when attention is swamped by other deficits in schizophrenia and the victim has difficulty retaining aspects of self or situation in working memory—disorders like thought insertion may occur. The subpersonal allocations necessary for self-ascription may periodically be blunted or stymied and ascription to another may occur.

Self-ascription to oneself as a thinking agent is an essential requirement if we are to know about ourselves as thinkers, to control and regulate our thinking, and to decide which lines of thought to pursue, as well as to observe and train ourselves to think more carefully and intelligently. Self-ascription is disordered in thought insertion. Thought insertion is puzzling in phenomenology and in subpersonal processing and purport. It is primed for ongoing ponder by philosophers, especially by those who, in Paul Churchland's (1989: 66) fortunate phrase, "prize the flux and content of our subjective phenomenological experience" but also appreciate the necessity of probing beneath phenomenology into the inner world of the mind/brain.

NOTES

I received help in writing this chapter from Colin Allen, Ralph Kennedy, Uriah Kriegel, Jennifer Radden, Peter Zachar, and audiences of philosophers and their guests at the University of California at San Diego and at the Claremont Graduate University. I am also indebted to G. Lynn Stephens.

1. "Blindsight" refers to the preserved ability (following damage to the primary visual cortex) of the visual system to extract information from the environment but in a manner that is not experienced as conscious. The pattern of preserved and impaired abilities varies from case to case but tends to involve such things as the detection and localization of light and the orientation, shape, and direction of movement of as stimulus. For a review of the blindsight literature, see Cowey and Stoerig (1991).

REFERENCES

Recommended readings are marked by an asterisk (*).

Braff, D. (1999) "Psychophysiological and Information-Processing Approaches to Schizophrenia." In D. Charney, E. Nestler, and B. Bunney (eds.), *Neurobiology of Mental Illness.* Oxford: Oxford University Press, pp. 258–71.

Brook, A. (2001) "The Unity of Consciousness." *Stanford Encyclopedia of Philosophy.* Available at http://plato.stanford.edu/entries/consciousness-unity/.

Brooks, V. (1986) *The Neural Basis for Motor Control.* New York: Oxford University Press.

Cahill, C., and Frith, C. (1996) "False Perceptions or False Beliefs? Hallucinations and Delusions in Schizophrenia." In P. Halligan and J. C. Marshall (eds.), *Method in Madness: Case Studies in Neuropsychiatry.* East Sussez, UK: Psychology Press, pp. 267–91.

*Campbell, J. (1999) "Schizophrenia, the Space of Reasons and Thinking as a Motor Process." *Monist* 82(4): 609–25.

Churchland, P. (1989) "Direct Introspection of Brain States." In P. Churchland (ed.), *A Neurocomputational Perspective.* Cambridge, MA: MIT Press.

Cowey, A., and Stoerig, P. (1991) "The Neurobiology of Blindsight." *Trends in Neuroscience* 14: 140–45.

Dainton, B. (2000) *Stream of Consciousness: Unity and Continuity in Conscious Experience.* London: Routledge.

Feinberg, I. (1978) "Efference Copy and Corollary Discharge: Implications for Thinking and Its Disorders." *Schizophrenia Bulletin* 4: 636–40.

*Frith, C. D. (1992) *The Cognitive Neuropsychology of Schizophrenia.* Hillsdale, NJ: Lawrence Erlbaum.

Frith, C. D., Blakemore, S.-J., and Wolpert, D. M. (2000) "Abnormalities in the Awareness and Control of Action." *Proceedings of the Royal Society of London* 355: 1771–88.

Fulford, K. W. M. (1989) *Moral Theory and Medical Practice.* Cambridge: Cambridge University Press.

Fulford, K. W. M. (1992) "Thought Insertion and Insight: Disease and Illness Paradigms of Psychotic Disorder." In M. Spitzer, F. Uehlein, M. Schwartz, and C. Mundt (eds.), *Phenomenology, Language and Schizophrenia.* New York: Springer.

*Gallagher, S. (2000) "Self-Reference and Schizophrenia: A Cognitive Model of Immunity to Error through Misidentification." In D. Zahavi (ed.), *Exploring the Self.* Amsterdam: John Benjamins, pp. 203–39.

Gelder, M. G., Gath, U., and Mayou, R. (1983) *Oxford Textbook of Psychiatry.* Oxford: Oxford University Press.

Graham, G. (2002) "Recent Work in Philosophical Psychopathology." *American Philosophical Quarterly* 39: 109–33.

Heil, J. (1992) *The Nature of True Minds.* Cambridge: Cambridge University Press.

Mellor, C. (1970) "First-Rank Symptoms of Schizophrenia." *British Journal of Psychiatry* 117: 15–23.

Place, U. T. (1999) "Ryle's Behaviorism." In W. O'Donohue and R. Kitchener (eds.), *Handbook of Behaviorism.* San Diego: Academic Press, pp. 361–98.

Place, U. T. (2000) "Consciousness and the Zombie Within: A Functional Analysis of the Blindsight Evidence." In Y. Rossetti and A. Revonsuo (eds.), *Beyond Dissociation: Interaction between Dissociated Implicit and Explicit Processing.* Amsterdam: John Benjamins, pp. 295–329.

Radden, J. (1999) "Pathologically Divided Minds: Synchronic Unity and Models of Self." In S. Gallagher and J. Shear (eds.), *Models of the Self*. Thoverton, UK: Imprint.

Sartorius, N., Jablensky, A., and Shapiro. R. (1977) "Two-Year Follow-up of Patients Included in WHO International Pilot Study of Schizophrenia." *Psychological Medicine* 7: 529–41.

Schneider, K. (1959) *Clinical Psychopathology*, 5th ed. New York: Grune and Statton.

Shoemaker, S. (1968) "Self-Reference and Self-Awareness." *Journal of Philosophy* 65: 555–67.

Shoemaker, S. (1986) "Introspection and the Self." In P. French, T. Uehling, and H. Wettstein (eds.), *Studies in the Philosophy of Mind*. Midwest Studies in Philosophy 10. Minneapolis: University of Minnesota, pp. 101–20.

Stephens, G. L., and Graham, G. (1994) "Self-Consciousness, Mental Agency, and the Clinical Psychopathology of Thought Insertion." *Philosophy, Psychiatry, and Psychology* 1: 1–10.

*Stephens, G. L., and Graham, G. (2000) *When Self-Consciousness Breaks: Alien Voices and Inserted Thoughts*. Cambridge, MA: MIT Press.

Stephens, G. L., and Graham, G. (2004) "The Delusional Stance." In K. W. M. Fulford, M. Chung, and G. Graham (eds.), *The Philosophical Understanding of Schizophrenia*. Oxford: Oxford University Press.

Wing, J. K. (1978) *Reasoning about Madness*. Oxford: Oxford University Press.

CHAPTER 7

MEMORY

The Nature and Significance of Dissociation

STEPHEN E. BRAUDE

DISSOCIATION is a topic that lends itself quite naturally (and perhaps all too easily) to philosophical speculation. The intriguing behavior and reports of subjects in both clinical and experimental settings can be dramatic and quite surprising. In dissociative fugue states, a person's memories and personality can disappear for a long time and be replaced by a new personality and set of dispositions. In dissociative identity disorder (DID; formerly multiple personality disorder), fairly robust systems of memories and dispositions can alternate (sometimes rapidly) and create the appearance that more than one person is inhabiting the same body. During systematized anesthesia (or negative hallucinations), highly hypnotizable subjects apparently fail to perceive not simply the experimenter but anything the experimenter does to the subject, including ordinarily painful interventions (e.g., needle pricks in the mucous membrane of the eye) and procedures that typically elicit involuntary responses (e.g., ammonia under the nose), even though subjects respond normally to those same procedures when administered by co-experimenters.

It's tempting, and even reasonable, to think that these phenomena point to important facts about the nature of the mind. But it's not easy to determine what those facts are. Clinicians and experimenters who speculate about these matters often don't realize how they import (sometimes questionable) abstract assumptions into their deliberations. As a result, the literature on dissociation offers philosophers many opportunities for conceptual clarification and analysis. Besides, until recently, philosophers have paid relatively little attention to the topic of dissociation. So, quite apart

from commenting on clinical and experimental reports (and the theoretical speculations they inspire), philosophers still have much to explore about the relevance of
dissociation to venerable issues in the philosophy of mind.

WHAT IS DISSOCIATION?

Although psychologists and psychiatrists have studied dissociative phenomena for a
long time, there is surprisingly little agreement about what dissociation is and about
which phenomena instantiate it. Historians of psychology usually credit Pierre Janet
with having originated the concept of dissociation (although he initially used the
term *désagrégation*) to pick out mental states that lack their customary integration or
associative links. Since then, the term "dissociation" has been used to denote a wide
variety of phenomena, drawn from the domains of psychopathology, experimental
psychology, and even everyday life (e.g., overlearned and automatic behaviors). Moreover, there is considerable confusion about the difference (if any) between dissociation and apparently similar or related concepts—in particular, repression, suppression, and denial.

Although space prohibits a comprehensive survey of attempts to characterize
dissociation, some general trends and common themes are easily discernible (see
Braude 1995 and Cardeña 1994 for details). For one thing, it's clear that the concept
of dissociation has evolved since Janet introduced it. Janet intended the concept of
dissociation to handle a distinctive and relatively limited class of psychopathological
phenomena. He considered dissociation to be a kind of weakness, a failure (in the
face of disturbing events) to synthesize or integrate parts of consciousness and thereby
maintain conscious unity. Janet's successors also recognized the apparent causal link
between trauma and dissociative pathology. But they tended to agree that the processes Janet was describing from cases of hysteria (now called conversion disorder)
or double consciousness were also at work in a broad range of nonpathological phenomena. And, along with that, they tended to view dissociation not as a weakness
but as a kind of capacity (not necessarily maladaptive) to sever familiar links between
mental states.

In a related development, researchers initially considered dissociated states to be
functionally *isolated*, not simply from conscious awareness but also from the mass of
ideas and dispositions with which they had formerly been associated. Moreover, they
believed that dissociated states could neither interfere with, nor be interfered with
by, ongoing mental processes or behavior. But, beginning with Messerschmidt's experiments in hypnotically divided attention (Messerschmidt 1927–28), that view has
been effectively undermined. Messerschmidt showed that even in automatic writing
there was some interference or leakage between conscious behavior and subconscious
tasks. Moreover, clinicians began reporting similar forms of interference—for exam-

ple, between alter identities in cases of DID. So experimental and clinical observations now converge in taking the dissociative barrier (whatever, exactly, it is) to be permeable.

Today, the primary debates over dissociation concern either (a) the inventory of phenomena to be regarded as dissociative or (b) whether the forms of dissociation differ in degree or in kind—and in particular, whether pathological dissociation is fundamentally different from nonpathological dissociation. But the literature on these topics shows little clarity or attention to underlying assumptions. In my view, the current debates might be resolved simply by attending to those underlying assumptions and then seeing whether we can lay down criteria of dissociation that conform to them. As a step in that direction, I offer the following observations and proposals.

First, there is widespread agreement that dissociation is not simply an occurrent psychological condition or state (i.e., the state of being dissociated) but also (contrary to Janet) something for which we have an aptitude or capacity. This seems to be a sensible move away from the position advocated by Janet, and it is continuous with the way we treat a great many other areas of human cognition and performance. Analogously, compassion, irony, patience, indignation, dishonesty, kindness, and sarcasm can be regarded as both occurrent states and corresponding capacities. So it seems reasonable to hold that dissociation is likewise one of many things (at least some) people are *able* to do. Let's call this the *capability assumption*. In fact, it's reasonable to think that the capacity to dissociate, *insofar as it's a capacity*, will be similar in broad outline to most other human capacities. Thus, even though dissociation presumably has distinctive features, we would expect it, qua capacity, to share features found generally in human (or just cognitive) capacities. Let's call this the *nonuniqueness assumption*.

Now capacities generally are things people express in different ways and to varying degrees. For example, the capacities for self-deception, intimidation, empathy, sensuality, or malice can range from extreme to very moderate forms, and they can be expressed in highly idiosyncratic ways. So it seems reasonable to assume that dissociation likewise assumes a variety of (possibly quite idiosyncratic) forms, that it can affect a broad range of states (both occurrent and dispositional), and that it spreads out along various continua (e.g., of pervasiveness, frequency, severity, completeness, and retrievability). Let's call this the *diversification assumption*.

Another important assumption allows us to distinguish dissociation from what we might call cognitive or sensory *filtering*. Although the term "filtering" has many meanings, in the sense that matters here it picks out a total blocking of information from a subject. Examples of this sort of filtering would be blindfolding, audio band-pass filtering, and local chemical anesthesia. These situations differ from (say) hypnotic anesthesia and negative hallucination, where subjects merely fail to experience consciously what they are nevertheless aware of subconsciously. So the relevant difference between filtering and dissociation is that in filtering, information never reaches the subjects (consciously or otherwise), whereas dissociation merely blocks subjects' conscious awareness that they have already registered certain information. Thus, the next important assumption is that the things dissociated from a person are always the person's own states. Let's call this the *ownership assumption*. Granted, it's common to say that information or data is dissociated. But, strictly speaking, what is dissociated are the subject's states: for example, volitions, knowledge, memories, dispositions, and sometimes even behavior (as in automatic writing).

The ownership assumption connects with a fifth (and very important) assumption. When a state is dissociated, it is not totally obliterated or isolated in principle (even if retrieving it is difficult in practice). Dissociated states may be subjectively hidden or psychologically isolated, but they are always potentially knowable, recoverable, or capable of reassociation. Thus, dissociation is a theoretically (but perhaps not practically) reversible functional isolation of one's own states from conscious awareness. Let's call this the *accessibility assumption*.

We should also note that the relation "*x* is dissociated from *y*" is *nonsymmetrical*, as in "*x* loves *y*" (even though *x* loves *y*, the latter may or may not love the former). We see this nonsymmetry clearly in cases of one-way amnesia in DID, or in *hidden observer* experiments where states of a hypnotically hidden observer may be dissociated from those of the hypnotized subject, even though the subject's states may not be dissociated from those of the hidden observer (see Hilgard 1986).

With these assumptions in mind, let's consider how to distinguish dissociation from a cluster of concepts easily confused with (but apparently closely related to) it. Probably the most important of these is the concept of repression. Although neither of these concepts is precise, we can effectively distinguish them so as to show that they mark off different (if slightly overlapping) classes of phenomena. In fact, they seem to rest on different presuppositions.

As Hilgard (1986) has noted, writers tend to employ different metaphors in describing the psychological barriers of repression and dissociation. Generally speaking, repressive barriers are described as horizontal, whereas dissociated barriers are described as vertical. As a result, repressed material is typically treated as psychologically (usually, emotionally) *deeper* than what we can access consciously. By contrast, dissociated states are not necessarily deeper than consciously accessible states.

This alleged difference connects with the different roles repression and dissociation ostensibly play in a person's psychological economy. Ordinarily, repression is linked to dynamic psychological forces and active mental defenses that inhibit recall. Granted, some writers similarly describe dissociation as a defense mechanism (primarily, one that produces amnesia), but that view seems both confused and needlessly restrictive (see Braude 1995; Cardeña 1994). In fact, paradigm cases of dissociation needn't involve any impairment of memory, and dissociation may be only fortuitously related to the exigencies of psychological survival. For example, systematized anesthesia does not affect memory, and posthypnotic amnesia can concern virtually any kind of material, whether important or unimportant.

Historically, the concept of repression is bound up with the psychoanalytic concept of a dynamic unconscious, which (among other things) acts as a repository for repressed material and access to which seems more indirect than access to a dissociated part of consciousness. According to the traditional and still standard view of repression, we learn about the unconscious through its byproducts (e.g., dreams or slips of the tongue), and expressions of unconscious material tend to be distorted, either symbolically or by means of more primitive primary-process thinking. So the received view is that repressed mental activities can only be inferred from their behavioral or phenomenological byproducts. By contrast, dissociated material can be accessed relatively directly, as in automatic writing, hypnosis, and interactions with alter identities in cases of DID. We can summarize this difference by saying that third- and first-person knowledge of dissociated—but not unconscious—states can be as direct as (respectively) third- and first-person knowledge of nondissociated states.

So we can say that if x is repressed for S (in this sense of "repressed"), then (a) S is not consciously aware of (or has amnesia for) x, and (b) third- and first-person knowledge of x is indirect as compared (respectively) with third- and first-person knowledge of both conscious and dissociated states (i.e., it must be *inferred* from its possibly distorted or primitive cognitive, phenomenological, or behavioral byproducts). Not surprisingly (and not alarmingly), this still leaves a variety of borderline cases—for example, amnesia for a memory we're motivated to forget but which can be recovered directly through hypnosis, or behavior that reveals hidden feelings but whose interpretation is clear even to the person exhibiting it (e.g., forgetting an appointment you prefer to avoid). In fact, in some cases the only difference between a repressed and a dissociated state may be the conceptual framework in terms of which it is treated clinically. For example, obsessional or compulsive behavior might be approached psychoanalytically, using indirect methods (e.g., free association) to uncover the reasons for the behavior. Or, it might be treated as a dissociative disorder, using hypnosis to reveal hidden memories lying at the root of the problem.

The concept of suppression is also a bit difficult to pin down, and certainly the term "suppression"gets used in various ways (often as a synonym for "repression"). To the extent that there is a standard view of the difference between suppression and repression, there seem to be two distinguishing features. First, "amnesia is absent in suppression, present in repression" (Hilgard 1986: 251), and second, suppression never results from unconscious activity. So suppression seems to be "a conscious putting-out-of-mind of something we don't want to think about" (Braun 1988: 5). So if we agree to use "suppression"in this fairly narrow technical sense, we can say that when x is suppressed for S, (a) S consciously diverts attention from x (i.e., puts x "out of mind"), and (b) S does not have amnesia for x.

Although Braun regards *denial* as yet another distinct point on a continuum of awareness (Braun 1988), I submit that if we define the relevant terms as I suggest here, a distinct category of denial is gratuitous. I propose instead that we consider analyzing the term "denial"in terms of repression, suppression, and dissociation. For example, one handy (if slightly oversimplified) approach would be the following. Let's suppose first that the difference between unconscious and subconscious mental states is that the former can be accessed only indirectly (as explained earlier), whereas the latter can be accessed relatively directly. Then we can regard repression as *unconscious denial*, dissociation as *subconscious denial*, and suppression as *conscious denial*.

With these considerations in mind, I offer the following provisional analysis of dissociation. We can then see how it bears on current debates about dissociation. Let's say "*x* is dissociated from *y*" just in case:

1. (a) *x* is an occurrent or dispositional state of a person *S*, or else a system of states (as in traits, skills, and alternate personalities), and (b) *y* is either a state or system of states of *S*, or else the person *S*.
2. *y* may or may not be dissociated from *x* (i.e., dissociation is a nonsymmetrical relation).
3. *x* and *y* are separated by a phenomenological or epistemological barrier (e.g., amnesia, anesthesia) erected by the subject *S*.
4. *S* is not consciously aware of erecting the barrier between *x* and *y*.
5. The barrier between *x* and *y* can be broken down, at least in principle.
6. Third- and first-person knowledge of *x* may be as direct as (respectively) third- and first-person knowledge of *S*'s nondissociated states.

Condition 1 takes the capability, ownership, and diversification assumptions into account, and condition 5 acknowledges the accessibility assumption. Since condition 4 requires *S* to erect the dissociative barrier either subconsciously or unconsciously, it provides a way of ruling out cases of suppression. Similarly, condition 6 rules out a large set of cases ordinarily classified as instances of repression.

Condition 3 is designed to rule out a large class of cases we would presumably not count as dissociative but in which *S*'s states seem to lie behind an epistemological barrier. In particular, this condition rules out many examples of conceptual naiveté and inevitable forms of self-ignorance. For example, *S* might desire or dislike something but lack the introspective or conceptual sophistication, or the relevant information, needed to recognize those states. So condition 3 rules out cases in which infants, small children, or naive or mentally challenged adults lack the conceptual categories to identify their own mental states. The epistemological barrier in these cases is not something they erect. Similarly, many conceptually sophisticated adults may fail to recognize they have certain mental states, either because they are insufficiently introspective or because they lack relevant information. For example, *S* might be unaware he detests the sound of a fortepiano because he has not yet heard enough examples for that disposition (or regularity in his preferences) to become clear. He might mistakenly think he dislikes only the one or two fortepianos he's heard. That is clearly not a case of dissociation, and condition 3 rules it out as well.

I believe this account of dissociation is sufficiently abstract and general to undergird and also correct the needlessly restrictive or overinclusive accounts one finds throughout the clinical and experimental literature. For example, Cardeña (1994) has identified several general approaches to the analysis of dissociation, many (or perhaps the most credible) of which can be seen as presupposing most of the conditions specified here. These approaches include taking dissociation to be (1) the absence of conscious awareness of impinging stimuli or ongoing behaviors; (2) the coexistence of separate mental systems or identities that should be integrated in the person's consciousness, memory, or identity; (3) ongoing behaviors or perceptions that are inconsistent with a person's introspective verbal report; and (4) an alteration of consciousness in which one feels disconnected from the self or from the environment. Moreover, the foregoing account also corrects some obvious shortcomings of the prevailing approaches—for example, that some instances of (3) would include as dissociative what are clearly cases of self-deception, cognitive dissonance or confusion, or outright ignorance or stupidity (say, a person's simply failing to grasp that simultaneously held beliefs are inconsistent). (For further details, see Braude 1995: ch. 4; Cardeña 1994.)

In any event, my proposed criteria of dissociation clearly countenance a large range of phenomena as instances. Naturally (and predictably), classic forms of pathological dissociation satisfy the criteria, including DID and dissociative fugue. Moreover, other familiar impressive phenomena likewise satisfy the criteria—for example, hypnotic amnesia, anesthesia or analgesia, and automatic writing. Perhaps more interesting, the criteria are apparently satisfied by a range of normal phenomena many want to regard as dissociative. These include, for example, blocking out the sound of ongoing conversation while reading (but being able to respond when your name is mentioned) and shifting gears and obeying traffic lights while driving but consciously focusing only on your conversation with your passenger. I consider it a virtue of these criteria that they undergird a variety of disparate intuitions about which phenomena are instances of dissociation. And that brings us to the next issue.

Probably the most hotly debated topic today about dissociation is whether normal, experimental, and pathological dissociation are all forms of a single phenomenon (let's call this the *inclusivity position*), or whether pathological and nonpathological dissociation differ in kind rather than in degree (the *exclusivity position*). Thus, the debate concerns the viability of the diversification assumption, according to which dissociation assumes (nonessentially) different forms and spreads out along a variety of relevant continua. Until recently, most clinicians and experimenters embraced the inclusivity position. But on the basis of some recent taxonometric analyses by Waller, Putnam, and Carlson, and a small number of subsequent studies by other investigators, some now claim that pathological and nonpathological forms of dissociation are sharply distinct categories, and they argue that it is a mistake to view normal and pathological dissociation as continuous (see, e.g., Putnam 1997; Waller et al. 1996; Boon and Draijer 1993; Ogawa et al. 1997).

But this recent endorsement of the exclusivity position seems unconvincing for several reasons. First, it's likely that the appearance of distinct classes or taxa of dissociative phenomena is simply an artifact of the categories and form of questions used in the questionnaire from which the data were gathered (Ruk, in press). But, quite apart from that, even if pathological and nonpathological forms of dissociation differ consistently and dramatically (so that many properties of the latter are never properties of the former), that *could not* by itself show that the two forms of dissociation were discontinuous. One of the assumptions apparently underlying the exclusivity view is that if the two forms of dissociation were continuous, one would expect to find a fairly even distribution of dissociative phenomena along a dissociative continuum. And because Waller et al. report finding two distinct clusters or taxa of phenomena, not the relatively smooth distribution to which they think the inclusivity view (or diversification assumption) is committed, they believe they have disconfirmed the inclusivity view.[1] However, it seems simply arbitrary to suppose that the distribution between normal and pathological dissociative phenomena must be smooth. In fact, uneven distributions are clearly compatible with treating all dissociative phenomena as continuous. At least some leading researchers recognize this (see, e.g., Nijenhuis 1999: 175f). For example, pathological lying and ordinary lying can easily be regarded as falling along various continua, even if the former can be sharply distinguished from the latter and even if there are relatively few examples of lying that fall between the extremes. Similar observations can be made about the differences between normal orderliness and pathological or compulsive orderliness, and between ordinary anxiety and panic attacks.

Moreover, I suspect that defenders of the exclusivity position set up a straw man when they state the inclusivity position. To say that normal and pathological dissociative phenomena are continuous is not to say that there is a *single* dissociative continuum along which those forms of dissociation are spread (unevenly or evenly). That's an absurdly simple and antecedently incredible formulation of the inclusivity position, and it's all too easy to overturn. Presumably, one can always select a list of allegedly relevant properties in such a way that the classes of normal and pathological dissociation appear to be disjoint. But on different characterizations of dissociation, or using different lists of relevant properties, the two forms of dissociation might turn out to overlap. Indeed, we saw that the criteria of dissociation I listed earlier countenance both normal and pathological forms of dissociation, and phenomena that satisfy those criteria clearly spread out (smoothly or otherwise) along the continua mentioned when I stated the diversification assumption (e.g., pervasiveness, frequency, severity).

The Humpty Dumpty Fallacy

So let's assume we have a reasonably clear idea of which phenomena count as examples of dissociation. What do those phenomena tell us about the nature of the mind? Of course, for many the main issue is whether human beings are deeply unitary or, alternatively, whether they are fundamentally multiple persons or colonies of lower-order selves (or humunculi). That issue is addressed elsewhere in this volume (but for large-scale treatments of the issue, see Braude 1995; Radden 1996; Saks and Behnke 1997; and Wilkes 1988; and for a recent and thoughtful survey, see Graham 2002). For now, we may focus on a related but more modest issue.

When the pioneers of hypnosis observed the phenomena of divided consciousness, they believed that their techniques *uncovered* aspects of mental functioning that were normally hidden. Specifically, they assumed that their therapeutic techniques disclosed a doubling of consciousness that had existed all along within their patients. So they supposed that their magnetic (hypnotic) techniques illuminated a normally hidden feature of our mental *structure* (Braude 1995; Crabtree 1993; Ellenberger 1970). Once nineteenth-century research into multiple personality had gotten under way, we find helpfully explicit statements of this assumption. For example, Ribot wrote, "Seeing how the Self is broken up, we can understand how it comes to be" (1887: 20). Later, Myers wrote, "Subjected continually to both internal and external stress and strain, its [i.e., the personality's] ways of yielding indicate the grain of its texture" (1903: 39).

These authors seem to be making a kind of historical or developmental claim — namely, that dissociative disorganization or splitting is a reversal or undoing of a prior functional organization or unity. So from the phenomena of dissociation, we should be able to infer the elements or organizing principles underlying that former unity. That is, we should be able to argue from postdissociative divisions of the self to the predissociative structures or divisions that made them possible. I've called this the *Principle of Compositional Reversibility* (or CR principle), and the fallacy it commits the *Humpty Dumpty Fallacy*.

This brief summary can't explore all the relevant issues here, but we can note the following. First, the CR principle has been articulated in both a weak and a strong form. The strong version (prevalent during the nineteenth century) holds that there is correlation (perhaps an identity) between the *particular* clinical or experimental entities produced dissociatively and the components of the predissociative self. So from our discovery of the former, we should be able to infer the existence of the latter. Let's call this the *token* CR principle. The weaker version asserts a correlation merely between the *kinds* of entities produced dissociatively and the *kinds* of things composing the predissociative self (see, e.g., Beahrs 1982; Watkins and Watkins 1979–80). Let's call this the *type* CR principle.

Both versions of the CR principle are fatally flawed, and although the details of their errors vary somewhat, the main problem is quite simple. Just because something is now in pieces, it doesn't follow that those pieces correspond to permanent or previously existing natural elements of that thing. Certainly, it's not a general truth that things always divide along some preexisting grain or that objects divide only into their historically original components.

Consider the token CR principle first. I can break a board in two pieces with an axe, but it doesn't follow that the board resulted initially from the uniting of those two parts. Moreover, some cases of splitting, such as cell division, are evolutionary and create entities that didn't exist previously. So if the token CR principle is true, it's not because it's an instance of a more general truth about the way things break up. It would have to be true in virtue of the special way the self divides.

But there is no reason to think that the self always breaks along a preexisting grain or structure, especially under extreme trauma or stress. In cases of DID we see alter identities that apparently form in response to *contingent* stressful situations, and those identities seem to be contingent *products* of a creative process of defense or adaptation. That's why some alters are animal identities, and it's why some are highly specialized (e.g., for cleaning toilets or taking enemas) or specifically impaired (e.g., blind or deaf). Moreover, a multiple's system of alters evolves over time, and sometimes it undergoes temporary integration and subsequent fundamental functional reorganization into a different system of alters. But then it becomes arbitrary to choose one temporal slice of a multiple's history and to claim that the alters at that time reveal the deep grain or structure of the predissociative self. It's much more reasonable to maintain that a multiple's array of alters *at any time* represents merely one of many possible dissociative solutions to problems in living.

A similar point works against the type CR principle, because a multiple's system of alters at different times may divide along quite different functional lines. So it would be arbitrary to select one set of alter *types* as representing the deep functional divisions of the predissociative self. Moreover, it's difficult to know what the type CR principle means and, in particular, to *which* types of postdissociative entities it should apply. Surely, not every type—for example, alters that prefer analog to digital sound, collect ostrich purses, or enjoy rap music. In fact, even if we identify types more conservatively, the type CR principle still seems committed to an absurdly inflated inventory of personality divisions. Suppose an alter identity emerged to deal with witnessing the murder of one's parents. Does that mean that there was a preexisting personality component of the type specifically suited to dealing with the murder of one's parents? And, if so, must we posit a distinct component waiting in the wings (so to speak) just in case the murder had been to the person's siblings, or in-laws, or next-door neighbors? Even if we say there needs only to be a component to deal with murder of any kind and to any person, does that mean we need to posit a component that could have been dissociated just in case the victims had been tortured instead, and another if they had been kidnapped, and another if they had merely been stalked?

It won't help advocates of a type CR principle to argue that there is (in part) only a small number of psychologically primitive types, and dissociative splits reveal them. Like descriptive categories of any sort, a set of personality or functional types represents one of any number of ways of slicing the psychological pie. There is no privileged (or perspective- or context-independent) inventory of psychological types or divisions into parts, just as there is no single correct or privileged answer to the questions "How many things are in this room?" and "How many events were there in World War II?"

Despite these considerations, some might think that some sort of CR principle *must* be true. Perhaps they would agree with Binet that "what is capable of division must be made up of parts" (1896: 348f). That is, perhaps they still believe that the self cannot be unitary, since if it were, DID and other dissociative phenomena would be impossible. But if they want to avoid the fatal flaws of the token and type CR principles, their only option would seem to be a *noncommittal* CR principle, analogous to the position called "anomalous monism" in the philosophy of mind. They might argue that there are, indeed, predissociative divisions of the self but that they don't correlate with postdissociative divisions. In other words, there would be a non-lawlike correlation between pre- and postdissociative divisions of the self, and we would not be able to infer features of the former from features of the latter.

Of course, this strategy seems thoroughly unenlightening, and if researchers subscribed to it, we might wonder why they would expect dissociation to yield great and *distinctive* insights into the nature of the mind or self. To see this, consider why partisans of a type CR principle regard the functional types of dissociative entities or states to be of theoretical interest. Obviously, we don't need angry or sexually promiscuous alter identities (say) to demonstrate that people have a predissociative capacity for anger or sexual promiscuity. So what reason do we have for focusing on *dissociative* anger and so on? What special fact about the predissociative self could we hope to learn from an angry alter? The answer, presumably, is that an alter of that type would tell us something about how the predissociative self came to be—that is, about the self's processes of organization and formation, or about the historically original components of the predissociative self. If that were not the case, dissociated anger would apparently tell us no more about our underlying mental *structure* than would nondissociative anger.

So advocates of the CR principle seem to hope that dissociative phenomena will illuminate the predissociative divisions of the self that made *those* phenomena possible. They seem to be looking for nontrivial lawlike connections between pre- and postdissociative divisions. But that means they have to decide between the fatally flawed token or type CR principles.

Quite apart from all these details, it should be clear that there was something wrong from the start about the strategy of inferring predissociative divisions of the self from postdissociative divisions. To argue successfully for the predissociative complexity of the self, one must show that it's required to handle *nondissociative* phenomena. Otherwise, one can always maintain plausibly that alter identities, hidden observers, and other dissociative splits are simply products of (rather than prerequisites for) dissociation. That is why some adopt a strategy, similar to Plato's, of inferring parts of the self merely from ordinary (but nondissociative) internal conflicts. Although I believe that strategy is also defective (see Braude 1995 for details), that's clearly a matter for another occasion. For now, we can be satisfied with a modest (but nevertheless important) conclusion: namely, that we seem unable to establish a nonunitary view of the self by appealing exclusively to dissociative phenomena.

NOTE

1. In the study by Ogawa et al. (1997), the assumption is slightly different, but just as questionable and (*mutatis mutandis*) subject to the same criticism. The researchers conducted a longitudinal study with young children at risk for traumatization. According to Nijenhuis, they found that the largest difference was between the clinical dissociative group and the normal group as a whole, which consisted of low- and high-dissociative normal subjects. They argued that if the clinical group were merely the high end of a distribution of dissociation scores, then one would expect that discriminant analyses would differentiate the low-normal group, the largest group, from the two smaller high-dissociation groups (Nijenhuis 1999: 174).

REFERENCES

Beahrs, J. O. (1982) *Unity and Multiplicity: Multilevel Consciousness of Self in Hypnosis, Psychiatric Disorder and Mental Health.* New York: Brunner/Mazel.

Binet, A. (1896) *Alterations of Personality.* New York: D. Appleton.

Boon, S., and Draijer, N. (1993) *Multiple Personality Disorder in the Netherlands.* Amsterdam: Swets and Zeitlinger.

Braude, S. E. (1995) *First Person Plural: Multiple Personality and the Philosophy of Mind,* rev. ed. Lanham, MD: Rowman and Littlefield.

Braun, B. G. (1988) "The BASK (Behavior, Affect, Sensation, Knowledge) Model of Dissociation." *Dissociation* 1(1): 4–23.

Cardeña, E. (1994) "The Domain of Dissociation." In S. J. Lynn and J. W. Rhue (eds.), *Dissociation: Clinical and Theoretical Perspectives.* New York: Guilford Press, pp. 15–31.

Crabtree, A. (1993) *From Mesmer to Freud: Magnetic Sleep and the Roots of Psychological Healing.* New Haven: Yale University Press.

Ellenberger, H. F. (1970) *The Discovery of the Unconscious.* New York: Basic Books.

Graham, G. (2002) "Recent Work in Philosophical Psychopathology." *American Philosophical Quarterly* 39: 109–34.

Hilgard, E. R. (1986) *Divided Consciousness: Multiple Controls in Human Thought and Action,* exp. ed. New York: Wiley-Interscience.

Messerschmidt, R. A. (1927–28) "Quantitative Investigation of the Alleged Independent Operation of Conscious and Subconscious Processes." *Journal of Abnormal and Social Psychology* 22: 325–40.

Myers, F. W. H. (1903) *Human Personality and Its Survival of Bodily Death.* London: Longmans, Green.

Nijenhuis, E. (1999) *Somatoform Dissociation.* Assen: Van Gorcum.

Ogawa, J. R., et al. (1997) "Development and the Fragmented Self: Longitudinal Study of Dissociative Symptomatology in a Nonclinical Sample." *Development and Psychopathology* 9: 855–79.

Putnam, F. W. (1997) *Dissociation in Children and Adolescents: A Developmental Perspective.* New York: Guilford Press.

Radden, J. (1996) *Divided Minds and Successive Selves.* Cambridge, MA: MIT Press.

Ribot, T. (1887) *Diseases of Personality.* New York: Fitzgerald.

Ruk, D. (In press) "Teorija Stephena Braude i Eksperimentalno Ispitvanje Mnogostrukosti Licnosti u Psihologiji [The theory of Stephen Braude and the experimental examination of DID in psychology]." *Pedagoska Stvarnost* [Pedagogic Reality].

Saks, E. R., and Behnke, S. H. (1997) *Jekly on Trial: Multiple Personality Disorder and Criminal Law.* New York: New York University Press.

Waller, N. G., Putnam, F. W., and Carlson, E. B. (1996) "Types of Dissociation and Dissociative Types: A Taxometric Analysis of Dissociative Experiences." *Psychological Methods* 1: 300–21.

Watkins, J. G., and Watkins, H. H. (1979–80) "Ego States and Hidden Observers." *Journal of Altered States of Consciousness* 5: 3–18.

Wilkes, K. V. (1988) *Real People: Personal Identity without Thought Experiments.* Oxford: Oxford University Press.

CHAPTER 8

....

BODY

Disorders of Embodiment

....

SHAUN GALLAGHER

METTE VAEVER

PROPONENTS of nondualistic philosophical theories—whether those in materialist traditions who argue that cognitive processes are identical with or reducible to brain functions, or those in the phenomenological tradition who argue that the experiencing subject is primarily a living body—could claim that in some sense all psychiatric disorders are bodily disorders. Psychiatric symptoms are generated insofar as something goes wrong with the brain or body (or both). This is a statement of objective etiology. In this chapter we are concerned primarily not with etiology but with understanding the structure and dynamics of bodily experiences in disorders where the body is not only the cause of the problem but also the locus or theme of the symptomatology.[1]

Disorders of embodiment in this sense are many and varied. Such disorders are of philosophical interest to the extent that they throw light on issues that concern the mind-body problem, the nature of the self, self-consciousness, action, free will, and our relations with others. In this chapter, while touching on many of these issues, we focus our analysis on how disorders of embodiment can affect the minimal self—the nonconceptual, prereflective sense of self that comes along with being an embodied and conscious being[2]—and its corresponding form of self-awareness, which is a basic and necessary aspect of more sophisticated forms of cognition and action.

To make any advances on these issues, however, one needs to distinguish among the wide variety of such disorders. To do this, we first survey some examples of pathologies in which the body is the primary or exclusive locus or theme of the disorder. We then consider bodily pathologies that appear to be part of or, in some cases, to constitute one of many symptoms of a more comprehensive disorder. To set these various cases in the framework of our analysis, we employ two distinctions that will help clarify the specific nature of individual bodily disorders: the first is a distinction between *body image* and *body schema*; the second is a distinction between *sense of ownership* and *sense of agency*. Both distinctions originate in phenomenological accounts of embodied action, but they also find empirical support in neuropsychological studies and are clearly reinforced in the pathological cases considered here.

PHENOMENOLOGICAL DISTINCTIONS

For our analysis we depend on the following distinction between body image and body schema.[3] A *body image* is constituted by intentional content, which is sometimes conscious (or can, in principle, be made conscious). Specifically, it consists of a system of perceptions, emotional attitudes, and conceptual beliefs that pertain to one's own body. A *body schema* is a close-to-automatic system of processes that constantly regulates posture and movement to serve intentional action. It is a system of sensory-motor capacities and activations that function without the necessity of perceptual monitoring. The difference between body image and body schema is like the difference between a *perception* (or conscious monitoring) of movement and the actual *accomplishment* of movement.

A body image can include mental representations, beliefs, and emotional attitudes where the object of such intentional states is one's own body. Studies that involve body image (e.g., Cash and Brown 1987; Gardner and Moncrieff 1988; Powers et al. 1987) frequently distinguish among three intentional elements:

1. A subject's *perceptual* experience of his/her own body
2. A subject's *conceptual* understanding (including folk and/or scientific knowledge) of the body in general
3. A subject's *emotional* attitude toward his or her own body

Conceptual and emotional aspects of body image are no doubt affected by various cultural and interpersonal factors, but in many respects their content originates in perceptual experience.

In contrast, the body schema involves sensory-motor capacities, abilities, and habits that enable movement and the maintenance of posture. It continues to operate, and in many respects operates best, when the intentional object of perception is something other than one's own body. Of course, a *perceptual awareness* of one's movement (body image) can be complexly interrelated with the *accomplishment* of one's movement, although not all movement requires such body awareness.

Body-schematic processes are not perceptions, beliefs, or feelings, but motor functions—tacit performances that play a dynamic role in governing posture and movement at the subpersonal level. In most instances, movement and the maintenance of posture are accomplished by body-schematic performances that are close to automatic. The normal adult, in order to move around the world, neither needs nor has a constant body percept. Rather, in the self-movement of most intentional activities the body-in-action tends to efface itself and to be experientially absent (see Gallagher 1986; Leder 1990). To the extent that one does become aware of one's own body in terms of monitoring or directing perceptual attention to limb position, movement, posture, pleasure, pain, kinesthetic experience, and so on, then such awareness helps to constitute the perceptual aspect of a body image. Such awareness may interact with body-schematic processes in complex ways, but it is not equivalent to a body schema itself.

Body-schematic control of movement can be precisely shaped by the intentional experience or goal-directed behavior of the subject. That is, although a body schema operates in a *close to automatic* way, its operations are not a matter of mere reflex. Neuropsychological studies show that if I reach for a glass of water with the intention of drinking from it, my hand, completely outside of my awareness, shapes itself in a precise way for picking up the glass. It shapes itself in conformity with my intention. In this sense, although body-schematic control is neither a form of consciousness nor a cognitive operation, it enters into and supports intentional activities.

In some situations, a body image may contribute to the controlled production of movement. The visual, tactile, and proprioceptive attentiveness that I have of my body may help me learn a new dance step, improve my golf swing, or imitate the novel movements of others.[4] In extraordinary pathological cases of deafferentation, where a subject who lacks the sense of touch and proprioception below the neck line may be described as lacking a body schema, control of movement may be gained by the use of a body percept that is strengthened by practiced use of vision and cognitive effort (Cole 1995; Gallagher and Cole 1995). Such cases of neuronopathic deafferentation constitute clear instances for one side of a double dissociation between body schema and body image.[5] The other side can be found in cases of unilateral neglect (discussed later in this chapter).

Before moving further into a discussion of pathological cases, we want to introduce a second conceptual distinction that will be helpful in accounting for different aspects of such cases. This distinction, between a *sense of ownership* (for the body or for action) and a *sense of agency* (for action), cuts across the previous distinction between body image and body schema in complex ways.[6] In the normal phenomenology of intentional action, the sense of agency and the sense of ownership coincide and are indistinguishable. The sense of agency is the prereflective sense that I am the initiator or source of the action. When I reach for a cup, my sense is that I am the one who generates the action. My sense of ownership is the prereflective sense that my body is the one that is moving in the action. Although in the case of intentional action it is difficult to distinguish between these senses, it is quite possible to distinguish them in the case of *involuntary* action. I may experience ownership of a movement—for example, I have a sense that I am the one who is moving or is being moved—but I may not have a sense of causing or controlling the movement—that is, no sense of agency. The agent of the movement is someone else who is pushing me from behind or who is manipulating my arm. It is also the case, as we will see, that in some pathologies of embodiment the sense of ownership is disrupted, while in others the sense of agency fails.

The sense of ownership and sense of agency are two aspects of prereflective self-awareness that help define the minimal self. A minimal self can be defined in contrast to a self that is extended beyond the short-term or "specious" present to include past thoughts and actions. It is the basic, current subject of experience, even if we strip away episodic or autobiographical memory (as in amnesia) or long-term sense for the future.[7] Although identity over time is a major issue in the philosophical definition of personal identity, the concept of the minimal self involves a more basic differentiation between self and nonself and is limited to that which is accessible to immediate and present self-consciousness.

Many disorders of embodiment disrupt the primary aspects of self-awareness that help constitute the minimal self. Specifically, some disorders of the body image involve varying degrees of problems with the sense of ownership; problems with the sense of agency always involve some aspect of the body schema. There are also complex hybrid disorders that can be defined in these terms. A study of these various disorders contributes to our philosophical understanding of how the minimal self is structured.

PATHOLOGIES THAT ARE PRIMARILY DISORDERS OF EMBODIMENT

We noted that in many situations when someone is engaged in world-directed activity, the body-in-action remains in large degree experientially absent. Implicit in this experiential absence, however, is a sense of ownership—a prereflective sense that it is my body that is engaged in activity. One may come to notice this experiential absence in a negative way, when the body suddenly appears inadequate to the task or as fatigued or ill, or when some other event calls one's attention to one's body—for example, if someone stares at you when you are engaged in some activity. In such cases, one may become aware that one's body has been functioning all along, beneath the threshold of explicit awareness. Of course, there are more positive ways in which one may become conscious of one's body—through self-inspection, by looking in the mirror, or in sexual arousal, for example. In such positive or negative cases, a subject experiences normal perceptual aspects of the body image, including a more explicit sense that the body in question is one's own.

In some psychiatric cases, a patient may suffer the loss of the experiential absence of the body-in-action in a way that results in some alteration in the sense of ownership. The body may be felt as something present but more like an alien object than like the experiencing subject. For example, in depersonalization disorder, patients may report that they feel detached from their body. In the Cotard delusion, subjects claim that they have died and that their body is decomposing. In such cases, however, the patients make it clear that it is their own body that is at stake — the sense of ownership is still intact, even if altered. These kinds of experiential disembodiments may be due to disturbances in affect, where partial or entire networks of affective processing may be destroyed (Gerrans 1999). As a result, with the loss of normal affect, the subject ceases to feel connected with her own body and comes to regard it as one object among others. This abnormal presence of the body is a curious form of *objective* self-consciousness. It alters a normal sense of ownership for the nonobjective body, a minimal self-awareness that forms an important element of the body image.

Disorders in the affective aspect of the body image can also account for pathologies like anorexia nervosa. Although there is general agreement that anorexia involves distortions of the body image, there is some debate about whether the distortions are affective or perceptual in nature. Some studies document perceptual distortions, while others find none (see, e.g., recent studies by Fernández-Aranda et al. 1999; Uys and Wassenaar 1996); some find neurological evidence for affective problems, while others focus exclusively on questions about body percept (see, e.g., Hennighausen et al. 1999; Seeger et al. in press). The lack of consensus in this type of debate points in a different and more productive direction: namely, toward a holistic view.

As recent studies in neuroscience suggest, one should avoid the Cartesian view of affect as something that operates independent of cognitive function (e.g., Damasio 1994). Disruptions in affect likely involve disruptions in perceptual and cognitive/conceptual dimensions, and vice versa. Indeed, a number of theorists, acknowledging anorexia as a "multidimensional disorder,"[8] approach the explanation of anorexia through an analysis of cultural and socially determined ideals of acceptable body shape. Susan Bordo (1993), for example, outlines three axes of culture that are expressed in anorexia. The *dualist axis* represents a Western conceptual tradition that reaches from Plato through Christianity to Descartes and beyond, and which conceptualizes the body as alien (the nonself), a limitation to be overcome, and vicious. The *control axis* expresses itself in the anorectic as her struggle to gain control over her life, a life over which, in most aspects, she has no control. By controlling her body, the anorectic gains a feeling of accomplishment she finds no place else. The *gender/power axis* reflects the cultural emphasis on slender and sexual bodies. These images and concepts of what constitutes an acceptable body are easily the source for large-scale dissatisfaction with one's body.

A holistic view, then, recognizes that all aspects of the body image—perceptual, affective, conceptual, social—are mutually implicated in disorders like anorexia. In regard to a sense of ownership, anorexia remains ambiguous. Like disorders that involve degrees of disembodied experience (depersonalization, the Cotard delusion), anorexia manifests itself as an ambiguous presence of the body as object. In some respects (on Bordo's dualist axis), the body appears as something alien; in other respects (on Bordo's control axis), a controlling ownership is apparent: it is something that can be brought under control and made to conform to a certain culturally determined concept.

In the disorders discussed so far, the feeling of alienation from the body does not advance to the point where the subject fails to acknowledge it as his or her own body. Some sense of ownership for the body is still in place. Other disorders involve more radical disruptions of the body image in which there is neither a sense of presence nor a sense of experiential absence that includes the normally tacit sense of ownership. After an injury of the right parietal cortex (often the result of stroke), for example, the left side of the body can literally disappear from the body image—a condition referred to as personal or unilateral neglect, a form of asomatognosia (see, e.g., Vallar et al. 1993). In some cases, there are complications from paralysis or anosognosia (denial of the condition). In unilateral neglect, patients fail to acknowledge one side of their body or simply ignore it (for instance, they fail to shave or dress that side). In such cases, subjects have no body image for the neglected side and may fail to register it perceptually, affectively, or even conceptually. Accordingly, they have no sense of ownership for that neglected side. In some cases, in fact, the body appears to the patient to belong to someone else. Patients often misidentify their arm or leg. They famously complain that there is a strange leg in their bed, or that they can't understand whose hand it is that is lying next to them.[9] In most cases, however, they pay no attention to that side of their body, and it seems not to belong to their embodied self-image.

Despite problems with the body image, there are reports of unilateral neglect cases in which the body schema seems clearly intact (Denny-Brown et al. 1952). Patients will use the neglected side of their body to dress, eat, or walk; their motor abilities for the neglected side remain operational and controlled. Precisely such cases, in a complementary way to cases of deafferentation mentioned earlier, provide evidence for the other side of the double dissociation of body image and body schema (Gallagher and Cole 1995).

A different sort of disruption of the minimal self can be caused by lesions that result in what is usually called Alien Hand Syndrome (AHS). AHS is often described as a clinical disorder in which the patient's hand performs actions that are beyond the patient's control. The actions can appear purposeful, although the patient claims the actions are involuntary. In addition, the involuntary movements may be accompanied by feelings of foreignness and sometimes the personification of the affected limb. Thus, Tow and Chua (1998) note that AHS includes "a feeling that the hand is foreign together with autonomous activity, as if the hand is driven by an external agent." Accordingly, Marchetti and Della Sala (1998) have made an important distinction between "Alien Hand Syndrome" and "Anarchic Hand Syndrome." Involuntary action of the hand, or "anarchic hand," involves a disruption in the sense of agency, although the subject may still acknowledge that it is his hand that is performing the action. Della Sala (2000) recounts that a patient at dinner, to her dismay, observed *her* left hand taking some leftover fishbones and putting them into her mouth. Another patient complained that *her* hand did what it wanted to do; she tried to control its autonomous behavior by hitting it violently or by shouting at it. In contrast, the *alien* hand involves a disruption in the sense of ownership for the bodypart—a form of asomatognosia—it may or may not engage in anarchic behavior.[10]

It is important to note that in Anarchic Hand Syndrome, patients do not have a delusion that someone else is *actually* performing the action; rather, it is *"as if"* someone else were controlling their own arm or simply that there is something wrong with their arm (Frith and Gallagher 2002; Gallagher and Marcel 1999; see reports in Tow and Chua 1998; Della Sala 2000).

AHS is sometimes associated with the split brain; it often involves lesions to the corpus callosum.[11] Accordingly, it could be taken to support the radical notion of self-dissociation sometimes proposed in relation to split-brain behavior. On the basis of such studies, it is sometimes proposed that there are two independent consciousnesses or personalities, one in each hemisphere. They are normally and pragmatically integrated into one self via the corpus callosum. Lesioning the corpus callosum allows a less dominant self to emerge on its own, and this results in AHS in some cases, as well as unusual performance on experimental tests. The interpretation of AHS in terms of the distinction between sense of ownership and sense of agency, however, offers a more conservative interpretation in regard to the minimal self. Specifically, rather than positing two relatively independent centers of self-consciousness, these pathologies involve a disruption of the minimal self in two conceptually precise ways. Either the sense of ownership is disrupted, producing Alien Hand Syndrome, or the sense of agency is disrupted, producing Anarchic Hand Syndrome. Neither of these conditions produces a second self that would take the perspective of the uncontrolled hand.

Problems with Embodiment in More Comprehensive Disorders

The examples discussed so far have been pathologies of embodiment in which the body has been the primary or exclusive locus or theme of the disorder. Schizophrenia, and conditions within the schizophrenia spectrum, represent a much more comprehensive and hybrid disorder in which problems of the minimal self and prereflective self-awareness are reflected in complex, often paradoxical, and intimately interrelated ways. Here we wish to focus on the structure and dynamics of the bodily experiences in the symptoms and pathologies of schizophrenia.

As with the disorders of anorexia, depersonalization, and the Cotard delusion, in schizophrenia there is also a *pathological experiential presence* of the body in what would otherwise be ordinary activities. In the disorders of the schizophrenia spectrum, it is sometimes the case that the normally tacit aspects of automatic body-schematic processes are transformed into explicit aspects. In some cases, a disruption in processes of action preparation (corresponding to neurological problems in the generation of motor commands and efference copy) may disrupt the sense of agency for such action and motivate a hyperreflexive focus on precisely these tacit aspects.[12] This, in turn, may lead to delusional interpretations of control—for example, attributions of the action to some other person.[13]

We noted earlier that when one moves around in the world, body-schematic functions are tacitly performed, and the body-in-action tends to efface itself. Only in special circumstances do we become conscious of these tacit performances of the body: for instance, when learning a new skill, like driving a car. In the beginning, the "driving-skills" are not lived performances; they do not work in an automatic way, and in some cases we may even describe it as "The car is driving me." Our sense of agency is not as sure as it ordinarily is. Overly attending to our bodily movements makes them seem almost mechanical, and in some way external. At such times, the advice given by experienced drivers, "Don't think about it, just do it," is impossible to follow. This sense of being unskilled, of "being outside the performance," makes one feel uneasy. Through practice, however, one begins to feel the car like an "extended body," part of our tacitly lived embodied performances, and we drive in virtually an automatic way. The sense of agency is built into such proficient action.

In conditions within the schizophrenia spectrum, the tacit aspects of bodily movement and bodily function become explicit for the experiencing subject. Instead of simply driving, walking, or breathing, for example, patients may start to think about the specific details of how they drive, walk, or breathe. They experience and verbalize the body-schematic processes that are normally tacit and automatic in everyday activity. For example,[14] a young male patient diagnosed with schizophrenia describes how he has to think about how to breathe; another reports that he has to think about how to walk, how to move his legs, how fast to walk, whether he should stick to the right or the left on the sidewalk, whether to look up or down when walking.

It seems that in these individuals, the normally tacit aspects of bodily movement are in some way disrupted; the subject no longer takes his bodily functions for granted and he is in a way detached from his own lived performances. The bodily functions are no longer lived but become mechanical, indirect, and reflected upon. In a case described by Parnas (2000), the patient, Robert, explains that when listening to music, he is somehow "internally watching" his own receptivity to the music, observing his own mind receiving or registering the musical tones. Robert in a way is witnessing his own sensory processes instead of living them; he is hyperreflexively experiencing his own experiencing.

The term "reflexive" refers to situations or processes whereby an agent or a self takes herself or some aspect of herself as her own object of awareness. Sass (1998, 2000) has termed the exaggerated way in which this occurs in schizophrenia "hyper-reflexivity." He argues that when these normally tacit dimensions of embodied activity become explicit, they can no longer perform the grounding, orienting, and consti-tuting functions that only processes that remain in the background can play.

In schizophrenia, the hyperreflexivity that objectifies and alienates the body may be manifested as a disruption in the sense of agency or in the sense of ownership. In the Bonn Scale for the Assessment of Basic Symptoms within the spectrum of schizophrenia (BSABS; Gross et al. 1987, Danish version 1995), a patient is cited as saying: "Sometimes I can't sense my own body. The sense of having a body ... normally one does sense one's body." Another patient says: "I simply don't have any body sensation anymore, no feeling of the body still belonging to me. I sense that I'm sitting here, but it is an alien feeling." Here we see a disruption in the sense of ownership because of the hyperreflective objectification of the body, in which the body seems to become an absolute object, losing its lived aspect in the process.

In delusions of control, as in the psychotic experience of thought insertion, schi-zophrenics experience a loss in the sense of agency for actions, although no loss in the sense of ownership (Gallagher 2000; Graham and Stephens 1994). Thus, patients report that their own body is moving, but not under their control: "I want to go to the room, but go away from it. I'm simply not sure where my legs are going" (BSABS 1995). Or, "When I reach for the comb it is my hand and arm which move ..., but I don't control them. I sit watching them move and they are quite independent, what they do is nothing to do with me" (Mellor 1970: 18). Disruptions like these in the sense of self-agency may lead to delusional interpretations of who is controlling the action. In contrast to the experiences of those with Anarchic Hand Syndrome, schi-zophrenics experience the loss in the sense of agency not simply "as if" someone else were moving their body but literally as if someone or something were making them move, a patient reports, for example: "The force moved my lips. I began to speak. The words were made for me" (Frith 1992: 66).

Disruptions in the basic structures that constitute the minimal self, and the grounding function of tacit experience, is often described by the schizophrenic sub-ject as a feeling of loss of touch with the world, a detachment from the world. A young female patient stated: "There is a wall all the way around me, I can see the objects, but I can't take the objects in." This detachment can be manifest not just in relation to the material world of objects but also as a distance involving intersubjective relations. The same woman reports:

> I don't know how to say things, and I always think double: What does the
>   other person think, when I say this?
> I am different from everybody, I feel wrong and I am not a part of it.
> I don't say the right things, I am acting, it is a play, and I try so hard that I fall
>   over.

I am not interested in other people, and I can't put myself in their place, it
    makes me a bad person.
I live in my head a lot, I drift away, thoughts come up, and I think of them, I
    am not listening, I just say yes and no.

This suggests that pathologies that disrupt embodied aspects of the minimal self may
have an effect on our experiences of others. This may have important relevance for
understanding autism, as well as schizophrenia. Autism is often regarded as a developmental disorder that affects a person's theory of mind — that is, the person's ability
to understand and to relate to others. Although this is often analyzed in a mentalistic
framework, in which capacities for understanding others are portrayed as capacities
for understanding the beliefs and intentions contained in the other person's mind, a
less mentalistic and more embodied approach may be justified.

There is good evidence that a subject's understanding of another person's actions
and intentions depends to some extent on a mirrored reverberation in the subject's
own motor system. When I observe someone else performing a certain action, or
imagine myself doing that action, the neuronal patterns that are activated in my
premotor cortex, SMA, and other brain areas are in large part the same neuronal
patterns that are activated when I perform action myself.[15] The neurology of intersubjective perception, then, suggests that problems with our own motor or body-
schematic system could significantly interfere with our capacities for understanding
others. It has been demonstrated that just such problems exist in autistic children
between ages 3 and 10 (see Damasio and Maurer 1978; Vilensky et al. 1981) and even
before that, in infants who are later diagnosed as autistic. Teitelbaum et al. (1998)
studied videos of infants who were diagnosed as autistic around age 3. Movement
disturbances were observed in all of the infants as early as age 4–6 months, and in
some from birth. These include problems in lying, righting, sitting, crawling, and
walking, as well as abnormal mouth shapes. They involve delayed development, as
well as abnormal motor patterns, for example, asymmetries or unusual sequencing
in crawling and walking.[16] Accordingly, following the logic of motor reverberation in
intersubjective perception, we should not be surprised to find that developmental
problems involving body-schematic functions, and therefore possible disruptions in
the development of the minimal self, may have an effect on the autistic child's ability
to understand the actions and intentions of others.

CONCLUSION

We reviewed a number of pathologies that involve disorders in which the body is the
primary or exclusive locus or theme of the disorder. These include depersonalization,
the Cotard delusion, anorexia nervosa, unilateral neglect, deafferentation, Alien Hand

Syndrome, and Anarchic Hand Syndrome. Each of these disorders involves problems with body image or body schema (or both), and in many cases such problems affect aspects of the embodied minimal self—specifically, the sense of ownership or the sense of agency for action. We also considered bodily pathologies that appear to be part of or, in some cases, to constitute one of many symptoms of more comprehensive disorders such as schizophrenia and autism. In this context, we suggested that some disorders of embodiment that affect the minimal self can also have important effects on intersubjective experience and likely need to be taken into account in working out any adequate explanation of such illnesses.

NOTES

1. Within the scope of this chapter it is not possible to discuss all such disorders. Disorders that we do not discuss, such as conversion hysteria, somataform disorder, and gender dysphoric disorder, deserve further analysis.

2. A cognitive version of the minimal self is suggested by Strawson (1997); a more embodied version is proposed in Damasio's (2000) notion of a "core" self.

3. Current usage of the terms *body image* and *body schema* in the psychological and medical literatures is relatively confused. For a review, and for arguments in favor of a conceptual distinction, see Gallagher (1995, 2001).

4. Various experiments show that visual awareness of one's own body can correct body-schematic functions (Gurfinkel and Levick 1991). For example, visual perception of the wrist, elbow, or shoulder can recalibrate motor performance that has been distorted by the effects of prismatic goggles (Paillard 1991). Focused attention, or the lack of it, on specific parts of the body may alter postural or motor performance (e.g., Fisher 1970; Winer 1975).

5. In psychology, a double dissociation is a good way to show that two things are actually distinct. If there is a real distinction between X and Y, then to identify one kind of case where there is X but not Y, and another kind of case where there is Y but not X, constitutes good evidence for that distinction.

6. The distinction between sense of ownership and sense of agency correlates phenomenologically with the distinction made by Graham and Stephens (1994) between "attributions of subjectivity" and "attributions of agency." Graham and Stephens explain these attributions, however, as the product of an introspective inference. In contrast, we understand the senses of agency and ownership to be experiential aspects, prereflectively implicit in action. They are generated in the subpersonal processes of the body schema, and specifically in the pre-action (forward) processes of motor preparation and the sensory feedback that results from the action (see Gallagher 2000).

7. The notion of a minimal self is developed by a number of authors; see, for example, Strawson (1997); Gallagher (2000). Damasio (2000) calls it the "core self." It is closely related to what Neisser (1988) calls the "ecological self." Evidence that it exists from birth can be found in developmental studies (see, e.g., Gallagher and Meltzoff 1996).

8. Garfinkel and Garner, cited in Bordo (1993: 140)

9. There are many reports like this. Some are more complicated than others. Feinberg (2001) reports on one patient, a 64-year-old construction worker with a right-hemisphere stroke, paralysis of his left arm, and anosognosia. Although he was told that he was in hospi-

tal, the patient insisted he was at his job site. He claimed that his mother-in-law was actually in the hospital and had had a stroke. When Feinberg lifted the patient's paralyzed left arm and asked what it was, the patient replied: "My mother-in-law's hand. Someone's hand."

10. Indeed, this was the original definition of AHS, and the test for it was "failure to identify an upper limb as one's own on palpating it behind the back or with the eyes closed" (Fisher 2000). In many cases, anarchic hand and alien hand occur together in complex ways (see, e.g., Inzelberg et al. 2000).

11. At the neurological level one can distinguish between frontal AHS and collasal AHS. Frontal AHS involves lesions in the supplementary motor area (SMA), a region that is often associated with volition. Thus, in some respects, frontal AHS can be associated with Anarchic Hand Syndrome, involving a disruption of the *sense of agency* for movement. *Callosal AHS*, in contrast, involves lesions to the corpus callosum. But here one needs to distinguish the specific area of the corpus callosum involved. Lesions in the anterior callosum may accompany damage to the SMA; lesions to the posterior callosum may accompany damage to the parietal cortex. The latter may account for the asomatognosia of alien hand experience. One should be cautious about defining correlations between the neurological distinction (frontal vs. collasal) and the clinical distinction (anarchic vs. alien), however; see Marchetti and Della Sala 1998).

12. We say "motivate" in order to avoid any claim for causality, both in relation to the disorder of schizophrenia itself and in relation to the development of the schizophrenic symptoms. One can experimentally disrupt the sense of agency, but that will not necessarily cause a schizophrenic interpretation in nonschizophrenic subjects, although it tends to do so in schizophrenics. We do not here discuss whether the hyperreflexivity (discussed later) is to be considered compensatory, consequential, or more basic.

13. Part of the explanation for delusions of control must be found on the subpersonal, neurological level (for example, see the work of Frith 1992; Frith and Done 1988; Frith et al. 2000); another important part of any successful explanation will involve phenomenological and personal-level accounts (see Gallagher 2000; Graham and Stephens 1994; Parnas 2000; and Sass 1998, 2000).

14. When no other reference is made, the examples stem from clinical research done at the Psychiatric Department, Hvidovre Hospital, Denmark, under the direction of Josef Parnas.

15. See Grezes and Decety (2001); Blakemore and Decety (2001). Positron emission tomography (PET) and functional magnetic resonance imaging (fMRI) studies show significant overlap among action observation, execution, and simulation in the supplementary motor area (SMA), the dorsal premotor cortex, the supramarginal gyrus, and the superior parietal lobe. Grezes and Decety suggest that other nonoverlapping areas may be responsible for distinguishing our own agency from the agency of others (also see Ruby and Decety 2001).

16. One of the authors (M.V.) is involved in an ongoing long-term study that promises to clarify similar developmental phenomena in schizophrenia. In the Copenhagen Infant Follow-up Study (CIFS), investigators (Parnas, Lier, Gammeltoft, and Vaever) are analyzing videotapes of motor patterns and conducting other neurodevelopmental assessment (Griffith's Scale) of 50 high-risk children of schizophrenic parents. The children were videotaped at regular intervals from the age of 6 months to 3 years. Assessments of attention, social referencing, and attachment were performed at appropriate ages. These children, now 11–13 years old, are currently being reassessed with a variety of psychopathological, behavioral, and neurocognitive measures.

REFERENCES

Blakemore, S-J., and Decety, J. (2001) "From the Perception of Action to the Understanding of Intention." *Nature Reviews: Neuroscience* 2: 561–67.

Bordo, S. (1993) *Unbearable Weight: Feminism, Western Culture, and the Body.* Berkeley: University of California Press.

Cash, T. F., and Brown, T. A. (1987) "Body Image in Anorexia Nervosa and Bulimia Nervosa: A Review of the Literature." *Behavior Modification* 11: 487–521.

Cole, J. D. (1995) *Pride and a Daily Marathon.* Cambridge, MA: MIT Press; originally London: Duckworth, 1991.

Damasio, A. (1999) *The Feeling of What Happens: Body and Emotion in the Making of Consciousness.* New York: Harcourt Brace.

Damasio, A. (1994) *Descartes' Error: Emotion, Reason, and the Human Brain.* New York: G. P. Putnam.

Damasio, A. R., and Maurer, R. G. (1978) "A Neurological Model for Childhood Autism." *Archives of Neurology* 35: 777–86.

Della Sala, S. (2000) "Anarchic Hand: The Syndrome of Disowned Actions." *Creating Sparks: The BA Festival of Science.* Available at www.creatingsparks.co.uk.

Denny-Brown, D., Meyer, J. S., and Horenstein, S. (1952) "The Significance of Perceptual Rivalry Resulting from Parietal Lesion." *Brain* 75: 433–471.

Feinberg, T. E. (2001) *Altered Egos: How the Brain Creates the Self.* Oxford: Oxford University Press.

Fernández-Aranda, F., Dahme, B., and Meermann, R. (1999) "Body Image in Eating Disorders and Analysis of Its Relevance." *Journal of Psychosomatic Research* 47(5): 419–28.

Fisher, C. M. (2000) "Alien Hand Phenomena: A Review with the Addition of Six Personal Cases." *Canadian Journal of Neurological Sciences* 27: 192–203.

Fisher, S. (1970) *Body Experience in Fantasy and Behavior.* New York: Appleton-Century-Crofts.

Frith, C. D. (1992) *The Cognitive Neuropsychology of Schizophrenia.* Hillsdale, NJ: Lawrence Erlbaum Associates.

Frith, C. D., and Done, D. J. (1988) "Towards a Neuropsychology of Schizophrenia." *British Journal of Psychiatry* 15: 437–43.

Frith, C., and Gallagher, S. (2002) "Models of the Pathological Mind." *Journal of Consciousness Studies* 9(4): 57–80.

Frith, C. D., Blakemore, S-J., and Wolpert, D. (2000) "Explaining the Symptoms of Schizophrenia: Abnormalities in the Awareness of Action." *Brain Research Reviews* 31: 357–63.

Gallagher, S. (2001) "Dimensions of Embodiment: Body Image and Body Schema in Medical Contexts." In S. K. Toombs (ed.), *Handbook of Phenomenology and Medicine.* Dordrecht: Kluwer Academic Publishers, pp. 147–75.

Gallagher, S. (2000) "Self-reference and Schizophrenia: A Cognitive Model of Immunity to Error through Misidentification." In D. Zahavi (ed.), *Exploring the Self: Philosophical and Psychopathological Perspectives on Self-experience.* Amsterdam: John Benjamins, pp. 203–39.

Gallagher, S. (1995) "Body Schema and Intentionality." In J. Bermúdez, N. Eilan, and a. J. Marcel (eds.), *The Body and the Self.* Cambridge, MA: MIT Press, 225–44.

Gallagher, S. (1986) "Body Image and Body Schema: A Conceptual Clarification." *Journal of Mind and Behavior* 7: 541–54.

Gallagher, S., and Cole, J. (1995) "Body Schema and Body Image in a Deafferented Subject." *Journal of Mind and Behavior* 16: 369–90.

Gallagher, S., and Marcel, A. J. (1999) "The Self in Contextualized Action." *Journal of Consciousness Studies* 6(4): 4–30.

Gallagher, S., and Meltzoff, A. (1996) "The Earliest Sense of Self and Others: Merleau-Ponty and Recent Developmental Studies." *Philosophical Psychology* 9: 213–36.

Gardner, R. M., and Moncrieff, C. (1988) "Body Image Distortion in Anorexics As a Nonsensory Phenomenon: A Signal Detection Approach." *Journal of Clinical Psychology* 44: 101–7.

Gerrans, P. (1999) "Delusional Misidentification As Subpersonal Disintegration." *Monist* 82(4): 590–608.

Graham, G., and Stephens, G. L. (1994) "Mind and Mine." In G. Graham and G. L. Stephens (eds.), *Philosophical Psychopathology*. Cambridge, MA: MIT Press, pp. 91–109.

Grezes, J., and Decety, J. (2001) "Functional Anatomy of Execution, Mental Simulation, Observation, and Verb Generation of Actions: A Meta-analysis." *Human Brain Mapping* 12: 1–19.

Gross, G., Huber, G., Klosterkötter, J., and Linz, M. (1987) *Bonner Skala für die Beurteilung von Basissymptomen (BSABS: Bonn Scale for the Assessment of Basic Symptoms)*. Berlin: Springer Verlag.

Gurfinkel, V. S., and Levick, Y. S. (1991) "Perceptual and Automatic Aspects of the Postural Body Scheme." In J. Paillard (ed.), *Brain and Space*. Oxford: Oxford University Press, pp. 147–162.

Hennighausen, K., Enkelmann, D., Wewetzer, C., and Remschmidt, H. (1999) "Body Image Distortion in Anorexia Nervosa: Is There Really a Perceptual Deficit?" *European Child and Adolescent Psychiatry* 8: 200–6.

Inzelberg, R. et al. (2000) "Alien Hand Sign in creutzfeldt-Jakob Disease." *Journal of Neurology, Neurosurgery and Psychiatry* 68: 103–4.

Leder, D. (1990) *The Absent Body*. Chicago: University of Chicago Press.

Marchetti, C., and Della Sala, S. (1998) "Disentangling the Alien and Anarchic Hand." *Cognitive Neuropsychiatry* 3(3): 191–207

Mellor, C. S. (1970) "First Rank Symptoms of Schizophrenia." *British Journal of Psychiatry* 117: 15–23.

Neisser, U. (1988) "Five Kinds of Self-knowledge." *Philosophical Psychology* 1: 35–59.

Paillard, J. (1991) "Knowing Where and Knowing How to Get There." In J. Paillard (ed.), *Brain and Space*. Oxford: Oxford University Press, pp. 461–81.

Parnas, J. (2000) "The Self and Intentionality in the Pre-Psychotic Stages of Schizophrenia." In D. Zahavi (ed.), *Exploring the Self*. Amsterdam: John Benjamins, pp. 115–47.

Powers, P. S., Schulman, R. G., Gleghorn, A. A., and Prange, M. E. (1987) "Perceptual and Cognitive Abnormalities in Bulimia." *American Journal of Psychiatry* 144: 1456–60.

Ruby, P., and Decety, J. (2001) "Effect of Subjective Perspective Taking during Simulation of Action: A PET Investigation of Agency." *Nature Neuroscience* 4(5): 546–50.

Sass, L. (2000) "Schizophrenia, Self-experience, and the So-Called Negative Symptoms." In D. Zahavi (ed.), *Exploring the Self*. Amsterdam: John Benjamins, pp. 149–82.

Sass, L. (1998) "Schizophrenia, Self-consciousness and the Modern Mind." *Journal of Consciousness Studies* 5: 543–65.

Seeger, G., Braus, D. F., Ruf, M., Goldberger, U., and Schmidt, M. H. (2002) "Body Image Distortion Reveals Amygdala Activation in Patients with Anorexia Nervosa: A Functional Magnetic Resonance Imaging Study." *Neuroscience Letters* 326(1): 25–28.

Strawson, G. (1997) "The Self." *Journal of Consciousness Studies* 4(5/6): 405–28.

Teitelbaum, P. Teitelbaum, O., Nye, J., Fryman, J., and Maurer, R. G. (1998) "Movement Analysis in Infancy May Be Useful for Early Diagnosis of Autism." *Proceedings of the National Academy of Sciences* 95: 13982–87.

Tow, A. M., and Chua, H. C. (1998) "The Alien Hand Sign: Case Report and Review of the Literature." *Annals Academy of Medicine Singapore* 27(4): 582–85.

Uys, D. C., and Wassenaar, D. R. (1996) "The Perceptual and Affective Components of Body Image Disturbances in Anorexic and Normal Females." *South African Journal of Psychology* 26(4): 236–42.

Vallar, G., Antonucci, G., Guariglia, C., and Pizzamiglio, L. (1993) "Deficits of Position Sense, Unilateral Neglect and Optokinetic Stimulation." *Neuropsychologia* 31: 1191–1200.

Vilensky, J. A., Damasio, A. R., and Maurer, R. G. (1981) "Disturbances of Motility in Patients with Autistic Behavior: A Preliminary Analysis." *Archives of Neurology* 38: 646–49.

Winer, G. A. (1975) "Children's Preference for Body or External Object on a Task Requiring Transposition and Discrimination of Right-Left Relations." *Perceptual and Motor Skills* 41: 291–98.

CHAPTER 9

IDENTITY

Personal Identity, Characterization Identity, and Mental Disorder

JENNIFER RADDEN

THE expression "personal identity" refers to the customary unity and integration we expect of lived experience and personality. In a long philosophical tradition, strict numerical identity was attributed to all persons. More recent theorizing has accepted a merely relative continuity and allowed that identity admits of degree; it has challenged the metaphysical status of traditional accounts, as well as the standpoint from which they are established, and, with the advent of postmodernism, has denied any unity or coherence to the self whatsoever, regarding conceptions of self-identity as a product of Western modernity.

Mental disorder inevitably challenges traditional ideas about personal identity since, as the notion of disorder suggests, it can profoundly alter and transform its sufferer, disrupting the smooth continuity uniting earlier and later parts of subjectivity and, viewed from the outside, of persons and lives. Episodes of mental disorder expunge and distort memories and change cognitive function, beliefs, and values; they alter capabilities, personality, mood, emotional style, and response. They disrupt normal psychological functioning of all kinds and interrupt lives in ways that are often devastatingly far reaching. (Distinguished by their unchanging nature, trait-based personality disorders are exempt from some forms of disruption and alteration; nonetheless, conditions such as borderline personality disorder and dissociative identity disorder are marked by patterns of disrupted agency and subjectivity.) Mental disorder is not alone in bringing such transformations. But while religious and ideological conversion, societal upheaval, and some injury and illness can have similar effects, the changes wrought by mental disorder are perhaps distinguished by their almost unfailingly unexpected, unbidden, and unwelcome nature.

Some psychopathology has drawn the particular attention of philosophers by the extreme and recurrent nature of the diachronic discontinuities and synchronic disunities it exhibits, and the present discussion is focused on those conditions. A secondary but significant element of personal change that often comes with mental disorder results from therapeutic intervention. Issues of personal identity are also raised when, for therapeutic or more superficial and "cosmetic" ends, a person's disposition, capabilities, moods, and behavioral responses are affected by, for example, psychopharmacological agents (Kramer 1993).

These conceptions of personal identity are closely bound to other metaphysical categories and concepts such as agency, autonomy, personhood, and responsibility. The unity and coherence attributed to and constitutive of persons, it has traditionally been asserted, is what renders persons the rightful subjects of praise, blame, reproach, and similar reactive attitudes. This link with other moral and metaphysical concepts means that the challenges to personal identity inherent in mental disorder provide some guide to mental health ethics, to the practical and policy issues concerning the treatment of the mentally ill, and to the moral and legal status of actions undertaken by, and on behalf of, them. Two of these have prompted extensive philosophical analysis and are discussed here. One is the ascription of moral (and legal) responsibility for crimes carried out as the result of or during an episode of mental disorder, particularly when, in the most extreme case, the person apparently houses multiple selves or alters and stands accused as one of these for the deed of another. A second ethical context is the one in which advance-care directives are issued by a person anticipating the changes wrought by an episode of mental disorder.

Personal identity theories involve reidentification of persons through time: what metaphysical posits or persisting traits provide grounds for the judgment the same person endures between T^1 and T^{2-n}. Another sense of the identity of persons, which also has bearing on mental disorder, involves the traits that comprise personality and, more particularly, the self-concept. This is distinguished as characterization identity.

In what follows, theories of personal identity are introduced and some of their ethical and normative consequences are examined in relation to two particular disorders, dissociative identity disorder and manic depression. In addition, theories of characterization identity and their relevance to psychopathology and therapeutic goals in psychiatry are briefly introduced.

PERSONAL IDENTITY AND MENTAL DISORDER

Theories of personal identity vary greatly, and the discontinuities and disunities of self or person so striking in mental disorder are more easily accommodated by some than others of these accounts (Radden 1995, 1996). If bodily continuity is not merely necessary but sufficient for personal identity, for example, no particular significance will be found in the disruptions wrought by mental disorder (see Williams 1973).

Nor will such disruptions affect a postmodernist rejection of any unified and coherent self, although the very presence of clinical cases of multiplicity in dissociative identity disorder and schizophrenia has been used to challenge as naive and conceptually incoherent the postmodernist valorizing of the fragmented self (Glass 1993). If multiple personality disorder and schizophrenia are extreme forms of what the postmodernists idealize, as Glass puts it, then "there is something terribly wrong in the postmodernist interpretation of what multiplicity or fragmentation of self means"; postmodern theory is cavalier about precisely that aspect of the self that enables it to organize, metabolize, and internalize the plurality of "becoming," yet, without that capacity, the self finds itself "overwhelmed by its various manifestations, its multiplicity" (Glass 1993: 8–9). (Similarly, it has been argued that [normal] diversity must be distinguished from [pathological] multiplicity; see Mullin 1995.)

The normal person in everyday contexts exhibits several kinds of continuity through time. As well as the continuation of the body through its spatiotemporal path, there is also continuity of enduring psychological states and dispositions, memory, the stream of consciousness, and persisting capabilities and skills. This continuity comports well with the traditional notion of a perfect numerical identity provided by a transcendental self or subject. In posing a challenge to customary notions of personal identity, psychopathology has not provided a refutation of traditional accounts. But it has forced those accounts to reveal the weight they place on such unobservable, metaphysical entities as transcendental selves.

Theories that replace this traditional conception with one of relative psychological continuity and connectedness derive from Hume. Such accounts argue that one or several of the relatively enduring, empirically observable sources of continuity ground our judgment that the same self or person persists through time. Emphasis has been placed on the causal connections linking the chains of empirical continuity (Shoemaker 1979; Parfit 1984). Theories such as Parfit's have as a consequence that the continuity or "survival" (which, on this account, has replaced the alleged identity in traditional accounts) admits of degree. In this respect they provide a way to at least describe the apparently fractured identities, selves, or lives found among the mentally disordered and to acknowledge that such discontinuities are possible. Parfit's account allows us not only to assign varying degrees of survival between earlier and later self slices (or selves), and thus between normal and pathological experiences and lives, but also to employ a survival threshold such that the same body might house more than one self. Thus, it provides for a language of successive and multiple selves that, while it may not be applicable to more unified lives, aids us in describing the radical fractures and apparent multiplicity associated with some mental disorder (Radden 1996).

MULTIPLICITY AND DISSOCIATIVE IDENTITY DISORDER

The case material here requires little introduction. Some philosophical work has been directed toward clarifying definitions and concepts (Braude 1996; Radden 1996; Flanagan 1996). Empirically and experientially understood, normal persons are not simple unities: they are complex, with multifarious plans, projects, and desires that are often in tension. They are "multiplex," in Flanagan's terminology, in contrast to the "multiple" selves of dissociative identity disorder (DID), who experience themselves or express their being "with different narrators who cannot grasp the connection between or among the narratives or narrative segments" (Flanagan 1996: 66). The epistemic relationships and attitudes among the selves that make up multiples and other confusions over self-ascription have been clarified by Braude's terminology: a state is indexical when a person *believes it to be* assignable to herself, but only autobiographical when a person *experiences it* as her own. Braude (1991) has argued that multiples alone comprise distinct "apperceptive centers"; the indexical and autobiographical states of each self are (respectively) largely nonautobiographical and nonindexical for the others. These pathologies have also been explored in relation to philosophical notions of personhood (Wilkes 1988). Four criteria arguably met in the multiplicity of some cases of DID include conditions of (1) separate agency (separate selves will have separate agendas); (2) separate personality (separate selves will exhibit distinct, nonagential personality traits); (3) continuity (separate selves will persist through time); and (4) disordered awareness (disordered awareness on the part of at least one self will result in disordered memory in the subject in excess of that found in normal people) (Radden 1996). Approaching from the other end, with tests for unity, Behnke and Sinnott-Armstrong (2000) have put forward less stringent conditions sufficient for two-person stages to belong to the same person: (a) they share the same functioning brain; (b) they share one or more experiential memories; (c) they have one or more experiential memory chains that converge on numerically the same experience; and (d) after appropriate therapy, they could have shared memories or experiential memory chains that converge on numerically the same experience.

Some theorizing denies the possibility of multiplicity; thus, neither DID nor any other case will fulfill the conditions for multiplicity (Clark 1996). Among those who define personal identity in such a way as to allow for the possibility of actual cases of multiplicity, however, there are degrees of support for the attribution of multiplicity to cases of DID. Some reject cases of DID as instances of multiplicity (Braude 1996; Brown 2001); others are somewhat more persuaded, though uncommitted (Rovane 1998; Radden 1996); still others appear convinced (Saks 1997). Nor do unified and multiple selves exhaust the range of possibilities here: thus, for example, Gunnarsson has argued that the alters of DID may be the subselves of the same or of distinct subjects, where one subject is distinct from another "when the first subject's commitments do not thereby commit the second one and when the first subject's stream of experience is therefore distinct from the second one's" (Gunnarsson 2001: 42).

Related discussions appeal to DID in determining the ontological status of selves. Here, clinical material has been employed to support a dizzying range of incompatible answers to the question of whether the self exists. Using Graham's classification, these fall into irrealist, anti-realist, or fictionalist accounts that assert that the self is a fiction based on the evidence of disorders such as DID (Wilkes 1988, 1991, 1992; Dennett 1988, 1991); Realist accounts assert that the self exists and identify a unifying self at work even in cases of DID (Braude 1996; Clark 1996); the "partition response" (Graham 2002: 30) holds that "some selves are real, others are unreal" and allows for the conclusion that DID robs the individual of self (Hardcastle and Flanagan 1999; Graham 2002). In a similar way, the question of what the self is, or is like, has been approached by appeal to DID (Graham 2002).

Skepticism about the disorder category itself has dogged theorizing here. The alleged etiology of DID implicates early trauma resultant from abuse followed by repression and dissociation, and one skeptical question concerns the status of the "memories" of such alleged abuse recovered through therapeutic intervention. Hacking's influential writing on the history of memory, dissociation, and the multiple self puts forward the provocative view that, rather than a kind of inner camera, recording determinate events, memory of motives and actions is somehow indeterminate in relation to the past, constructing as it goes. When we remember what we did, or what other people did, we may also rethink, reexperience, and re-describe the past. These re-descriptions may be perfectly true of the past, and yet, paradoxically, they may not have been true in the past: that is, not truths about intentional actions that made sense when the actions were performed (Hacking 1995). Hacking's subsequent writing employs the notion that mental disorders such as DID are "interactive kinds": categories and conditions affected not only by other cultural changes but also by their sufferers' awareness of themselves as so classified (Hacking 1999). The cultural construction of memory and of whole syndromes of mental disorder is a theme also found in the writing of Showalter (1997), who classifies multiple personality as one of several recent hysterical disorders. She argues that hysteria is a natural human response to conflict, anxiety, and distress. When, as today, a wide cultural exposure to a narrative or history invites recurrent psychogenic responses such as multiplicity, which appear to mimic each other because they are shaped by the same prevailing cultural narratives or histories, such "hystories" reach epidemic proportions, Showalter claims. Without questioning the distress that gave rise to it, both Hacking and Showalter cast doubt on the mechanisms of memory presupposed in the standard etiological account.

DID is strongly gender-linked, and the extent to which the recovered "memories" are those of women concerning abuse by male caregivers has invited an application of the new insights provided by feminist epistemology. Potter illustrates the way concepts like those of genuine and false memory are vulnerable to interpretation, and thereby likely influenced by social and political power relations (Potter 1996; Code 1996; Park 1997). Campbell has emphasized the relationship between memory and identity in her explanation of some of the particular ways women are discredited as rememberers when they accuse others of abuse (Campbell 1997). Attributions of "false memories" to women, she argues, are tantamount to attributions of false identities and identity disorders, so that "the intent of the charge of identity disorder is to question whether women can occupy self narrative positions that are testimonial. . . . The incest survivor . . . is not now someone who has survived incest. . . . She is someone who has a changed, false identity through false memory and consequently cannot testify to her own abuse" (Campbell 1997: 69, 72).

SUCCESSIVE SELVES AND MANIC DEPRESSION

Although they have received less philosophical attention than DID, manic depression and other cyclical or bipolar mood disorders also challenge the customary continuity we associate with normal multiplex persons; given a theory of personal identity hospitable to a metaphysics of successive selves, they arguably invite a description of the manic and depressed selves as more than mere aspects of a single identity. The radically differing states and traits associated with the manic and depressed phases of persons who suffer such conditions are in some cases as disruptive of the continuity of the person as are the shifts from one alter to another in DID. Taxonomically and clinically, the personality changes associated with the occurrence and course of mood and schizophrenic disorders differ importantly from the multiplicity of DID. The personality changes engendered by them are not central or defining symptoms; they are often more like effects of those symptoms, and clinically they may be of little significance. Nonetheless, they often represent transformations radical enough to warrant the title of successive and even recurrent selves. Returning to the criteria for multiplicity outlined earlier, the manic and depressive "selves" sometimes pursue distinct agendas and exhibit significantly different emotional and behavioral dispositions and propositional attitudes; moreover, these separate "selves" may be relatively permanent structures, lasting weeks, months, or even years; thus, they fulfill the continuity condition. In addition, they sometimes reveal forms of incomplete awareness and deficient memory that are at least comparable to, although different from, the lacunae that result from dissociation. Persons with mood disorders can exhibit distortions and selectivity of memory in striking excess of those associated with more continuous personal lives. At least when remembered from some distance in time, experiences do not feel like experiential memories as we usually understand them. Retrospectively, the person restored to his earlier personality and agent patterns, or something close to them, often regards the changes wrought in him during a past manic or depressed episode not simply as unsought, unwelcome, and unnatural but as alien.

ETHICAL AND NORMATIVE IMPLICATIONS: ADVANCE DIRECTIVES

Anticipating the transformations wrought by mental disorder, people have presumably always attempted to control their fate through the exercise of what has been called "future oriented" (Dresser 1984) or "precedent" autonomy (Dworkin 1993) by issuing directives as to their care and treatment; such advance-care directives are today known as psychiatric wills or Ulysses contracts. Someone envisioning the treatment resistance of an anticipated future manic phase might attempt to ensure that her later treatment refusals would be overridden, for example. These Ulysses contracts resemble the advance-care directives of those envisioning incapacitating physical or neurological damage and disease, although with particular features that distinguish them, such as the likely temporary nature of the anticipated condition and the fact that the competence of the later decision (to resist treatment, for example) frequently meets the threshold required of rational autonomy. The ethical question of whether such contracts should be honored in these cases has given rise to a philosophical literature in which questions of personal identity become central. Depending on theories of personal identity, honoring the earlier request and imposing treatment against the wishes of the patient during the manic phase can be seen as the enslavement of an earlier, more normal self over those of the later, manic self (Buchanan 1988; Buchanan and Brock 1989); if not as enslavement, then it can be seen as a form of unfairness that arbitrarily privileges the earlier over the later self (Radden 1996) and as permitted or even obligatory for caregivers as an expression of the person's autonomous decision to bind herself in advance (Feinberg 1986; Dresser 1984; Quante 1999). The quandary of the treater in deciding whether or not to honor the Ulysses contract has been described as an ethical dilemma, where imposing treatment in spite of the patient's current dissent is at once unwarrantedly paternalistic and respectful of the patient's autonomy (Quante 1999). Our ability to entertain second thoughts—to reconsider, adapt, and change direction in the light of a new piece of information or a telling experience — is deeply bound up with what makes us autonomous human beings and is as essential to the full and complete exercise of our freedom as is our ability to bind ourselves with a plan (Radden 1995).

Some have introduced the notion of authenticity here, arguing that the dilemma be resolved through privileging whichever manifestation of the patient's will is the more authentic one (Appelbaum 1982; Quante 1999). Authenticity wants for any agreed-upon and objective criterion for its application, however; a decision to privilege *persistence* of character traits as more authentic, for example, is belied by the way personal transformation that is voluntarily sought is valued as an expression of autonomy. A second approach allows for degrees of competence, and it privileges the decision that exhibits a greater degree of rationality (Quante 1999). Use of any but a threshold concept of competence for these purposes invites discriminatory judgment, however, and has been avoided for that reason (Buchanan and Brock 1889).

FURTHER IMPLICATIONS: RESPONSIBILITY FOR PAST DEEDS

In the long history of regarding insanity as an excusing condition, when attributions of moral and legal responsibility have been withheld because of the mental disorder of the perpetrator at the time of the wrongful deed, it has not been as the result of any unusual theory of personal identity but because of incapacities and deficits of psychological function. Indeed, it is rather the reverse: deontological and retributivist frameworks have depended on a form of methodological individualism. Thus, people are responsible for all actions they perpetrate precisely because of their numerical identity. The "one to a customer" rule (Dennett 1988) by which each body houses one person only throughout its lifespan ensures that that person is the author of all deeds perpetrated by his body.

In recent years, two contingencies have prompted analyses that challenge customary theories of personal identity and permit, even invite, a metaphysics of successive selves in relation to responsibility for past wrong deeds. Cases of DID arise where the perpetrator of the wrongdoing appears to be a different self or "alter" from the one accused, as well as being unaware of, and powerless to prevent, its commission. Those concerned over the injustice of attributing blame and according punishment have argued that other alters may be blameless, even though they share a body with those alters who perpetuated the wrongdoing (Saks 1995, 1997). Again, responses have been mixed here. The dispositive purposes of law and its fundamental reliance on methodological individualism appear to work against making use of such a metaphysics in deciding these cases (Feinberg 1986; Radden 1996). Moreover, recent attempts to define personal identity such as Behnke and Sinnott-Armstrong's (2000), noted earlier, are designed to preclude a "multiplicity" defense by establishing that a single person was responsible for the crime. (Not all discussion about the exculpating nature of DID appeals to the apparent lack of personal identity in these cases; thus, for example, Braude [1996] insists that it is the familiar criteria of control and rationality, rather than identity, that should guide our judgments here, and Thomasma [2000] identifies general criteria for directing responsibility from the patient toward the treating psychiatrist in DID cases. Related issues arise with the practice of altering, by the administration of psychotropic medications, defendants who would otherwise be unfit to stand trial due to mental disorder. Whether voluntarily or involuntarily imposed, a regimen that ensures a state of "chemical sanity" sufficient to stand trial or undergo execution threatens to try or punish one self for the crime of another, according to a successive-selves metaphysics [Graber and Marsh 1979; Radden 1989].)

The relationship between responsibility and personal identity outlined earlier gives cases such as these a particular methodological centrality in some discussions. When answers are sought to first-order moral questions concerning responsibility in these puzzling cases (should the defendant who suffers DID be excused from past crimes?), it has been proposed that intuitions as to whether the person on trial was the same person who committed the crime be treated—at risk of circularity—as guiding (MacIntosh 1969).

THERAPEUTIC GOALS AND PERSONAL IDENTITY

In a very particular way, therapy with DID usually involves attempts to reunify and integrate the disparate psychic parts of the patient, and these efforts have given rise to philosophical speculation about the customary unity found in more normal selves (Flanagan 1996; Clark 1996). More generally, as well, since such identity is presupposed in the widely sought therapeutic goal of autonomy, this emphasis on restoring or enhancing unity and coherence is sought in almost all, if not all, therapeutic endeavors in psychiatry. Whatever form of therapy (and whatever the disorder), the unification and integration of the person aptly describe its rationale and end. Recent narrative conceptions of identity make clear that such integration and unification are as much diachronic as synchronic, moreover. These conceptions represent the therapeutic project in terms of re-creating or restoring a linear and coherent narrative, its goal the "narrative repair of damaged identities" (Nelson 2001).

CHARACTERIZATION IDENTITY AND MENTAL DISORDER

When we speak of a person's identity, of self-identity, or of identity politics, a different notion of identity prevails. Various contrasts have been introduced to separate this second sort of identity. Schechtman (1996) speaks of identity as concerning *characterization* (in contrast to the *reidentification* sense of identity associated with traditional theorizing). A person's characterization identity is constituted by the content of her self-concept, which comes in the form of a self-narrative; the traits, actions, and experiences included in it are parts of her personal story. Quante (1999) marks the same contrast using the *personality* or *biographical* senses of identity in contrast to the *persistence* sense: the personality or biographical sense of identity concerns "the complex pattern of values, preferences, and beliefs, in which a person manifests who she is and wants to be" (366). The persistence of traits that allow for reidentification are presupposed by this second sense, since a person's personality characterization is itself a set of persisting traits. But the emphasis on reidentification and on the identity judgment that the same person persists is not uppermost here.

Rather than relying on a passive model of the person as subject of this characterization identity, recent theorizing emphasizes its active and creative construction by the "author" of the self "narrative." Characterization identity involves self-characterization, rather than characterization by others, then. That said, however, these narratives are not solely authored works, nor are they mere fabrications; personal identities are constituted by a complex interaction between first-, second-, and third-person perspectives (Nelson 2001).

With its emphasis on the enduring aspects of the patient's person and personality, much therapeutic endeavor in psychiatry is focused around characterization identity, broadly understood. Inquiries into who we have been, are, and want to become are at the heart of the therapeutic enterprise. These concerns, surfacing in and even in part defining psychiatric practice, are illustrated here with two examples. First is the diagnosis of gender identity disorder, which emphasizes one aspect of the broader self-concept: the patient's characterization of her identity as a gendered and sexed being.

Defined as a strong and persistent cross-gender identification accompanied by a persistent discomfort with one's assigned sex (APA 1994), gender identity disorder (GID) has become an increasingly common diagnosis; its estimated prevalence in the general population today has been placed at between 2 and 5 percent. Criticisms of this diagnosis rest on its reliance on socially constructed categories and norms, particularly strict gender dualism, and the "sex/gender/sexuality dimorphism" (Morgan 2002) which asserts that male and female, masculine and feminine, are exhaustive categories and that every individual's sex, gender, and sexuality are natural, singular, and invariant across his or her life. (See also Scheman 1997; Feder 1999; Nelson 2001; Holmes 2002.) Moreover, because parents of GID children have also been subject to psychiatric scrutiny as likely reinforcers of gender-dysphoric traits, and because GID has been identified as a precursor of homosexuality, this diagnostic category has been strongly criticized as an arbitrary psychiatric classification that serves to "reinforce, reinscribe, and legitimate problematic social norms with regard to masculinity and femininity" (Feder 1999). Other critics of GID have directed their attention to the puzzling focus of therapeutic intervention with these cases. The clinically correct story, in Hilde Lindeman Nelson's words, tries to have it both ways. It "represents sex-reassignment surgery as the moment when the transgendered person passes from being a woman to being a man, or vice versa, but since it also insists that "man" and "woman" are natural kinds, it denies that transgendered people could actually be the men or women they appear to be" (Nelson 2001: 126). This concept of passing, Nelson argues, positions those who do not conform to the norms as deviant and defective, stigmatizing them not only before but after reassignment surgery.

The symptoms of other disorders, such as schizophrenia, implicate characterization identity and the self-concept in a different way, and schizophrenia constitutes my second example. Reporting on the morbid or delusional selfhood in schizophrenia, Cutting (2000) notes the commonness of delusions concerning misidentification and misclassification of self (e.g., I am my father), self as a different sort of person (I am a witch, God, or an animal), and self with some distinct qualitative change (e.g., supernatural powers, altered sexual orientation or gender, altered genealogy, altered mental status, altered biography). More generally, as recent phenomenological studies show, schizophrenic subjectivity centers around questions of characterization identity and even personal identity (see Zahavi 2000). Though we can only speculate why this should be so, philosophical categories and questions of identity seem to be mirrored in the pathological obsession.

CONCLUSION

The ruptures and discontinuities associated with much mental disorder challenge traditional, orderly notions of personal identity and invite the more flexible framework provided by neo-Humean accounts such as Partfit's. Moreover, because personal identity is tied to the categories of agency, autonomy, personhood, and responsibility, the challenges to personal identity posed by mental disorder affect practical and policy issues, two of which—the ascription of moral and legal responsibility for crimes carried out as the result of or during an episode of mental disorder and psychiatric advance-care directives—were discussed here. Finally, "identity," in the sense sometimes distinguished as characterization identity, is also a key category in psychiatry. It is central to much clinical endeavor; it is directly implicated in disorders such as gender identity disorder and the therapeutic approaches that condition is believed to dictate (although, as we have seen, serious concerns over the arbitrary social norms on which they are solely based apparently taint the category of GID); and, last, it is a recurrent theme in schizophrenic subjectivity.

REFERENCES

American Psychiatric Association (1994) *Diagnostic and Statistical Manual of Mental Disorders*, 4th ed. Washington, DC: American Psychiatric Association.

Appelbaum, P. (1992) "Case Studies: Can a Subject Consent to a 'Ulysses Contract'? Commentary." *Hastings Center Report* 12(4): 27–28.

Behnke, S., and Sinnott-Armstrong, W. (2000) "Responsibility in Cases of Multiple Personality Disorder." In James Tomberlin (ed.), *Action and Freedom*. Philosophical Perspectives, 14. Malden, MA: Blackwell Publishers.

Braude, Stephen E. (1991) *First Person Plural: Multiple Personality and the Philosophy of Mind*. London: Routledge.

Braude, Stephen E. (1996) "Multiple Personality and Moral Responsibility." *Philosophy, Psychiatry and Psychology* 3(1): 37–54.

Brown, M. T. (2001) "Multiple Personality and Personal Identity." *Philosophical Psychology* 14: 435–47.

Buchanan, A. (1988) "Advance Directives and the Personal Identity Problem." *Philosophy and Public Affairs* 17(4): 277–302.

Buchanan, A., and Brock, D. (1989) *Deciding for Others: The Ethics of Surrogate Decision Making*. New York: Cambridge University Press.

Campbell, S. (1997) "Women, 'False' Memory, and Personal Identity." *Hypatia* 12(2): 51–82.

Clark, S. R. L. (1996) "Minds, Memes and Multiples." *Philosophy, Psychiatry and Psychology* 3: 21–28.

Code, L. (1996) "Commentary on Potter's Loopholes, Gaps, and What Is Held Fast: Democratic Epistemology and Claims to Recovered Memories." *Philosophy, Psychiatry and Psychology* 3: 255–60.

Cutting, J. (2000) "Questionable Psychopathology." In Dan Zahavi (ed.), *Exploring the Self: Philosophical and Psychopathological Perspectives in Self-Experience*. Amsterdam: John Benjamins, pp. 243–55.

Dennett, D. C. (1988) "Why Everyone Is a Novelist." *Times Literary Supplement*, 16–22 September, p. 1016.

Dennett, D. C. (1991) *Consciousness Explained*. Boston: Little, Brown.

Dresser, R. (1984) "Bound to Treatment: The Ulysses Contract." *Hastings Center Report* 14(3): 13–16.

Dworkin, R. (1993) *Life's Dominion:An Argument about Abortion and Euthanasia*. London: HarperCollins.

Feder, E. (1999) "Gender Identity Disorder, Children's Rights, and the State." In Uma Narayan and J Bartkowiak (eds.), *Having and Raising Children: Unconventional Families, Hard Choices, and the Social Good*. University Park: Pennsylvania State University Press.

Feinberg, J. (1986) *The Moral Limits of the Criminal Law*, Vol. 3: *Harm to Self*. Oxford: Oxford University Press.

Flanagan, O. (1996) *Multiple Identity, Character Transformation, and Self-Reclamation*. New York: Oxford University Press.

Freyd, J. (1996) *Betrayal Trauma: The Logic of Forgetting Childhood Abuse.* Cambridge, MA: Harvard University Press.

Glass, James M. (1993) *Shattered Selves: Multiple Personality in a Postmodern World.* Ithaca: Cornell University Press.

Graber, G., and Marsh, F. (1979) "Ought a Defendant Be Drugged to Stand Trial?" *Hastings Center Report* 9(Feb.): 8–10.

Graham, G. (2002) "Recent Work in Philosophical Psychopathology." *American Philosophical Quarterly* 39: 109–33.

Gunnarsson, L. (2002) "The Many I's of Eve." Unpublished ms.

Hacking, Ian (1995) *Rewriting the Soul: Multiple Personality and the Sciences of Memory.* Princeton: Princeton University Press.

Hacking, Ian (1999) *The Social Construction of What?* Cambridge, MA: Harvard University Press.

Hardcastle, V., and Flanagan, O. (1999) "Multiplex vs. Multiple Selves: An Assessment of Multiple Personality Disorder." *Philosophy, Psychiatry and Psychology* 3: 37–54.

Holmes, M. (2002) "Questioning Genival Determinism and Sexual Dualism: intersexuality, identity and ideology." Unpublished ms.

Kramer, Ian (1999) *Listening to Prozac.* New York: Viking.

MacIntosh, J. J. (1969) "Memory and Personal Identity." In J. J. Macintosh and S. Coval (eds.), *The Business of Reason.* London: Routledge and Kegan Paul.

Morgan, K. (2002) "Gender Police: Biomedicine and the Social Construction of Gender Disabilities and Disorders." Unpublished ms.

Mullin, A. (1996) "Selves, Diverse and Divided: Can Feminists Have Diversity without Multiplicity?" *Hypatia* 10(4): 1–31.

Nelson, H. L. (2001) *Damaged Identities, Narrative Repair.* Ithaca, NY: Cornell University Press.

Parfit, D. (1984) *Reasons and Persons.* Oxford: Oxford University Press.

Park, S. M. (1997) "False Memory Syndrome: A Feminist Philosophical Perspective." *Hypatia* 12(2): 1–50.

Potter, N. (1996) "Loopholes, Gaps, and What Is Held Fast: Democratic Epistemology and Claims to Recovered Memories." *Philosophy, Psychiatry and Psychology* 3: 237–54.

Quante, M. (1999) "Precedent Autonomy and Personal Identity." *Kennedy Institute of Ethics Journal* 9(4): 365–81.

Radden, Jennifer (1989) "Chemical Sanity and Personal Identity." *Public Affairs Quarterly* 3: 64–79.

Radden, Jennifer (1995) "Second Thoughts: Revoking Decisions over One's Future." *Philosophy and Phenomenological Research* 54(4): 787–801.

Radden, Jennifer (1996) *Divided Minds and Successive Selves: Ethical Issues in Disorders of Identity and Personality.* Cambridge, MA: MIT Press.

Rovane, C. (1998) *The Bounds of Agency.* Princeton, NJ: Princeton University Press.

Saks, Elyn (1995) "The Criminal Responsibility of People with Multiple Personality Disorder." *Psychiatric Quarterly* 66(2): 119–31.

Saks, Elyn (with Stephen Behnke) (1997) *Jekyll on Trial: Multiple Personality Disorder and Criminal Law.* New York: New York University Press.

Schechtman, M. (1996) *The Constitution of Selves.* Ithaca, NY: Cornell University Press.

Scheman, N. (1997) "Queering the Center by Centering the Queer: Reflections on Transsexuals and Secular Jews." In D. Meyers (ed.), *Feminists Rethink the Self.* Boulder: Westview Press.

Shoemaker, S. (1979) "Identity, Properties, and Causality." In Peter French, Theodore Edward Uehling, and Howard Wettstein (eds.), *Studies in Metaphysics*. Midwest Studies in Philosophy, No 10. Minneapolis: University of Minnesota Press.

Showalter, E. (1997) *Hystories*. New York: Columbia University Press.

Spanos, N. (1996) *Multiple Identity and False Memories: A Sociocognitive Perspective*. Washington, DC: American Psychological Association.

Szasz, T. (1982) "The Psychiatric Will: A New Mechanism for Protecting Persons against "Psychosis" and Psychiatry." *American Psychologist* 37: 762–70.

Thomasma, D. (2000) "Moral and Metaphysical Reflections on Multiple Personality Disorder." *Theoretical Medicine and Bioethic* 21(3): 235–60.

Wilkes, K. (1988) *Real People: Personal Identity through Thought Experiments*. Oxford: Clarendon Press.

Wilkes, K. (1991) "How Many Selves Make Me?" In D. Cockburn (ed.), *Human Beings*. Cambridge: Cambridge University Press.

Wilkes, K. (1992) "Psyche and the Mind." In M. Nussbaum and A. Rorty (eds.), *Essays on Aristotle's 'De Anima.'* Oxford: Oxford University Press.

Williams, B. (1973) *Problems of the Self: Philosophical Papers, 1956–1972*. Oxford: Clarendon Press.

Zahavi, D. (ed.) (2000) *Exploring the Self: Philosophical and Psychopathological Perspectives in Self-Experience* Amsterdam/Philadelphia: John Benjamins.

CHAPTER 10

DEVELOPMENT

Disorders of Childhood and Youth

CHRISTIAN PERRING

CHILD and adolescent psychiatry is a relatively young field within psychiatry; one historian dates its start to the end of World War II (Showalter 2000: 461; see also Showalter 1994 for a discussion of earlier periods in the field). While the field has some differences from the rest of psychiatry, including arguably less emphasis on nosology and genetics, for example, it nevertheless reflects many of the trends in psychiatry. So there is a great deal of overlap between the philosophical issues that arise in child and adolescent psychiatry and those that arise for the rest of psychiatry. There has been very little discussion by philosophers of ethical, conceptual, meta-physical, or epistemological topics in the study of psychopathology in children and adolescents. In this chapter, I focus on philosophical issues that arise in particularly notable or interesting ways for the field.

I divide the chapter into four main sections. The first covers ethical concerns about recent trends in the treatment of child and adolescent psychiatric disorders; the second covers more general approaches to understanding the duties of physicians in diagnosing and treating the mental health problems of children and youth; the third discusses some of the debate over theories of the psychological development and the nature of the child's mind; and the fourth and final section briefly addresses how some issues in the debates over the definition of mental disorder and the foun-dation of nosology play out in the case of disorders of children and youth.

I should note that there are several topics that I do not discuss at all. These include controversies about the veracity of children's testimony concerning their abuse by family members, the rights of children and adolescents to mental health care, ethical and policy issues in the education of children with cognitive deficits and learning disorders, and the moral and legal responsibility of youth with mental disorders for their behavior. My neglect of these topics does not stem from any judgment about their lack of importance but is due to limitations in space, a dearth of philosophical debate on those topics, or my own lack of familiarity with the relevant philosophical literature.

ETHICAL ISSUES IN THE TREATMENT
OF CHILDREN AND YOUTH

There are good reasons to believe that many of the mental disorders of children and adolescents are going untreated and that, at the same time, other children and adolescents are receiving inappropriate treatment.

In 2000, the Surgeon General of the United States published a report arising from a Conference on Children's Mental Health. The report argues that "the nation is facing a public crisis in mental health for infants, children, and adolescents" (U.S. Public Health Service 2000: 11). While in any given year it is estimated that 10 percent of children and adolescents suffer from mental illnesses that cause some level of impairment, only one in five receives any treatment. It is estimated that as many as 1 percent of preschoolers have major depressive disorder (Son and Kirchner 2000). Furthermore, the World Health Organization estimates that childhood neuropsychiatric disorders will rise by more than 50 percent by 2020. There are clear indications that childhood mental illness is on the rise. For example, one study showed that children and young adults are more anxious than their counterparts in the 1950s (Twenge 2000).

On the other side of the coin, considerable concern has been expressed over the rising rates of children who are taking psychotropic medication, especially at early ages:

- Approximately 5 million children in the United States take at least one psychiatric drug (Diller 2002: 9).
- According to DEA statistics, production of Ritalin increased by more than 700 percent between 1990 and 1998 (Diller 2002: 9).
- From 1988 to 1994, in the United States, prescriptions for antidepressants to children increased by 300 to 500 percent. Prescriptions for SSRI medication (of which Prozac is the best-known example) increased 19-fold. In 1994, between 1.3 and 1.9 percent of children were prescribed an antidepressant (Zito et al. 2002).

- There are many reports of preschool children taking psychotropic medication. One study found that, in 1995, in the United States, among two- to four-year-old children, 1.2 percent were taking stimulants (such as Ritalin), 0.3 percent were taking antidepressants, and 0.1 percent were taking neuroleptics (normally used in adults to treat psychosis). About 15,000 two-year-olds were receiving psychotropic medication in 1995. These were significant increases from just four years earlier (Zito et al. 2000; see also Coyle 2000). Another news report claimed that 40,000 children ages 5 or younger were taking antidepressants (Price 1998).

The rise in psychotropic medication use in children may be entirely justified medically and ethically, of course, especially given the evidence that the rates of childhood mental illness are increasing dramatically. If there is a legitimate concern over the use of medication, there must be an argument that it is not medically necessary or appropriate or that alternative treatments are better.

One of the main concerns about medication derives from the fact that often there is little evidence that the medication is effective. Most of the medication used in the United States on children and adolescents is "off-label." Medications are normally tested on adults with particular illnesses, and the U.S. Food and Drug Administration (FDA) gives approval for such use. However, it is possible for physicians to prescribe an FDA-approved medication for any use they deem fit. It is widely acknowledged that there is a great need for more testing of the efficacy, safety, and long-term effects of psychotropic medication in children, and what studies exist often indicate no significant benefit from medications. (See, for example, Graham 1999; Son 2000; State 2002; American Academy of Child and Adolescent Psychiatry 2001.) As several commentators have suggested, it may well be that physicians tend to prescribe unproven medications for treatment in response to pressure from health insurance companies or managed-care companies seeking to reduce the costs of treatment or from parents who want a "quick fix" for their child's problems; the response may even arise from changes in cultural expectations. (See Perring 1997; Diller 1998, 2002; DeGrandpre 1999.)

Yet, it is also worth noting that in some cases medication appears to be the best treatment option for childhood mental disorders. For example, despite claims to the contrary by psychiatric critics (the most vocal of whom is Breggin 2001, 2002), a growing body of evidence indicates that stimulants are the best treatment for at least a large proportion of children with ADHD (Goldman et al. 1998; Anastopoulos 1999; MTA Cooperative Group 1999).

Of course, the data behind these disputes require careful interpretation, and a full analysis of the issues would require far more detail than I provide here. What is important for our purposes here is that the ethical issues concerning psychopharmacological treatment of children and adolescents are basically empirical. The proper treatment is whatever is safest and most effective, and this is decided by scientific study.

ETHICAL ISSUES IN DIAGNOSING AND TREATING CHILD AND ADOLESCENT MENTAL DISORDERS

Physicians and psychologists treating young people face a wide variety of ethical issues in their practices. Treating a child very often requires dealing with the child's family and can also involve schools and social services. I focus this discussion around the issue of what rights children and adolescents have to choose or refuse treatment with or without parental consent.

The work that has been done in medical ethics concerning children has tended focus on issues of informed consent and proxy consent. It is clear that children and adolescents are sometimes judged competent to make some decisions. This has received a fair amount of attention in the legal literature, and, although our topic is ethics, it is instructive to examine some of the legal issues. In Britain, the decision in the 1985 *Gillick* case has been especially important in recognizing children's legal rights. Lord Scarman said:

> The common law has never treated [parental] rights as sovereign or beyond review and control. Nor has our law ever treated the child as other than a person with capacities and rights recognized by law. . . . Parental rights yield to the child's right to make his own decisions when he has reached sufficient understanding and intelligence to be capable of making up his own mind. (Quoted in Daniels and Jenkins 2000: 16 and Graham 1999: 305)

Dickenson and Fulford point out (2000: 200) that the justices did not provide criteria for determining what should count as sufficient understanding and intelligence but add that Lord Scarman included "the emotional and familial implications of the decision in addition to cognitive criteria."

Berg et al. write that, concerning the United States, "in many states, statutes exist permitting older children validly to authorize the administration of certain limited kinds of medical care (e.g., treatment for mental illness, substance abuse, venereal disease, pregnancy), or there may be a common law basis for permitting mature minors to consent to medical care" (2001: 97). They suggest, though, that this may not be because these older children are judged competent but because "minors will be less likely to seek medical care for these particular conditions if parental consent were required." Nevertheless, Berg et al. suggest standards for determining incompetence that apply equally to children and adults (98–109). They distinguish between general incompetence (e.g., advanced dementia) and specific incompetence, and they outline five main elements that can be involved in judging competence: the ability to make a decision, to understand the facts, to appreciate the risks, to have some kind of reasonable method for decision making, and, most controversial, the rationality of the decision itself.

Moving back to the ethical arena, some consensus exists that children may be competent to make decisions concerning their health care in certain instances. The main debate is what standards to use. A good deal of literature indicates that children are more capable of understanding what is involved in medical decisions than is often supposed. For example, research by Weithorn and Campbell (1982) indicates that 14-year-olds are as competent as 18- and 21-year-olds. (See Dickenson and Jones 1995 for careful argument that the differences between young people and adults have been exaggerated in recent British legal decisions.)

A sustained philosophical discussion of children's competence is made by Buchanan and Brock (1990), who argue that "children's well-being depends less on their individual preferences and more on the objective conditions necessary to foster their development and opportunities than does the well-bring of adults" (1990: 228). The value of self-determination for adults lies largely in their determining their own values, but this is less true for children. The capacity to make decisions for oneself needs to be nurtured in children, not because as children they have the right to self-determination but so they can become self-determining adults.

Buchanan and Brock also note that even if children are competent to make decisions, their parents may yet have a legitimate interest in making the decision for the child (232). One argument for this is that parents have the right and duty to promote their child's well-being, and even competent decision makers can act against their own best interest. Thus, when children choose against their own best interest, parents may have the right to override such decisions. Furthermore, parents are directly affected by the treatment chosen for the child, and this arguably also entitles them to participate in the decision making. It has also been argued that parents have some right to raise their children according to their own standards and values.

This last line of argument is taken up by Engelhardt (1996: 326), who emphasizes that children incrementally gain the capacity to understand and appreciate the choices available to them and, from this, states that there are no sharp boundaries between competence and incompetence. It is very difficult to find the right balance between the rights of parents and those of their maturing children, and Engelhardt concludes that "there is no understanding of parenting or guardianship that does not involve a particular vision of beneficence, of which there are many" (329). He argues, then, that different moral communities are entitled to make different decisions concerning these matters. (For the only book-length discussion of children's autonomy in health care decision making, see Ross 1998.)

Having a mental disorder is quite likely to impair one's judgment, and so children with mental disorders may be less competent than other children. It is also clear, however, that people with mental illnesses very often are competent to give informed consent to treatment. Note that for adults with mental illnesses, the practice of most Western societies is to impose treatment on those adults only if they pose a probable danger to themselves or others. Of course, there is much debate over what should count as probable danger. (For one discussion of this, see Buchanan and Brock 1990: ch. 7.) But it is clear that in our standard practices, children can be compelled by their parents to receive treatment for mental disorders even when their condition does not pose any serious immediate danger to themselves or others. Families could not compel adults with comparable problems to receive treatment for them. This suggests that, for children with mental illnesses, it is their status as children, rather than their status as a people with mental illnesses, that is the main ground for paternalism.

So far, we have discussed only whether parents have the authority to override their children's wishes concerning medical treatment, but we also need to consider the role of the health professional in her interaction with the family. Clearly, if a child or an adolescent with a mental disorder is reluctant to participate in the treatment favored by the clinician and the parents, the situation is delicate. Thoughtful work has been done on the usefulness of getting adult patients to participate in their treatment and the problems involved, especially in mental health treatment, when the patient is alienated from the clinician (see for example Winick [1994]), and, presumably, this is also true for children. Clinicians need to be skillful and sensitive when dealing with such delicate situations, and family therapy may be called for. Being a good clinician certainly requires awareness of these issues, but it is not clear that there are any special ethical concerns here.

While we have outlined some of the ethical issues involved in parents' overriding their child's wishes concerning mental health treatment, we are still far from being in a position to provide substantive guidelines about how to deal with particular cases. We should note that there is in the medical ethics literature a thriving discussion of the extent to which it is possible to derive concrete conclusions from general ethical schemes when dealing with the complexities of particular cases. Real-life cases typically bring with them a daunting complexity of issues, and many ethical considerations come into play. There is certainly no algorithm that will provide concrete recommendations from very general considerations, and some have expressed doubts whether general ethical theories have the ability to provide concrete answers to real-life controversies.

Unfortunately, we have made limited progress in regard to the question whether we are able to say when older adolescents should be able to choose or refuse treatment with or without parental consent. We have not broached the case where parents are united with their children against the opinions of mental health professionals, and, even in cases of conflicts between parents and children, we are far from having substantive and helpful ethical guidelines about how clinicians should proceed. This is a large and largely unexplored area, although it does overlap a great deal with other areas in medical ethics and the philosophy of psychiatry. I have explored only the tip of the iceberg. We should not expect any easy answers, but we can hope for invigorating philosophical debates. Even if this exploration fails to provide definite answers to difficult questions, it can at least point out concerns to which we should be sensitive when dealing with real cases.

THEORIES OF CHILD DEVELOPMENT AND PSYCHOPATHOLOGY: THE CONNECTION WITH PHILOSOPHY

Philosophers have been very interested in theories of child development and psychopathology for a variety of reasons. In this section, I catalog some of the literature, with only brief discussion.

Perhaps the first philosophical concern with children came from the study of knowledge and thus the question whether we are born with innate knowledge or whether all our knowledge derives ultimately from our experience, and this debate can be traced back to ancient Greek philosophy. Much of the debate has focused on whether it is possible to explain our acquisition of ideas, knowledge, and skills using the empiricist hypothesis. John Locke discusses children's knowledge of mathematics in his argument against innate ideas (Locke 1975: book I, ch. II, sec. 16), and the debate continues to this day, with Jesse Prinz defending empiricism concerning the acquisition of concepts and also discussing infants' understanding of mathematics (Prinz 2002: 185–87). Locke also discusses children with defects in the mind with reference to his theory of knowledge and, in particular, points out our ignorance of real essences. He argues that such children are at least as much monsters as children with physical defects and that there is no reason to think they have rational souls. To modern ears his use of language is offensive when he talks of a "drivelling, unintelligent, intractable changeling" (Locke 1975: book IV, ch. IV, sec. 16), and these days the philosophical debate concerning the nature of children with severe mental disorders is framed in very different language. It also addresses different questions.

Cognitive and emotional deficits are of particular interest in modern philosophy of mind because they can serve as important test cases for different views of the nature of mind. While the debate is complex, the central issue is whether in our ordinary interactions with other people we use a theory to understand their behavior. If it exists, this theory is generally given the name "folk psychology." Some deny this "theory" theory and argue instead that we use skills of pretending and simulating to predict and understand the behavior of other people. Defenders of the simulation theory point out that, while children with Down syndrome are poor theorists generally, they are relatively sophisticated in their understanding of other people, and they argue that this is good evidence for not using a theory of folk psychology to understand other people. While some theorists have claimed that autistic children lack a theory of folk psychology (Baron-Cohen et al. 1985), others have disputed the evidence and argued that, in fact, it favors the simulation theory (Gordon and Barker 1994). For a fuller account of these issues, see Gordon (2002) and Ravenscroft (2002).

Other work with philosophical relevance has been done on theories of childhood psychological development that is critical of the ideological underpinnings of the theories or the social consequences. The best example of this is the feminist criticisms of Freud's psychosexual theories generally, and his theory of female infantile sexuality and identity formation in particular (e.g., Freud 1925). Freud's theories were controversial from the start, and many disputed the evidential base of psychoanalytic theory before philosophers of science scrutinized the issue. Simone de Beauvoir's (1952) criticisms of psychoanalysis have been particularly influential. Some feminists have used psychoanalysis to criticize patriarchal childrearing practices and the resultant formation of female identity (see Chodorow 1978). Also, a great deal of scholarly discussion centers on hysteria, a relatively frequent psychoanalytic diagnosis of young women, at least among certain groups in late-nineteenth-century Vienna. The case of Dora has gained particular attention; see, for example, the works collected in Bernheimer (1990). Using a nonpsychoanalytic approach, Carole Gilligan, in her book *In a Different Voice* (1982), has been especially influential with her powerful criticisms of Kohlberg's ideas on the moral development of children and adolescents. Notwithstanding this notable scholarly work, limited attention has been paid by feminist theory to child and adolescent psychopathology, and feminist bioethics has paid little attention to psychiatry in general (for a presentation of recent discussion on this topic, see Martin 2001). The most notable recent feminist discussion of the mental illnesses of youth has focused on eating disorders, linking the pathology to the patriarchal nature of society and the unrealistic norms of beauty that are promoted in popular media (see Bordo 1993; Brumberg 1988). In the past decade, there has been a vigorous debate among social commentators influenced by or reacting against feminism concerning the mental problems of young people and the possible social causes (see Pipher 1994; Pollack 1998; Hoff Sommers 2000).

Other research in psychology and sociology has linked childhood development and psychopathology to class and culture. Erikson (1963), strongly influenced by psychoanalysis, was of major importance in analyzing the notion of American identity; while his work is not primarily critical in its stance, it lent itself to a critical analysis of capitalist culture and its treatment of children within the privacy of the nuclear family (see, for example, Poster 1978). Similarly, R. D. Laing's work on schizophrenia in young people and the role of the family in the illness can be used toward a wider critique of contemporary culture. Even if Laing's theories about schizophrenia are wrong, his approach to understanding the relation between the individual child or adolescent and the rest of society may nevertheless be important. (See Laing and Esterson 1964; Laing 1969; and Burston 2000: ch. 4.) Work in medical sociology on attention-deficit disorder and juvenile delinquency has also drawn connections between the individual child and the nature of society, often with a critical attitude toward the categorization of mental illness in children (see, for example, Conrad 1980).

The Concept of Mental Disorder in Children and Adolescents

Although within child and adolescent psychiatry, the issue of nosology has not been the focus of most research, important work has been done and disputes over diagnostic categories have arisen. The field has often expressed dissatisfaction concerning the DSMs, and often cited for its importance is a 1966 publication on disorders of childhood by the Group for the Advancement of Psychiatry, which "stressed the intermingling of normal development within a spectrum of normality and pathology, as well as the multiple meanings of symptoms" (Schowalter 2000: 468). In theoretical psychiatry, philosophy, and medical ethics, a great deal of recent work has been done on the concept of mental disorder (for a review of the literature, see Perring 2002). The ideal goal of the debate is to establish a well-grounded, clear, and helpful analysis of mental disorder that will settle disputes about controversial categories of mental disorder such as homosexuality, paraphilias, psychopathy, and various kinds of addiction. The analysis would apply to all mental disorders, including those of children and adolescents. There has certainly been a dispute concerning the legitimacy of certain kinds of diagnosis in child psychiatry; some critics have suggested, for example, that ADHD is overdiagnosed and that young boys are by nature hyperactive.

Without entering into the details of the debate over the nature of mental illness, it is worth making one point of central importance concerning disorders of childhood and youth. Borduin et al. (1999: 498) emphasize, "there is now substantial evidence to suggest that children's emotional and behavioral disorders are often linked with relational problems in their family, peer, and school systems." Furthermore, they explicitly link this observation to trenchant criticisms of the existing classification schemes for mental disorders of children and adolescents, since *The Diagnostic and Statistical Manual of Mental Disorders,* 4th ed. (DSM-IV; APA 1994) and The International Classification of Disease, 10th ed. (ICD-10; WHO 1992), while acknowledging the existence of relational problems, give them very little attention and assign them a negligible role in diagnosing mental disorders. The theoretical models for understanding relational problems are primarily social learning theories, family systems theories, and a multisystemic therapy approach. In these models, the fundamental unit is the family or larger system, rather than the individuals who make up the unit. There can be a mutually reinforcing relation between children's mental problems and the attitudes and behavior of their parents. For example, children who experience low parental warmth are at risk for developing depressive disorders, and some parents may become less emotionally warm to their depressed children (see Borduin et al. 1999: 504).

Some approaches to classification would draw different conclusions from the relational nature of many childhood mental disorders. For example, Horwitz, drawing on the work of Wakefield, argues systematically for the view that mental disorders must be "dysfunctions of some internal psychological mechanism" (2002: 22). While he pays very little attention to the case of children, it seems to follow straightforwardly from his view that he would agree that many of the conditions currently treated as mental disorders of children are not in fact mental disorders at all. Thus, childhood mental illness could be a central issue in the debate over psychiatric nosology.

CONCLUSION

In this chapter, I surveyed some of the main ways that philosophical and ethical issues arise in child and adolescent psychiatry. I hope I have shown that this is a rich area for further philosophical study, raising issues that are both important and complex and bringing together a variety of different debates that are not often seen as connected.

REFERENCES

Ackerman, Terrence F., and Strong, Carson (1989) A Casebook of Medical Ethics. New York: Oxford University Press.

Agich, George J. (1997) "Toward a Pragmatic Theory of Disease." In James M. Humber and Robert F. Almeder (eds.), What Is Disease? Totowa, NJ: Humana Press, pp. 219–46.

American Academy of Child and Adolescent Psychiatry (2001) Prescribing Psychoactive Medication for Children and Adolescents, Policy Statement 41. Available online at http://www.aacap.org/publications/policy/ps41.htm

American Psychiatric Association (1994) Diagnostic and Statistical Manual of Mental Disorders, 4th ed. (DSM-IV). Washington, DC: American Psychiatric Association.

American Psychiatric Association (2000) Diagnostic and Statistical Manual of Mental Disorders, 4th ed., Text Revision (DSM-IV-TR). Washington, DC: American Psychiatric Association.

Anastopoulos, Arthur D. (1999) "Attention-Deficit/Hyperactivity Disorder." In Sandra D. Netherton et al. (eds.), Child and Adolescent Psychological Disorders: A Comprehensive Textbook. New York: Oxford University Press, pp. 98–117.

Arras, John D., and Steinbock, Bonnie (1999) Ethical Issues in Modern Medicine, 5th ed. Mountain View, CA: Mayfield.

Baron-Cohen, Simon, et al. (1985) "Does the Autistic Have a 'Theory of Mind'?" Cognition 21: 37–46.

Beauchamp, Tom L. (1999) "The Philosophical Basis of Psychiatric Ethics." In Sidney Bloch et al. (eds.), Psychiatric Ethics, 3rd ed. New York: Oxford University Press, pp. 25–48.

Beauchamp, Tom L., and Childress, James F. (2001) Principles of Biomedical Ethics, 5th ed. New York: Oxford University Press.

Berg, Jessica W., et al. (2001) Informed Consent: Legal Theory and Clinical Practice, 2nd ed. New York: Oxford University Press.

Bernheimer, Charles (1990) *In Dora's Case: Freud-Hysteria-Feminism,* 2nd ed. New York: Columbia University Press.

Bolton, Derek (2000) "Alternatives to Disorder." *Philosophy, Psychiatry, and Psychology* 7(2): 141–153.

Bordo, Susan (1993) *Unbearable Weight.* Berkeley: University of California Press.

Borduin, Charles M., et al. (1999) "Relational Problems: The Social Context of Child and Adolescent Disorders." In Sandra D. Netherton et al. (eds.), *Child and Adolescent Psychological Disorders: A Comprehensive Textbook.* New York: Oxford University Press, pp. 498–519.

Breggin, Peter (2001) *Talking back to Ritalin: What Doctors Aren't Telling You about Stimulants for Children,* rev. ed. Cambridge, MA: Perseus Books.

Breggin, Peter (2002) *The Ritalin Fact Book What Your Doctor Won't Tell You about ADHD and Stimulant Drugs.* Cambridge, MA: Perseus Books.

Brumberg, Joan Jacobs (1988) *Fasting Girls: The Emergence of Anorexia Nervosa as a Modern Disease.* Cambridge, MA: Harvard University Press.

Buchanan, Allen E., and Brock, Dan W. (1990) *Deciding for Others: The Ethics of Surrogate Decision Making.* New York: Cambridge University Press.

Burston, Daniel (2000) *The Crucible of Experience: R. D. Laing and the Crisis of Psychotherapy.* Cambridge, MA: Harvard University Press.

Chodorow, Nancy (1978) *The Reproduction of Mothering: Psychoanalysis and the Sociology of Gender.* Berkeley: University of California Press.

Conrad, Peter (1980) "On the Medicalization of Deviance and Social Control." In David Ingleby (ed.), *Critical Psychiatry: The Politics of Mental Health.* New York: Pantheon, pp. 102–19.

Coyle, Joseph T. (2000) "Psychotropic Drug Use in Very Young Children." *Journal of the American Medical Association* 283(8): 1059–60.

Daniels, Debbie, and Jenkins, Peter (2000) *Therapy with Children: Children's Rights, Confidentiality and the Law.* London: Sage.

de Beauvoir, Simone (1952) *The Second Sex.* New York: Knopf.

DeGrandpre, Richard (1999) *Ritalin Nation: Rapid-Fire Culture and the Transformation of Human Consciousness.* New York: W. W. Norton.

Dickenson, Donna, and Fulford, Bill (2000) *In Two Minds: A Casebook of Psychiatric Ethics.* Oxford: Oxford University Press.

Dickenson, Donna, and Jones, David (1995) "True Wishes: The Philosophy and Developmental Psychology of Children's Informed Consent." *Philosophy, Psychiatry and Psychology* 2(4): 287–303.

Diller, Lawrence H. (1998) *Running on Ritalin: A Physician Reflects on Children, Society, and Performance in a Pill.* New York: Bantam.

Diller, Lawrence H. (2002) *Should I Medicate My Child? Sane Solutions for Troubled Kids with — and without — Psychiatric Drugs.* New York: Basic Books.

Douchette, Ann (2002) "Child and Adolescent Diagnosis: The Need for a Model-Based Approach." In Larry E. Beutler and Mary L. Malik (eds.), *Rethinking the DSM: A Psychological Perspective.* Washington, DC: American Psychological Association, pp. 201–20.

Edwards, Rem B. (1997) *Ethics of Psychiatry: Insanity, Rational Autonomy, and Mental Health Care.* Amherst, NY: Prometheus Books.

Engelhardt, H. Tristram (1996) *The Foundations of Bioethics,* 2nd ed. New York: Oxford University Press.

Erikson, Erik (1963) *Childhood and Society,* 2nd ed. New York: W. W. Norton.

Freeman, John M., and McDonnell, Kevin (2001) *Tough Decisions: Cases in Medical Ethics*, 2nd ed. New York: Oxford University Press.

Freud, Sigmund (1953–74) *Some Psychological Consequences of the Anatomical Distinction between the Sexes*. Standard Edition of *The Complete Psychological Works of Sigmund Freud*. Edited and translated by James Strachey. London: Hogarth Press, vol. 19, pp. 243–58. Originally published in 1925.

Gert, Bernard et al. (1997) *Bioethics: A Return to Fundamentals*. New York: Oxford University Press.

Gilligan, Carole (1982) *In a Different Voice: Psychological Theory and Women's Development*. Cambridge, MA: Harvard University Press.

Goldman, Larry S., et al. (1998) "Diagnosis and Treatment of Attention-Deficit/Hyperactivity Disorder in Children and Adolescents." *JAMA* 279(14): 1100–1107.

Gordon, Robert (2002) "Folk Psychology as Simulation." In Edward N. Zalta (ed.), *The Stanford Encyclopedia of Philosophy* (spring ed.), available online at http://plato.stanford.edu/archives/spr2002/entries/folkpsych-simulation/

Gordon, Robert M., and Barker, John A. (1994) "Autism and the 'Theory of Mind' Debate." In George Graham and G. Lynn Stephens (eds.), *Philosophical Psychopathology*. Cambridge, MA: Bradford, pp. 163–81.

Graham, Philip (1999) "Ethics and Child Psychiatry." In Sidney Bloch et al. (eds.), *Psychiatric Ethics*, 3rd ed. New York: Oxford University Press, pp. 301–17.

Group for the Advancement of Psychiatry (1966) *Psychopathological Disorders in Childhood: Theoretical Considerations and a Proposed Classification*. GAP Report No. 62. New York: GAP.

Hoff Sommers, Christina (2000) *The War against Boys: How Misguided Feminism Is Harming Our Young Men*. New York: Simon and Schuster.

Horwitz, Allan V. (2002) *Creating Mental Illness*. Chicago: University of Chicago Press.

Hudziak, James J. (2002) "Importance of Phenotype Definition in Genetic Studies of Child Psychopathology." In John E. Helzer and James J. Hudziak (eds.), *Defining Psychopathology in the 21st Century: DSM-V and Beyond*. Washington, DC: American Psychiatric Association, pp. 211–30.

Iltis, Ana Smith (ed.) (2000) "Bioethics as Methodological Case Resolution: Specification, Specified Principlism and Casuistry." *Journal of Medicine and Philosophy* 25: 271–84.

Jensen, Peter S., and Members of the MTA Cooperative Group (2002) "ADHD Comorbidity Findings from the MTA Study: New Diagnostic Subtypes and Their Optimal Treatments." In John E. Helzer and James J. Hudziak (eds.), *Defining Psychopathology in the 21st Century: DSM-V and Beyond*. Washington, DC: American Psychiatric Association, pp. 169–92.

Kaysen, Susanna (1993) *Girl, Interrupted*. New York: Turtle Bay Books.

Kymlicka, Will (1996) "Moral Philosophy and Public Policy: The Case of New Reproductive Technologies." In L. W. Sumner (ed.), *Philosophical Perspectives on Bioethics*. Toronto: University of Toronto Press.

Laing, R. D. (1969) *The Politics of the Family and Other Essays*. New York: Vintage Books.

Laing, R. D., and Esterson, Aaron (1964) *Sanity, Madness and the Family: Families of Schizophrenics*. London: Tavistock Publications.

Locke, John (1975) *An Essay Concerning Human Understanding*. Oxford: Clarendon Press.

Martin, Norah (2001) "Feminist Bioethics and Psychiatry." *Journal of Medicine and Philosophy* 26(4): 431–41.

MTA Cooperative Group (1999) "A 14-Month Randomized Clinical Trial of Treatment

Strategies for Attention-Deficit/Hyperactivity Disorder." *Archives of General Psychiatry* 56: 1073–86.

Murphy, Dominic, and Woolfolk, Robert L. (2000) "The Harmful Dysfunction Analysis of Mental Disorder." *Philosophy, Psychiatry, and Psychology* 7(4): 241–52.

Pipher, Mary (1994) *Reviving Ophelia: Saving the Selves of Adolescent Girls.* New York: Putnam.

Perring, Christian (1997) "Medicating Children: The Case of Ritalin." *Bioethics* 11(3–4): 228–40.

Perring, Christian (2002) "Mental Illness." In Edward N. Zalta (ed.), *The Stanford Encyclopedia of Philosophy* (spring ed.). Available at http://plato.stanford.edu/archives/spr2002/entries/mental-illness/

Pollack, William (1998) *Real Boys: Rescuing Our Sons from the Myths of Boyhood.* New York: Random House.

Poster, Mark (1978) *Critical Theory of the Family.* New York: Seabury Press.

Price, Joyce Howard (1998) Experimenting on Children. *Insight* (November 23): 42.

Prinz, Jesse (2002) *Furnishing the Mind: Concepts and Their Perceptual Basis.* Cambridge, MA: MIT Press.

Ravenscroft, Ian (2002) "Folk Psychology as a Theory." In Edward N. Zalta (ed.), *The Stanford Encyclopedia of Philosophy* (spring ed.). Available at http://plato.stanford.edu/archives/spr2002/entries/folkpsych-theory/

Ross, Lainie Friedman (1998) *Children, Families, and Health Care Decision-Making.* Oxford: Clarendon Press.

Schowalter, John E. (1994) "The History of Child and Adolescent Psychiatry." In Robert Michaels et al. (eds.), *Psychiatry*, rev. ed. Philadelphia: J. B. Lippincott, vol. 2, pp. 1–13.

Schowalter, John E. (2000) "Child and Adolescent Psychiatry Comes of Age, 1944–1994." In Roy W. Menninger and John C. Nemiah (eds.), *American Psychiatry after World War II. 1944–1994.* Washington, DC: American Psychiatric Press, pp. 461–80.

Son, Sung E., and Kirchner, Jeffrey T. (2000) "Depression in Children and Adolescents." *American Family Physician* 62: 2289–2308, 2311–12.

State, Rosanne C., et al. (2002) "Mania and Attention Deficit Hyperactivity Disorder in a Prepubertal Child: Diagnostic and Treatment Challenges." *American Journal of Psychiatry* 159(6): 918–25.

Toulmin, Stephen (2001) *Return to Reason.* Cambridge, MA: Harvard University Press.

Twenge, Jean M. (2000) "The Age of Anxiety? Birth Cohort Change in Anxiety and Neuroticism, 1952–1993." *Journal of Personality and Social Psychology* 79: 1007–21.

U.S. Department of Health and Human Services (1999) *Mental Health: A Report of the Surgeon General.* Rockville, MD: U.S. Department of Health and Human Services, Substance Abuse and Mental Health Services Administration, Center for Mental Health Services, National Institutes of Health, National Institute of Mental Health.

U.S. Public Health Service (2000) *Report of the Surgeon General's Conference on Children's Mental Health: A National Action Agenda.* Washington, DC: Department of Health and Human Services.

Wakefield, Jerome C. (2002) "Spandrels, Vestigial Organs, and Such." *Philosophy, Psychiatry, and Psychology* 7(4): 253–69.

Weithorn, L., and Campbell, S. (1982) "The Competency of Children and Adolescents to Make Informed Treatment Decisions." *Child Development* 53: 1589–98.

Winick, Bruce J. (1994) "The Right to Refuse Mental Health Treatment: A Therapeutic Jurisprudence Analysis." *International Journal of Law and Psychiatry* 17(1): 99–117.

World Health Organization (1992) *International Classification of Disease*, 10th ed. ICD-10. Geneva: WHO.

Wurtzel, Elizabeth (1994) *Prozac Nation: Young and Depressed in America*. Boston: Houghton Mifflin.

Younger, Stuart J., and Arnold, Robert M. (2001) "Philosophical Debates about the Definition of Death: Who Cares?" *Journal of Medicine and Philosophy* 26(5): 527–37.

Zito, Julie Magno, et al. (2000) "Trends in the Prescribing of Psychtropic Medications to Preschoolers." *JAMA* 283: 1025–30.

Zito, Julie Magno et al. (2002) "Rising Prevalence of Antidepressants among U.S. Youths." *Pediatics* 109: 721–27.

PART II

ANTINOMIES OF
PRACTICE

CHAPTER 11

DIAGNOSIS/ ANTIDIAGNOSIS

JOHN Z. SADLER

A Chinese healer might interrogate a family for recurrent patterns of behavior and cycles of symptoms, then identify the patient's tongue as one of 37 clinical kinds. Traditional Indian clinicians, relying on all senses, often tasted the urine of suspected diabetics. Before Laennec's invention of the stethoscope, the French Victorian physician exercised the privilege of placing an ear between the breasts of breathless women. Doctors in the British Enlightenment thought observation and inference were the core of diagnosis. Hippocrates attended not just to the patient's expressions and narrative but to habits, home, work, even the seasons of the year. In order to understand fully the patient's ordeal, contemporary psychoanalysts consider what *is not* said as well as what *is* said. Paracelsus dismissed autopsy as revealing the nature of disease but elevated the chemical analysis of humors. The great Persian physician Al-Razi carefully observed the pulse but practiced careful reasoning as the key to good diagnosis. Bantu healers in Africa worked themselves into a frenzy in efforts to uncover the secret of illness. The Scandinavian family therapist sought to uncover clan myths and then collaboratively reinvent them (Ackerknecht 1982; Sigerist 1951 1961; Porter 1997, 2002).

The criticism, even rejection, of diagnosis in mental health care is a recent phenomenon in the history of medicine and the history of madness, even considered against psychiatry's own short history as a defined medical specialty. To understand the controversy about psychiatric diagnosis, understanding the peculiar ambiguities of the human experiences we call "mental disorders" is a useful starting point.

Four items of context can provide a modicum of this background understanding.

First, compared to the illnesses, injuries, and diseases of "physical" medicine, mental disorders have a history of stigmatization as long as the recorded history of madness itself (Dain 1994; Fabrega 1990, 1991; Porter 2002). While the social phenomenon of stigma has waxed and waned in severity throughout history, the vilification of the mad has been a historical universal. In past centuries, the mentally ill were fettered by ankle irons and collars, and today even the seriously mentally ill are blamed for their failures: they face explicit insurance discrimination; are portrayed in popular media as criminally dangerous on the one hand and comically inept on the other; and often live in cardboard boxes underneath bridges, like trolls, which they are sometimes called. Stigmatization as a social phenomenon, then, provides a cultural atmosphere that permeates and reinforces other social phenomena surrounding these unfortunate human experiences called "mental illness."

Stigma is no doubt fed by the second background feature to be presented here. This feature involves the ambiguities around personal responsibility and volition posed by mental illness. When we are injured or become physically ill, particular social expectations kick in. As Talcott Parsons (1958) explained, the sick are excused from their usual social responsibilities: an ill person can go home and rest, seek treatment, not be judged because he is grumpy or impatient, and so forth. In Western industrialized societies, our illnesses are, by and large, not our fault or choice and society tends to forgive some of our usual responsibilities. Further, as the philosopher-psychiatrist Bill Fulford (1989, 1994) notes, physical illness is something, in the main, "done to" me, not something "I do" as an agent. Even in the case where our physical illness has been precipitated by our foolishness or willful indulgences, once we are sick or injured, our affliction is, in an important sense, out of our hands.

In the case of mental illness, however, it is often, perhaps usually, not clear when "I do" the illness and when the illness is "done to me." While some casual observers may be convinced that the hallucinations of schizophrenia are "done to" the patient, whether the lack of motivation and passivity of such people are the consequences of the disorder or the responsibility of the afflicted is less clear. In the case of the personality disorders, most people, even psychiatrists, would contend that, for instance, the egocentrism, pomposity, and contempt for others exhibited by the narcissistic character are fully the responsibility of the person. So psychiatry contends with a complex set of human phenomena that defy easy categorization as "responsible conduct," or as "blameworthy," or as "sick" (see Wilson and Adshead, Chapter 20 in this volume).

Ambiguities about moral responsibility, in turn, are fed by a third background feature of psychiatric diagnosis. That feature concerns an even more general feature of the phenomena we call mental disorders, which is the relation between the self and mental illness. Nonpsychiatric physicians may consider, quite seriously, the self, the psyche, or the "whole person" in their ministrations to the sick, but the self is never the foreground of their efforts; rather, the internist and surgeon focus on the diseased or injured organ/structure/physiological system. The internist is legitimately concerned with helping his hypercholesterolemic patient with lifestyle and dietary changes, and the surgeon is legitimately concerned with prudent exercises for preventing re-injury of the repaired knee joint, but these concerns are not in the phenomenological foregrounds of their practices; their focus is on diagnosing, medicating, and surgically intervening. For psychiatry, however, the phenomenological foreground *is* the self, the psyche, even, perhaps, the whole person. However crucial they are to the psychiatrist, the body and the brain are never the center of the affliction as lived and, even today, not the center of the mental disorder as diagnosed. Broken legs are never psychiatry's first concern, and broken hearts are relevant only as a metaphor for spirit, affect, and the personal ordeal. Because the psychiatrist's focus is on the psychic foreground and not the somatic background (Leder 1990) of human life, the psychiatrist's phenomenal domain happens to be the same as the one that makes humans distinctly different from other animals: the sense of self; the ability to reflect on and modify one's own thought and behavior; and the capacity to imagine, experience, even create alternative worlds. Even in the seeming "bodily" intervention of prescribing a psychoactive medication, a pill doesn't simply correct some somatic balance; more than this, it *alters* the way the patient thinks, feels, or acts. Other doctors may act upon the body, but the psychiatrist acts upon the soul. And it is the rich evaluative complexity of the self—the seat of evaluations, preferences, changes of mind, wishes, poetry, and passion—that sets the stage for the ambiguities of diagnosis (Sadler in press).

The fourth background feature of psychiatric diagnosis concerns how mental disorders and their component features are valued. The patient with schizophrenia may also happen to be a gifted artist. If this is true, what shall we treat? Are her artistic expressions "just" a manifestation of illness, or even related to her illness? Relatively few conditions in medicine and surgery elicit ambivalent attitudes about them (people want to be rid completely of colds, broken bones, suppurating wounds, and angina pectoris), but it is common for mental disorders to have positive, even desirable aspects for patients (e.g., the increased energy of mania, the sympathy of others for the hypochondriac, the euphoria of intoxication in addiction) and even for other people or society at large. Because mental disorders are commingled with the multivalent self, any given feature of the disorder is open to challenge as positive or negative, asset or liability, impairment or inspiration, pain or pleasure. Moreover, as Ian Hacking (1999) has noted, mental disorders as part of the self are subject to reflexivity and self-modification—what he calls "looping effects." Diagnosis does not just address the self; it also addresses a self engaged in the continuous modification and reinventing of itself. Who the patient "is" is under constant modification, and whichever mental disorder the person "has" is revised in concert with the self. Psychiatric diagnosis, in turn, becomes a moving target, and mental disorders mutate within a complex biocultural interchange.

The stakes of all these considerations are raised when we consider the fifth and final item in the contextual background, which is the social power of psychiatry. Most Western societies, puzzled like the rest of us by all the features of mental disorders that I have described, have afforded psychiatrists a unique place, not just as healers but also wielders of considerable social and interpersonal power. Such power extends in multiple directions. For instance, psychiatrists may involuntarily (coercively) seclude, and treat, their patients with the full arm of the law at their side. The diagnosis and treatment of a mental disorder may cause a government employee to lose his security clearance, provide the opportunity for obtaining needed assistance, or instigate employment discrimination—or even all of these. Parents appeal to psychiatrists for advice about child rearing. Psychotherapy patients appeal to psychiatrists (legitimately or not) for guidance about whether to marry or divorce or whether to get a job or stay at home, about who is right and who is wrong, and even about what kind of person to be.

A clinical procedure as universal as diagnosis is both a literal and a symbolic instrument of this power. Diagnosis operates as a literal instrument when it fulfills a concrete requirement for services, confinement, reimbursement, or opportunity. It operates as a symbolic instrument in parallel: when, for instance, societies treat the diagnosed differently than the undiagnosed, when the diagnosis means more, as it so often does, than the name of the condition to be treated.

Dorland's Medical Dictionary defines diagnosis as "(1) The art of distinguishing one disease from another. (2) The determination of the nature of a case of disease" (Taylor 1988 p. 461). The etymology is mostly Greek, *gnosis* meaning "investigation" or "knowledge" and *dia-* meaning "thorough" or "apart." This suggests that diagnosis is a thorough investigation or knowledge-gaining procedure, perhaps one that involves a taking apart or a breaking down into smaller components. One of the foremost diagnosticians of twentieth-century American psychiatry, Robert L. Spitzer, provides his own etymology, tongue firmly in cheek, that of *agnosis*, meaning "not knowing," and *di* meaning "two," so "diagnosis" means "doubly ignorant"!

But conventional use of the term "diagnosis" betrays that it is both a noun and a verb, a proclamation and a process people do. "What's his diagnosis?" "What's your approach to diagnosis?" are both common questions in clinical parlance, as well as in psychiatric research settings. The dual meanings of diagnosis-as-epistemic-act and diagnosis-as-a-denotative-signifier are important in understanding the debates to follow.

A consideration of our opening historical and cross-cultural considerations may reveal a richer sense about diagnosis. What are some of the common phenomenological features of diagnosis that are disclosed by these diverse clinical traditions? Further, what do these features suggest in terms of developing a concept of elegant diagnostic practice (e.g., an aesthetics of diagnosis)? As is discussed later, the latter idea of diagnostic elegance, of "proper" diagnosis, is important in appraising diagnostic practices, and by implication, diagnostic concepts.

Diagnosis as Characterization

The Chinese practitioner, like the Western psychiatrist, intends to characterize the patient's distress as an example of a more general phenomenon. By transforming a particular malady into a general exemplar, the characterizations of diagnosis set the stage for the scientific investigation of disease, disorder, and distress (Grinnell 1992). Instead of a singular and ineffable phenomenon, diagnosis permits the consideration of the malady as an identifiable and measurable condition in a group of individuals, subject to empirical assessment and consensual review by an epistemic community — that is, diagnosis permits scientific inquiry, indeed, is a condition upon which scientific investigation of illness depends. Diagnosis as characterization undergirds the colossal enterprise of psychiatric research. Characterization is the basis for one of the most common ordinary uses of "diagnosis": that is, diagnosis-as-signifier. Characterization permits the naming of, and the defining identity of, the singular malady, rendering it into an object for consideration, comparison, explanation, and control. But simply naming a malady is not enough, as both Chinese and Enlightenment physicians teach us. The characterization must cohere with a pattern of features, a complex of related attributes which then co-occur or recur in "cycles." Such characteristic forms or presentations of illness (syndromes) provide the benchmarks for clinical scientists to establish validity (Gorenstein 1992). Validity assures that diagnoses (the named disorders) are not the specious manifestation of the doctor's whim or fancy but, instead, are relatively uniform expressions of nature or culture. As Hippocrates, the Bantu, and the Scandinavian family therapist suggest, such patterns or cycles of phenomena can occur in almost any experiential domain. Having good diagnostic practices suggests a need for an openness to diverse experience; that is, it suggests an important *aesthetic* for diagnosis — namely, that diagnosis should provide a simpler characterization of complex phenomena. In this sense, every diagnostic semantic or diagnostic act is, and should be, a reduction or a simplification, much like any generalization involves a reduction or a simplification. Moreover, the sense of diagnosis-as-characterization makes it hard to imagine that anyone attempting to do clinical work could simply dispense with diagnosis, any more than one could dispense with language, the mother of cultural signification and the reducer par excellence of undifferentiated, raw experience. So, while many may reject this or that denotation of psychiatric illness (anorexia nervosa, schizophrenia, hysteria, demonic possession, enmeshed families), it is difficult to dismiss diagnosis as a primordial epistemic act.

DIAGNOSIS AS DISCLOSURE

The diagnostician's work is framed by the healing task. However, the patient may not apprehend the source of the malady or may not have the tools or techniques to heal herself. In either case, clinical diagnosis requires a looking beyond the self-evident toward a more profound or complex understanding of the malady. In other words, the patient's appeal to the diagnostician's expertise is practically grounded on the patient's inability to heal herself. The diagnostician must, then, reinterpret the malady in terms suitable to the therapeutic options available. The expertise offered by the healer often resides in the ability to see beyond the surface—that is, to apprehend a hidden or obscure facet of the illness. The Indian physician tastes the urine of the suspected diabetic because he knows that this is not part of the patient's routine. The psychoanalyst attends to what is not said because such omissions point toward a painful understanding that the patient does not, or does not wish to, possess. The Bantu healer seeks an altered consciousness to reveal what is not accessible to ordinary consciousness. Paracelsus, wary of the misleading tomfoolery of even visceral appearances, relied on the analysis of chemicals in bodily fluids. Diagnosis discloses that which is not evident, and such disclosure implies a *second aesthetic* of diagnosis: that of penetrating beneath the surface appearances, being skeptical of the "received view," a duty to reinterpret the patient's experience anew, to think outside the box. Diagnosis-as-disclosure renders the clinician akin to the philosopher and the detective.

Diagnosis as Embedded Observation

A primary tool of the diagnostician is observation, and, as we've seen already, the observation may include the full range of human expression, as well as the context of human expression. Diagnostic observation involves a framing of the context, and, as Hippocrates, the Scandinavian family therapist, and the Bantu healers teach us, the relevant context may come from anywhere: from within the bodily interior; from spiritual or supernatural domains; from the natural environment; or from human communication, expressions, artifacts, and myths (Jaspers 1963). This understanding suggests a *third aesthetic* of diagnosis, one involving the proper balance between receptivity to multiple contexts and reducing illness complexity: that is, balancing an openness to experience and observation with the rigors of characterization.

Diagnosis as Relevance

Etymology to the contrary, diagnosis has come to mean more than thorough knowledge. Diagnostic knowledge is driven by a particular practical and moral impetus, that of doctoring or healing. In contrast to other epistemic tasks like science or philosophy, the epistemic task of diagnosis is framed by its relationship to the task of the clinic, that of caring and curing. The moral justification, then, for diagnostic action is based less on the value of knowledge in isolation and more on diagnostic contributions to healing and the provision of comfort to the troubled or the suffering. In this sense, diagnosis is saturated with a particular morality, and the denotative categories of diagnosis are undergirded with these moral tasks of the clinic. But, in order to provide comfort or healing, the clinician must take effective practical action, and so diagnosis is framed by the therapeutic imperative as well. Given these explicit moral purposes, just any kind of knowledge will not do: the knowledge given by diagnosis must be *relevant to* the moral and practical demands of therapy because diagnosis is a purposeful knowing. The art and skill exhibited by the clinician in forging knowledge and moral purpose into effective action constitutes the *fourth aesthetic* of diagnosis.

DIAGNOSIS AS PRIVILEGE

The practical/moral frame of diagnosis has a further element, illustrated by Laennec's motivations to invent the stethoscope. In Victorian Europe, the idea of laying an ear between naked French breasts was justifiable, even thinkable, only through the provision of aid to a woman in dire distress. Probing the intimate details of people's lives and bodies is a privilege that, like all privileges, has particular responsibilities attached. The clinician is obligated to not misuse this privilege and knowledge and to apply these gifts only for furthering the patient's welfare; such is the ethos of the profession of medicine (Flexner 1915). This privilege today is articulated as duties and ethics, so that diagnosis-as-act involves respecting the people who are disclosing their most private truths, and diagnosis-as-denotation involves ensuring that, as a tool, the diagnostic category performs its function well. Privilege, then, implies a *fifth aesthetic*, that of respecting the patient in diagnostic practices.

DIAGNOSIS AS RATIONALITY

We noted earlier that understanding and treating illness is not always self-evident, that diagnosis involves a disclosure of the puzzle of illness. The riddle of illness implies that diagnosis requires not only observation but also interpretation. But the interpretation of illness manifestations characteristic of diagnosis are not just any kind of interpretation—that is, they are not mystical, intuitive, or self-reflexive interpretations or matters of taste.

The interpretation of illness manifestations, especially for clinical beginners or of maladies that are stubborn or elusive, is deliberative and rational, as noted by Al-Razi and the physicians of the British Enlightenment. The rationality of diagnosis is a curious one, however, related to the two senses we have already noted, diagnosis-as-signifier and diagnosis-as-act. Diagnostic rationality eludes characterization as simple theoretical or technical rationality, where simple truths are sought through (today's) scientific research, research that characterizes the aggregate of illnesses and not the uniquely ill individual. Diagnosis also exhibits features of practical rationality, whose features select actions toward particular practical goals, namely caring and curing (Phillips 2002). Stated differently, no serious diagnostician today would wish to dispense with scientific knowledge relevant to diagnosis—that is, to dispense with the elements of theoretical rationality—nor would a wise clinical practitioner wish to dispense with practical rationality, which would govern the application of theoretical knowledge to the goals of the clinic. The enigmatic rationality of diagnosis generates some of its most nagging philosophical problems, rivalries between particularism and universalism (Mezzich et al. 1996), between nomothetic and idiographic science (Sadler and Hulgus 1994), between theoretical and practical reason (Berger 1996; Phillips 2002), and between understanding (*Verstehen*) and explanation (*Erklären*) (Jaspers 1963; Wiggins and Schwartz 1997a, 1997b). Such ambiguities are reflected in the difficulties in articulating and practicing the fourth aesthetic of diagnosis, that of coalescing knowledge and moral purpose into effective action.

DIAGNOSIS AS RITUAL

The permutations of diagnostic interpretation almost universally have their own standards and norms. The strangeness of the Bantu diagnostic practices noted in the opening of this discussion suggest "ritual" to Western observers, but clinical ritual is not unique to traditional or third world societies. Indeed, ritual is part and parcel of clinical diagnostic training and practice in the West; it is manifested through history taking, examination of physical and mental status, and consideration of differential diagnosis, and it is even "inscribed into tablets" through structured diagnostic interviews, diagnostic manuals, and DSM decision trees (American Psychiatric Association 1994). The rituals of diagnosis suggest a *sixth* and complex normative *aesthetic*: that diagnosis should be rigorous, accountable, thorough, consistent, and the like. We might summarize these multifaceted diagnostic virtues as "clinical faithfulness"—to the "data," to the patient, to traditions, to the clinical context, to science, and to the other aesthetics of diagnosis.

Philosophical and rhetorical critiques of psychiatric diagnosis have, in past decades, tended to be derived from general critiques of psychiatry. For instance, if one is to pose, like Thomas Szasz (1961), a metaphysical view that characterizes mental disorders as only disease metaphors and not literal diseases, then psychiatric classification is a nominalistic systematization of such metaphorical diseases, closer to the nominalistic classification of books in libraries or groceries in the supermarket than to the biological (naturalistic) classification of species. If one views the sole purpose of psychiatry as the regulation of deviance and the securing of power, then diagnosis is merely one of the tools of such social machinations.

Critiques based on twentieth-century antipsychiatry themes fall into four motifs, though the four are not crisply distinct: labeling, medicalization, reductionism, and power. Each motif interrelates with others, depending on the author and the particular viewpoint. A more recent critical thread concerning psychiatric diagnosis, itself often critical of so-called antipsychiatry, concerns how diagnosis and classification reflect particular values. Such value-based critiques seek not just to expose the evaluative aspects of diagnosis but to reform or suggest the substitution of other value commitments, choices, or even systems (for instance, substituting the medical ethos of mental health care for other evaluative frameworks; see Charland, chapter 4 in this volume). So the general conceptual critiques of psychiatric diagnosis then can be loosely arranged as exhibiting five motifs: labeling, medicalization, reductionism, power, and values. As we shall see, each of these resonates in various ways with the meanings and functions of diagnosis as sketched in this discussion.

LABELING

In the 1960s and 1970s, some social thinkers articulated a view that emphasized the social-regulatory function of labeling, where social orders were created and maintained on the basis of the characterization of individuals in the society (Scheff, 1966, 1970, 1986; Sarbin 1967; Sarbin and Kitsuse 1994). Such "labeling" of people (like the mentally ill) then supplemented, even supplanted, the regulation of deviance by more overt or explicit social mechanisms, such as laws, education, and government agencies. Psychiatry was the paradigm example of such supplementary regulatory institutions, and the critical concern was that, because psychiatry's regulatory function was often implicit and its powers so great, it was prone to abuse and self-serving interests; indeed, the very notion of psychiatry came to be associated with regulation of deviance. In recent years, this critique has extended to explicit diagnostic systems like the DSM (*Diagnostic and Statistical Manual of Mental Disorders*) and ICD (*International Classification of Disease*) (see Sadler 2002a) classifications, where the proliferation of the numbers of mental disorders, along with the widespread use and public acceptance of these classifications, is interpreted as the expression of an expanding hegemonic social agenda for the regulation of deviance. The labeling theorists' critiques raise ongoing philosophical difficulties with the psychiatricnosological task: "How are we to characterize mental disorders? As expressions of culture? Of nature?" "If psychiatric labeling serves state or social interests, then what becomes of the moral task of psychiatric-medical healing?" "Are mental disorders clinical, moral, political, or some combination?"

MEDICALIZATION

The notion of medicalization, derivative upon reductionism, is that complex human phenomena are articulated or reduced into the terms of medicine and the clinic. For instance, if we consider the complex personal, cultural, biological, and political phenomenon of menstruation and focus instead on "premenstrual dysphoric disorder," we have redefined the larger phenomenon into an epistemologically, politically, ontologically, and implicitly more value-and theory-laden phenomenon, one that is explicitly medical at its conceptual core. We have "medicalized" menstruation; it becomes a referent to putative disease. As a second example, if we view the propensity to crime as primarily (or even merely substantively) a biogenetic phenomenon manipulable by genetic and neuropharmacological interventions, we have "medicalized" crime. The medicalization critique, then, addresses the motivations, functions, and consequences of psychiatric medicalization, the latter in large part formalized through explicit attempts to classify and diagnose mental disorders. In the case of the ever-expanding nomenclature of the DSM and ICD classifications, more and more domains of human experience come to be defined in reference to their associated "psychopathologies." Under a medicalization critique, the diagnosis and classification of mental disorders progresses toward a diagnosing and classifying of human life itself. Depending on the author and viewpoint, such medicalization critiques of psychiatry can focus on the marginalizing of other cultural views or discourses about the phenomena, may focus on the sociopolitical functions and motivations of medicalization, or may incorporate other themes (Ingleby 1982; Kovel 1980, 1982; Nissim-Sabat, 2001; Potter 2001; Russell 1994; Rothblum et al. 1986). These wide-ranging critiques can impugn psychiatric diagnosis as a kind of cultural imperialism, a tool of colonization, a factor in the repression of women's rights or equality, or simply the expression of self-interested capitalist greed through the expansion of the health care market share.

The philosophical questions raised by psychiatric medicalization include these: "In what senses, if any, should medicopsychiatric formulations of human distress prevail over other formulations?" "In particular, what is the proper role for medical formulations of human distress?" "How should medical formulations of human distress be constrained?" "What does medicalization do to our image of humanity?"

REDUCTIONISM

In philosophy of science, *reduction* often refers to the epistemological process of understanding complex phenomena in simpler terms (Schaffner 1994), here part of the epistemic charge of diagnosis. *Reductionism*, however, particularly in reference to discussions about psychiatric diagnosis, takes on a negatively connoted evaluative meaning, where the epistemological necessity of selective attention and interpretation is caricatured into a remote semblance of the phenomenon at hand. Here, the experience of depression becomes "little more" than a serotonin deficit. The reductionist critique of recent classifications like the DSMs or ICDs was articulated decades ago by psychoanalytic critics (e.g., Schimel 1976), but it has been echoed by critics of various theoretical stripes (e.g., Gergen et al. 1996; Kraus 1994; Mishara 1994), as well as by philosophers and cultural theorists (Gergen 1990; Harris and Schaffner 1992; Schaffner 1994; Margolis 1994).

Antireductionist critics of psychiatric diagnosis are concerned that focusing on simple, generalizable elements in helping distressed people dehumanizes them and transforms them into objects of theoretical manipulation instead of seeing them as peer-agents to be collaborated with. These general concerns may be voiced in various ways: as claims that diagnosis "silences" the dialogue, political or interpersonal, or marginalizes the social nature of mental disorders, or, as we'll see later, facilitates the perpetuation of power structures.

Considerations of reductionism in psychiatric diagnosis generate manifold philosophical problems: "If we overlook or set aside aspects of clinical phenomena, how can we be assured that our understanding and explanation of them are correct?" "What is the moral and humane significance of parsing out and objectifying human experience?" "If the psychiatrist's task is to interpret the patient's experiences anew, isn't reductionism the very undermining of this task of interpretation?"

POWER

The significance of psychiatric power has already been described, and the relationships among labeling, reduction, and medicalization have already been suggested. For Szaszians, psychiatric power reduces to that of a proxy for the state; such proxy governance exercises its power over its subjects unidirectionally, and the psychiatrist who declares a diagnosis is an example of the denial of civil liberty. This dynamic, along with Szasz's explicit political alliances, give the Szaszian account of psychiatric power a politically Libertarian flavor. Critics of psychiatry and psychiatric diagnosis from the left (e.g., Kovel 1980, 1982; Sedgwick 1982; Skene 2002; Foucault 1970, 1980,

1987, 1990) see psychiatric power as participating in a complex multidirectional interplay of various personal, social, economic, and political power structures. For instance, while involuntary hospitalization may deny, at least temporarily, key civil liberties, psychiatric treatment may ultimately liberate the impoverished schizophrenic person to pursue the American Dream, or, alternatively, to work as a Marxist proletarian to undermine capitalism and pursue the revolution. Psychiatric diagnosis, then, participates in the interplay of social and interpersonal power in various ways. As noted earlier, psychiatric diagnosis may close off opportunity in some sectors of society (through stigma and other mechanisms), but it is also the occasion for economic opportunity and social assistance. In the hands of philosophers like Foucault (1990), however, power, including psychiatric power, embraces more than mere economic or political power; it takes on metaphysical power as well, influencing how we understand ourselves, how we think, and what the "nature of things" is. Under Foucault's rubric, whether psychiatric diagnosis is liberating, enslaving, or something in between depends on the complex interplay of social and metaphysical "forces."

The critique of psychiatric power raises its own cluster of philosophical issues: "What is, and should be, the role of psychiatric diagnosis within society at large?" "How should mental health clinicians be accountable to the social impact of their diagnostic efforts?" "What is the function and importance of psychiatric criticism?"

VALUES

A more recent—and, if numbers of philosophical publications are indicative, perhaps the currently predominant—strand of philosophical appraisals of psychiatric diagnosis might be characterized as critiques of the values involved in psychiatric diagnosis and classification. The values critics by and large have assimilated both the efforts of mainstream psychiatric diagnostic classification efforts (like the World Health Organization's ICD manual and the American Psychiatric Association's DSMs) and those of the antipsychiatry-based critiques from the 1960s, 1970s, and 1980s discussed earlier. Generally sympathetic to the psychiatric and mental-health enterprise, the values theorists might be construed as taking a middle ground. Perhaps more accurately, values theorists could be viewed as taking alternative grounds, as the fundamental political/economic premises of antipsychiatry or critical theory (e.g., Libertarianism, Marxism) are not necessarily endorsed, and values theorists tend to center their perspective on conceptual/philosophical, not political or social, grounds.

The values critics of psychiatric diagnosis are quite wide ranging in their discussions, often, unlike many of their predecessors, considering particular diagnostic categories and practices and generally digging more deeply into the nitty-gritty of clinical practice and scientific research. Values theorists in the most general sense are concerned with *revealing* the evaluations or value judgments involved in psychiatric diagnosis and classification, in perhaps *revising* the various values involved in psychiatric diagnosis and classification, and even, on occasion, *rethinking* or substituting alternative value choices, value structures, or value commitments, as reflected in diagnostic systems and diagnostic practices. Values theorists exhibit a wide range of interests, from (a) considering the normative functions of diagnosis (Agich 1994; Sadler et al. 1994, 2000; Radden 1994; Sadler in press), to (b) analyzing metaphysical assumptions in diagnosis (Zachar 2000; Hacking 1999; Sadler in press), to (c) defining the relations of social values to other sorts of values in diagnosis (Sadler 2002a, in press; Wakefield 1992a, 1992b), to (d) considering how value commitments are implemented in the process of developing diagnostic systems (Sadler 2002b, in press), to (e) studying the logic of evaluation as reflected in diagnostic categories and diagnostic criteria (Fulford 1989, 1999, 2002). At present, values theorists' viewpoints are still very much in the making, rendering a historical perspective premature.

How can psychiatric diagnosis, and its controversies, be understood? In general, psychiatric diagnosis should be understood within the richness of its meanings, uses, ethics, and aesthetics. Careful scrutiny of ongoing discourses about psychiatric diagnosis often reveals that the "diagnosis" concept is considered only in part and not in its full complex meaning. Ironically, rhetoric around psychiatric diagnosis often has a reductionistic flavor of its own. In this sense, many critiques of psychiatric diagnosis have a straw-person quality—that of painting one dimension of diagnosis, omitting others, and then criticizing the single dimension or aspect.

One can find numerous examples of these sorts of omissions. For instance, rejections of formal diagnostic systems such as the DSMs or ICDs may be founded on notions of diagnosis-as-signifier only; diagnosis here is presented as a distorted, reductionistic oversimplification of the clinical encounter and a patient's life. In the extreme, diagnosis may be presented as a danger that should be rejected completely (Gergen et al. 1996). However, if one considers diagnosis-as-epistemic-act more carefully, such arguments fall away, as the problem becomes one of prudence in applying the aesthetics of diagnostic practice—that is, ensuring that the second aesthetic of diagnosis is respected (the revelatory aspects of diagnosis), along with the third aesthetic of diagnosis (balance between characterization and context), the fifth aesthetic (respecting the patient), and the sixth (faithfulness). These aesthetics tend to temper the distortions of an epistemic reductionism through regulating the practice elements, not the denotative elements, of diagnosis. Elegant diagnostic practice situates the reduction of denotative diagnosis within a richer context of clinical work.

As a second example, insensitivity to the social power of diagnosis may result from viewing diagnosis only as a medicalized denotative signifier and not as an epistemic act. If we reify our diagnostic categories into infallible truths (or merely into good scientific generalizations) that underlie natural processes, then we risk overlooking the moral impact diagnosis has on people's lives, as well as the function of diagnosis in society. In so doing, we fail to respect the fourth and sixth aesthetics (respecting people and faithfulness/accountability).

As a third example, critiques of psychiatric diagnosis might be founded on the marginalization of diagnosis; diagnosis is seen as simply irrelevant in taking care of human psychological distresses (see, for instance, Kirk and Kutchins's 1992 review of psychoanalytic views of DSM diagnosis). But this would be to ignore (naively) the first aesthetic of diagnosis, to characterize well, and runs the risk of ignoring the second and third (interpreting experience anew and balancing openness and rigor, respectively).

What often remains after considering the assorted meanings of psychiatric diagnosis is its proper place in society. This question, of course, is one for political and moral philosophy, social policy, and government. The question of meaningful, moral, and effective sociopolitical action regarding mental health care has a reach beyond the individual doctor-patient encounter, beyond diagnosis as act and signifier, and it will be a source of ongoing debate for years to come (Radden 2002).

REFERENCES

Ackerknecht, E. H. (1982) A Short History of Medicine, rev. ed. Baltimore: Johns Hopkins University Press.

Agich, G. J. (1994) "Evaluative Judgments and Personality Disorder." In J. Z. Sadler, O. P. Wiggins, and M. A. Schwartz (eds.), Philosophical Perspectives on Psychiatric Diagnostic Classification. Baltimore: Johns Hopkins University Press.

American Psychiatric Association (1994) Diagnostic and Statistical Manual of Mental Disorders (DSM-IV). 4th ed. Washington, DC: American Psychiatric Association.

Berger, Louis (1996) "Toward a Non-Cartesian Psychotherapeutic Framework: Radical Pragmatism as an Alternative." Philosophy, Psychiatry, and Psychology 3(3): 169–84.

Bernstein, Richard J. (1985) Beyond Objectivism and Relativism: Science, Hermeneutics, and Praxis. Philadelphia: University of Pennsylvania Press.

Dain, N. (1994) "Reflections on Antipsychiatry and Stigma in the History of American Psychiatry." American Journal of Psychiatry 45(10): 1010–15.

Fabrega, Horacio Jr. (1990) "Psychiatric Stigma in the Classical and Medieval Period: A Review of the Literature." Comprehensive Psychiatry 31(4): 289–306.

Fabrega, Horacio Jr. (1991) "The Culture and History of Psychiatric Stigma in Early Modern and Modern Western Societies: A Review of Recent Literature." Comprehensive Psychiatry 32(2): 97–119.

Flexner, Abraham (1915) "Is Social Work a Profession?" Proceedings of the National Conference of Charities and Correction, 42nd Annual Meeting, Baltimore, MD, May 12–19, 1915. Chicago: National Conference of Charities and Correction.

Foucault, M. (1970) The Order of Things: An Archeology of the Human Sciences. New York: Vintage.

Foucault, M. (1980) Power/Knowledge. Translated by C. Gordon. New York: Pantheon.

Foucault, M. (1987) Mental Illness and Psychology. Translated by A. Sheridan. Berkeley: University of California Press.

Foucault, M. (1990) History of Sexuality. Translated by R. Hurley. New York: Vintage.

Fulford, K. W. M. (1989) Moral Theory and Medical Practice. Cambridge: Cambridge University Press.

Fulford, K. W. M. (1994) "Closet Logics: Hidden Conceptual Elements in the DSM and ICD Classifications of Mental Disorders." In J. Z. Sadler, O. P. Wiggins, and M. A.

Schwartz (eds.), *Philosophical Perspectives on Psychiatric Diagnostic Classification*. Baltimore: Johns Hopkins University Press.

Fulford, K. W. M. (1999) "Nine Variations and a Coda on the Theme of an Evolutionary Definition of Dysfunction." *Journal of Abnormal Psychology* 108(3): 412–20.

Fulford, K. W. M. (2002) "Report to the Chair of the DSM-VI Task Force from the Editors of *PPP* on 'Contentious and Noncontentious Evaluative Language in Psychiatric Diagnosis.' " In John Z. Sadler (ed.), *Descriptions and Prescriptions: Values, Mental Disorders and the DSMs*. Baltimore: Johns Hopkins University Press, pp. 323–62.

Gergen, Kenneth J. (1990) "Therapeutic Professions and the Diffusion of Deficit." *Journal of Mind and Behavior* 11(3–4): 353–67.

Gergen, Kenneth J., Hoffman, Lynn, and Anderson, Harlene (1996) "Is Diagnosis a Disaster? A Constructionist Trialogue." In F. W. Kaslow (ed.), *Handbook of Relational Diagnosis and Dysfunctional Family Patterns*. New York: Wiley, pp. 102–18.

Gorenstein, E. E. (1992) *The Science of Mental Illness*. New York: Academic Press.

Grinnell, F. (1992) *The Scientific Attitude*, 2nd ed. New York: Guilford.

Hacking, I. (1999) *The Social Construction of What?* Cambridge, MA: Harvard University Press.

Harris, H., and Schaffner, K. (1992) "Molecular Genetics, Reductionism, and Disease Concepts in Psychiatry." *Journal of Medicine and Philosophy* 17(2): 127–53.

Ingleby, D. (1982) "The Social Construction of Mental Illness." In P. Wright and A. Treacher (eds.), *The Problem of Medical Knowledge: Examining the Social Construction of Medicine*. Edinburgh: Edinburgh University Press.

Jaspers, K. (1963) *General Psychopathology*. Translated by J. Hoenig and Marian W. Hamilton, with a new foreword by Paul R. McHugh. Baltimore: Johns Hopkins University Press.

Kirk, S. A., and Kutchins, H. (1992) *The Selling of DSM: The Rhetoric of Science in Psychiatry*. Hawthorne, NY: Aldine de Gruyter.

Kovel, J. (1980) "The American Mental Health Industry." In D. Ingleby (ed.), *Critical Psychiatry: The Politics of Mental Health*. New York: Pantheon, pp. 72–101.

Kovel, J. (1982) Book Review of *Diagnostic and Statistical Manual of Mental Disorders, Edition III*. *Einstein Quarterly Journal of Biology and Medicine* 1(2): 103–4.

Kraus, A. (1994) "Phenomenological and Criteriological Diagnosis: Different or Complementary?" In J. Sadler, O. P. Wiggins, and M. A. Schwartz (eds.), *Philosophical Perspectives on Psychiatric Diagnostic Classification*. Baltimore: Johns Hopkins University Press, pp. 148–60.

Leder, Drew (1990) *The Absent Body*. Chicago: University of Chicago Press.

Margolis, Joseph (1994) "Taxonomic Puzzles." In J. Sadler, O. P. Wiggins, and M. A. Schwartz (eds.), *Philosophical Perspectives on Psychiatric Diagnostic Classification*. Baltimore: Johns Hopkins University Press, pp. 104–28.

Mezzich, Juan E., Kleinman, Arthur, Fabrega, Horacio, and Parron Delores, L. (1996) *Culture and Psychiatric Diagnosis: A DSM-IV Perspective*. Washington, DC: American Psychiatric Press.

Mishara, A. L. (1994) "A Phenomenological Critique of Commonsensical Assumptions in DSM-III-R: The Avoidance of the Patient's Subjectivity." In J. Sadler, O. P. Wiggins, and M. A. Schwartz (eds.), *Philosophical Perspectives on Psychiatric Diagnostic Classification*. Baltimore: Johns Hopkins University Press, pp. 129–47.

Nissim-Sabat, M. (2001) Review of *Psychiatry, Psychoanalysis, and Race*. *Philosophy, Psychiatry, and Psychology* 8(1): 45–59.

Parsons, Talcott (1958) "Definitions of Health and Illness in the Light of American Values and Social Structure." In E. G. Jaco (ed.), *Patients, Physicians, and Illness*. Glencoe, IL: Free Press, pp. 165–87.

Phillips, James (2002) "Technical Reason in the DSM-IV: An Unacknowledged Value." In J. Z. Sadler (ed.), *Descriptions and Prescriptions: Values, Mental Disorders, and the DSMs*. Baltimore: Johns Hopkins University Press, pp. 76–95.

Porter, Roy (1997) *The Greatest Benefit to Mankind: A Medical History of Humanity*. Oxford: Oxford University Press.

Porter, Roy (2002) *Madness: A Brief History*. Oxford: Oxford University Press.

Potter, Nancy (2001) "Key Concepts: Feminism." *Philosophy, Psychiatry, and Psychology* 8(1): 61–71.

Radden, Jennifer (1994) "Recent Criticism of Psychiatric Nosology: A Review." *Philosophy, Psychiatry, and Psychology* 1(3): 193–200.

Radden, Jennifer (2002) "Psychiatric Ethics." *Bioethics* 16(5): 397–411.

Rothblum, E. D., Solomon, L. J., and Albee, G. W. (1986) "A Sociopolitical Perspective of DSM-III." In T. Millon and G. L. Klerman (eds.), *Contemporary Directions in Psychopathology: Towards the DSM-IV*. New York: Guilford, pp. 167–89.

Russell, D. (1993) "Psychiatric Diagnosis and the Interests of Women." In J. Z. Sadler, O. P. Wiggins, and M. A. Schwartz (eds.), *Philosophical Perspectives on Psychiatric Diagnostic Classification*. Baltimore: Johns Hopkins University Press, pp. 246–58.

Sadler, John Z. (ed.) 2002a. *Descriptions and Prescriptions: Values, Mental Disorders, and the DSMs*. Baltimore: Johns Hopkins University Press.

Sadler, John Z. (2002b) "Values in Developing Psychiatric Classifications: A Proposal for DSM-V." In John Z. Sadler (ed.), *Descriptions and Prescriptions: Values, Mental Disorders, and the DSMs*. Baltimore: Johns Hopkins University Press, pp. 301–22.

Sadler, John Z. (In press) *Values and Psychiatric Diagnosis*. Oxford: Oxford University Press.

Sadler, J. Z., and Hulgus, Y. F. (1994) "Enriching the Psychosocial Content of a Multiaxial Classification." In J. Z. Sadler, O. P. Wiggins, and M. A. Schwartz (eds.), *Philosophical Perspectives on Psychiatric Diagnostic Classification*. Baltimore: Johns Hopkins University Press, pp. 261–78.

Sadler, J. Z., Hulgus, Y. F., and Agich, G. J. (1994) "On Values in Recent American Psychiatric Classification." *Journal of Medicine and Philosophy* 19: 261–77.

Sadler, J. Z., Hulgus, Y. F., and Agich, G. J. (2001) "Hindsight, Foresight, and Having It Both Ways: A Rejoinder to R. L. Spitzer." *Journal of Nervous and Mental Disease* 189(8): 493–97.

Sarbin, T. R. (1967) "On the Futility of the Proposition That Some People Be Labeled "Mentally Ill." *Journal of Consulting Psychology* 31(5): 447–53.

Sarbin, T. R., and Kitsuse, J. I. (1994) *Constructing the Social*. London: Sage.

Schaffner, K. F. (1994) "Psychiatry and Molecular Biology: Reductionistic Approaches to Schizophrenia." In J. Sadler, O. P. Wiggins, and M. A. Schwartz (eds.), *Philosophical Perspectives on Psychiatric Diagnostic Classification*. Baltimore: Johns Hopkins University Press, pp. 279–94.

Scheff, T. J. (1966) *Being Mentally Ill: A Sociological Theory*. Chicago: Aldine.

Scheff, T. J. (1970) "Schizophrenia as Ideology." *Schizophrenia Bulletin* 2: 15–19.

Scheff, T. J. (1986) "Accountability in Psychiatric Diagnosis: A Proposal." In T. Millon and G. Klerman (eds.), *Contemporary Directions in Psychopathology: Toward the DSM-IV*. New York: Guilford, pp. 265–77.

Schimel, John (1976) "The Retreat from a Psychiatry of People." *Journal of the American Academy of Psychoanalysis* 4: 131–35.

Sedgwick, P. (1982) *Psycho Politics*. New York: Harper and Row.

Sigerist, Henry E. (1951) A *History of Medicine*. Vol. 1: *Primitive and Archaic Medicine*. Baltimore: Johns Hopkins University Press.

Sigerist, Henry E. (1961) A *History of Medicine*. Vol. 2: *Early Greek, Hindu, and Persian Medicine*. Baltimore: Johns Hopkins University Press.

Skene, Allyson (2002) "Rethinking Normativism in Psychiatric Classification." In J. Z. Sadler (ed.), *Descriptions and Prescriptions: Values, Mental Disorders, and the DSMs*. Baltimore: Johns Hopkins University Press, pp. 114–27.

Szasz, T. S. (1961) *The Myth of Mental Illness: Foundations of a Theory of Personal Conduct*. New York: Hoeber-Harper.

Taylor, Elizabeth (ed.) (1988) *Dorland's Illustrated Medical Dictionary*, 27th ed. Philadelphia: W. B. Saunders.

Wakefield, J. (1992a) "Disorder as Harmful Dysfunction: A Conceptual Critique of DSM-III-R's Definition of Mental Disorder." *Psychological Review* 99(2): 232–47.

Wakefield, J. (1992b) "The Concept of Mental Disorder: On the Boundary between Biological Facts and Social Values." *American Psychologist* 47(3): 373–88.

Wiggins, Osborne P., and Schwartz, Michael A. (1997a) "Edmund Husserl's Influence on Karl Jaspers's Phenomenology." *Philosophy, Psychiatry, and Psychology* 4(1): 15–36.

Wiggins, Osborne P., and Schwartz, Michael A. (1997b) "Karl Jaspers." In L. Embree, E. A. Behnke, D. Carr et al. (eds.), *Encyclopedia of Phenomenology*. Dordrecht: Kluwer Academic, pp. 371–76.

Zachar, Peter (2000) "Psychiatric Disorders Are Not Natural Kinds." *Philosophy, Psychiatry, and Psychology* 7(3): 167–82.

CHAPTER 12

UNDERSTANDING/ EXPLANATION

JAMES PHILLIPS

UNDERSTANDING and explanation are not innocent terms used interchangeably in psychiatric discourse. They are technical terms that represent two opposed approaches to a comprehension of human behavior. In this chapter I begin with a preliminary explication of the terms, then offer a case history to exemplify their application in psychiatry, and finally review the further development of the terms since their initial articulation.

The categories of understanding and explanation were introduced in the late nineteenth century by the German philosopher Wilhelm Dilthey.[1] He was reacting to the dominance of the physical sciences in contemporary intellectual life and to the prevailing thought that all disciplines needed to model themselves on the physical sciences to secure adequate scientific grounding. Dilthey sought to secure for the human disciplines such as history and psychology (the *Geisteswissenschaften*) a unique methodology that would be different from but on par with the methodology of the natural sciences (the *Naturwissenschaften*). Dilthey formulated the methodological difference around the distinction between explanation (*Erklären*) and understanding (*Verstehen*): "We *explain* nature, but we *understand* psychic life" (Dilthey 1924 [1894]: 144). According to Dilthey, the natural sciences treat nature as objects and forces that can be explained through causal laws. The goal of such sciences is the establishment of such general, causally formulated laws. The scientist "knows" his object from the outside and remains alien to the object. In contrast, human studies such as history and psychology have for their "object" the human subject, which they "know" from the inside. The scientist *explains* through causal connections; the historian or psychologist *understands* through the interpretation of the meaning structures she finds in the text or other person. I can know the inner life of another person because I also am a person. I understand the other just as I understand myself, through the network of meanings associated with the behavior of each (Dilthey 1989 [1883]). Because the result of this understanding is not a causal law but, rather, an interpretation of meaning, understanding always involves interpretation, and the two terms are often used interchangeably. The art (or science) of interpretation is also known as hermeneutics, and thus the methodology of the human sciences is referred to both as understanding and as hermeneutics.

Hermeneutic methodology as developed by Dilthey generated a series of concerns that are unique to hermeneutic understanding and that distinguish it from natural scientific methodology. All of these concerns can readily be applied to the field of psychiatry. One concern is a focus on the individual. While natural science is interested in the individual only as an instance of the general law, the emphasis in hermeneutic understanding is the opposite. In the psychiatric encounter, we focus on the individual before us and use the discipline's generalizations only to aid in understanding the individual patient. A second concern is a focus on the historical and psychological context of the author or agent. In attempting to interpret a historical agent or literary text, we understand the agent or text in terms of the historical and psychological text in which it emerged. Likewise, in the psychiatric encounter, we place the presenting problem or symptom in biographical and social context. Finally, a unique dimension of hermeneutic methodology is the notion of the hermeneutic circle or round. Every level of hermeneutic investigation — whether literary text, historical monument, historical agent, or psychiatric patient — involves an understanding in terms of part-whole meaning structures that is quite different from the causal analysis of the physical sciences. In the interpretation or analysis of a novel, for instance, a chapter is understood in terms of the whole novel, while at the same time the novel as a whole is understood in terms of the individual chapters. We do not say that the chapters "cause" the novel or that the novel "causes" the chapters; rather, we understand and interpret each in relation to the other. We follow a similar procedure in understanding a psychiatric patient: we understand the particular symptom or problem in terms of the entire life, and we understand the life in terms of those individual symptoms, problems, and countless other particulars. The coherence of a life is a coherence of meaning structures, for which the hermeneutic methodology of part-whole understanding is quite applicable.

Finally, in this introduction to hermeneutic understanding, it is important to appreciate that for Dilthey hermeneutic understanding does not take place, as is often thought, through introspection, intuition, or empathy. Rather, it is the nature of human life to express itself, and understanding in the human sciences involves the interpretation of the objectifications of inner life. Hermeneutics is thus the method of interpreting and understanding human expression. To quote Dilthey:

> We can distinguish the human studies from the sciences by certain, clear, characteristics. These are to be found in the attitude of mind, already described, which moulds the subject-matter of the human studies quite differently from that of sci-

entific knowledge. Humanity seen through the senses is just a physical fact which can only be explained scientifically. It only becomes the subject-matter of the human studies when we experience human states, give expressions to them and understand these expressions. The interrelation of life, expression and understanding, embraces gestures, facial expressions and words, all of which men use to communicate with each other; it also includes permanent mental creations which reveal their author's deeper meaning, and lasting objectifications of the mind in social structures where common human nature is surely, and for ever, manifest. The psycho-physical unit, man, knows even himself through the same mutual relationship of expression and understanding; he becomes aware of himself in the present; he recognizes himself in memory as something that once was; but, when he tries to hold fast and grasp his states of mind by turning his attention upon himself, the narrow limits of such an introspective method of self-knowledge show themselves; only his actions and creations and the effect they have on others teach man about himself. So he gains self-knowledge by the circuitous route of understanding. . . . A discipline only belongs to the human studies when we can approach its subject-matter through the connection between life, expression and understanding. (Dilthey 1976: 175–76)

In this passage Dilthey refers to the expressions of human life as "gestures, facial expressions and words." We need add to his list only the symptoms and signs of psychiatric illness, and we have placed psychiatry within the gambit of hermeneutic understanding. We do not, then, intuit the mental state of the patient; we understand and interpret the meaning of his presentation, whatever that complex of words, gestures, and emotional expressions may be.

A CASE HISTORY

Let us now test out these notions of understanding and explanation in the context of a case history. The patient, Mrs. D, is a 45-year-old married mother of two. She had shown a tendency toward depression for much of her adult life and presented in this, her first psychiatric encounter, in a full-blown depression. She described a familiar array of symptoms: depressed mood, guilt, anhedonia, negative thinking, loss of energy and motivation, and suicidal ideation. The immediate precipitant for the depression was the psychiatric hospitalization of one of her adolescent children, a 15-year-old daughter who was herself depressed and who had made a suicide gesture. Mrs. D experienced this as a confirmation of her bad mothering and felt deeply responsible for her daughter's problems. In the initial sessions, further dimensions of her history unfolded. She had grown up in a bleak factory town in a family in which her parents were locked in a bad marriage and were both depressed, and her father was alcoholic. He was a minimally successful midlevel manager in the local factory who considered himself a failure and who dealt with his depression through drinking and withdrawing from the family. Mrs. D was a successful student and seemed in her adolescent years to surmount her background and get on with her life. She graduated from college with a degree in accounting, obtained a good job in the city where she attended college, and married a couple years after graduation. Her husband was an easygoing, affectionate man who did not make demands that the patient, somewhat constricted emotionally, could not meet. Mrs. D experienced a first major setback when, a couple years into her marriage, she had to undergo a hysterectomy for a significant, but not cancerous, medical condition. This event thwarted the couple's plans for having children, and after a period of seemingly appropriate mourning and depression on the patient's part, the couple decided to adopt children. They did the adoptions through a local agency and knew little of the biologic parents except that their daughter's mother had been something of a wayward girl. The children's early years were mostly uneventful, although the daughter showed a tendency toward hyperactivity and aggressiveness that was a poor fit with Mrs. D's sober style. In retrospect, it appeared that through these years Mrs. D harbored many ambivalent feelings concerning the adoptions and concerning her daughter's biologic parentage and character. When this girl reached adolescence, she began showing a combination of conduct-disordered and depressive symptoms. Mrs. D was ill equipped to deal with this situation, and much conflict between mother and daughter ensued. The problems culminated in the psychiatric hospitalization of her daughter and Mrs. D's clinical depression.

There were multiple aspects to Mrs. D's treatment. She was clearly a candidate for antidepressant medication and welcomed it. The medication had a clear mood-improving effect but made only a minor dent in her negativistic character style. Although feeling better after several weeks of medication, she still considered herself responsible for a life that had gone bad. It was only in psychotherapy sessions extended over many months that Mrs. D's attitudes began to change. These therapeutic discussions revealed her unwarranted assumption of personal responsibility for the hysterectomy; her ambivalent feelings toward her adopted daughter as the flawed reincarnation of a morally bad, biologic mother; and, of course, her sense of having to repeat the bleak life of her parents. Her relationship with me involved an expectation that I would follow in the footsteps of her parents and agree with their fatalistic, negative attitude toward life. Needless to say, the treatment did not make Mrs. D a different person. But she did emerge from the clinical depression, and she did in the end have a more balanced attitude toward life and a better, more realistic attitude toward her children.

In trying now to comprehend Mrs. D.'s condition in the conceptual framework of understanding and explanation, we are confronted with a phenomenon for which Dilthey has not prepared us. His statement—"We *explain* nature, but we *understand* psychic life"—indicates that causal explanation is directed at nature, while understanding is the method for dealing with human psychic life.[2] But Mrs. D, like any patient, is both meaning *and* natural process. She then requires both understanding *and* explanation. It is not difficult to locate the dimensions of understanding and explanation in our comprehension of this woman's condition and the treatment. Mrs. D showed clear indications of a genetic and constitutional predisposition toward depression, and the antidepressant medication certainly targeted her biomedical vulnerability. Explanation in terms of causal analysis readily fits this aspect of the treatment: antidepressants working on neuroreceptors and receptor sites in brain mood centers cause an alternation in the patient's mood. At the same time, the meanings that she gave to life events — her sense of being condemned to repeat her parents' life, her attitude toward the hysterectomy, her ambivalence toward her adopted children — also played a role in the genesis of her depression and in the treatment. The latter did not merely involve giving her pills; it also involved understanding *her* understanding of her life and helping her to correct that understanding in a beneficial way.

Sorting out the dimensions of understanding and explanation in this case history — as, again, in most case histories — is yet more complicated. On the one hand, Mrs. D's constitutional predisposition to depression, her altered brain state, did not simply "cause" an altered mood; to some degree her altered brain and altered mood "caused" her to think about the world in a different way, to give depressed meanings to her experiences. Thus, the causal dimension of explanation invades the dimension of meaning. On the other hand, the meanings with which she framed her life experiences themselves had a causal effect on her mood. This is the basis of the cognitive therapy of depression. Thus, while it remains very useful to distinguish the understanding of meaning and the explanation of causes, we must also recognize the deep interpenetration of these two dimensions in our analysis of any human being.

FURTHER DEVELOPMENTS

The further development of the understanding/explanation approach to the human studies has been complex. Over the course of the twentieth century, the field of hermeneutics has been developed by, among others, Hans-Georg Gadamer (1975 [1960]), Jürgen Habermas (1971 [1968]), Peter Winch (1990), Georg von Wright (1971), Karl-Otto Apel (1984), Paul Ricoeur (1974 [1969], 1981), and Charles Taylor (1985).[3] Max Weber introduced the methodology of *Verstehen* into sociology (Diggins 1996: 110–31), and under his influence Karl Jaspers introduced the conceptual framework of understanding and explanation into psychiatry with his landmark publication, *General Psychopathology* (1963 [1946]). In that work Jaspers devoted a major section to *verstehende Psychologie* (the psychology of meaningful connections). Jaspers broadened the range of explanation in psychology and psychiatry, arguing that, while understanding is limited to meaningful connections, causal analysis can penetrate anywhere. He wrote: "It is a mistake to suggest that the psyche is the field for understanding while the physical world is the field for causal explanation. Every

concrete event—whether of a physical or psychical nature—is open to causal explanation. There is no limit to the discovery of causes and with every psychic event we
always look for cause and effect" (1963 [1946]: 305). Furthermore, in a condition such
as schizophenia, Jaspers found that understanding (the psychology of meaningful
connections) reaches a limit; the patient's utterances are "ununderstandable," and
the condition falls primarily into the realm of causal analysis.[4]

The Jasperian tradition has continued into the present in the work of Schwartz
and Wiggins (1987; Schwartz et al. 1989) and in that of McHugh and Slavney (1998).
These theoreticians have tended, like Jaspers, to separate psychiatric conditions that
require a causal, disease-oriented explanation from those that lend themselves to an
interpretative understanding of meaning structures. Like Jaspers, they recognize the
overlapping of understanding and explanation in most psychiatric conditions. Mc-
Hugh and Slavney, for instance, while distinguishing the disease concept (requiring
causal explanation) from the life-story perspective (requiring interpretative understanding), write that "our understanding of *disease* and its course need not blind us
to the *life story* source of the psychological responses of the patient who suffers from
it" (1998: 62).

Another area in which the understanding/explanation distinction has been debated is psychoanalysis. Freud had wanted a scientific status for psychoanalysis, and
early psychoanalytic theoreticians argued for that distinction. George Klein (1976)
and Merton Gill (1976) were psychoanalytic theoreticians who first challenged psychoanalysis's status as a natural science and argued that it had more to do with the
understanding of meaning and purpose than with causal analysis.[5] Another stage in
the rethinking of psychoanalysis was carried out by philosophers Jürgen Habermas
(1971 [1968]), Karl-Otto Apel (1967), and Paul Ricoeur (1970 [1965]). Each argued for
the hermeneutic (and thus *Verstehen*) status of psychoanalysis, although each also
argued that psychoanalysis has cause-like features. For Ricoeur, the patient is someone involved in a network of meanings who is, at the same time, caught up in a field
of cause-like forces—someone who is to be treated both like a text to be interpreted
and like an organism subject to causal mechanisms. A final and recent stage in
psychoanalytic thinking is the adoption by psychoanalysts themselves of the language
of hermeneutics. Roy Schafer (1983, 1992) stands out as the preeminent psychoanalytic theoretician who has forcefully articulated the hermeneutic view of psychoanalysis. Finally, what may be considered an "official" announcement of the death of
psychoanalysis as an explanatory, causal science was the 1994 issue of the *International
Journal of Psycho-Analysis* (Tuckett 1994), titled "The Conceptualization and Communication of Clinical Facts in Psychoanalysis," on the occasion of the seventy-fifth
anniversary edition of the journal. In this 300-page issue, there was widespread agreement that psychoanalytic "facts" are meanings to be interpreted, not objects to be
observed and causally explained.[6]

Further developments in the course of understanding and explanation in contemporary psychiatry require an appreciation of the transformation of these concepts
through the work of Thomas Kuhn (1970, 1977). With his groundbreaking work, *The
Structure of Scientific Revolutions*, first published in 1962, Kuhn challenged the stan-

dard, positivist notion of science as a unified structure that develops in an incremental, progressive manner. He contrasts such "normal science" with "revolutionary science" that challenges the prevailing "paradigm" with a new one—a new way to do science and to solve the problems left unsettled by the older paradigm. Since Dilthey's concept of *Erklären* was based on the traditional, positivist notion of science, it is inevitable that the Kuhnian revolution would challenge the Diltheyan, nineteenth-century view of explanation. Just as understanding always involves interpretation—and the inevitability of multiple perspectives and interpretations—so now the sciences are caught in the same interpretative vortex: different perspectives on how to interpret a text; different perspectives on how to do science. The philosopher Richard Rorty, in his *Philosophy and the Mirror of Nature* (1979), drew out the broader implications of Kuhn's revolution and redefined hermeneutics as no longer the interpretative methodology specific to the human studies but, rather, as a discipline for dealing with the incommensurability of perspectives in any domain. He distinguished "normal discourse," in which there is agreement about terms and rules of adjudication, and "abnormal discourse," in which such agreement does not exist. Hermeneutics, then, is simply the effort to communicate in the face of incommensurability of perspectives or languages.

The consequence of this development in contemporary psychiatry is a further collapse of the straightforward distinction between understanding and explanation. We have already spoken of the interpenetration of understanding and explanation in psychiatry; now we must add that the causal, explanatory dimension is itself subject to differing interpretative perspectives. Advances in neuroscience and psychopharmacology have led psychiatry in a causal/explanatory direction, but the proliferation of theories and treatments points to the absence of a unified scientific model of psychiatric illness. Further, neuroscience and its findings of neuroplasticity have also lent support to the notion that psychotherapy and its work with the patient's meaning structures have an effect on the brain. Our understanding of a condition like major depression, of such cases as that of Mrs. D, points to the interweaving of meaning and cause, understanding and explanation—as well as to the multiplicity of perspectives—in both the etiology and the treatment of the condition.

We witness the phenomenon of multiple perspectives and the interpenetration of understanding and explanation in the work of those who have theorized in this direction. One example is Engel's work with the biopsychosocial model (1977, 1980), in which he attempts to formulate the application of three perspectives in a comprehensive view of the patient. Another example is the work of Sadler and Hulgus (1991), in which they demonstrate how different theoretical orientations generate different data and treatments and how an ability to shift between models may lead to a more nuanced treatment.

Finally, the area of diagnosis—the progression from one Diagnostic and Statistical Manual (DSM) to the next and the many controversies over nosology—demonstrates both the conflict of perspectives over how to develop a scientific nosology of psychiatric disorders and the controversy over what the balance of meaning and cause should be in any particular diagnosis (Sadler et al. 1994). A fundamental issue in the nosology controversies is whether an atheoretical diagnostic system—the goal of the DSMs—is even possible. If, as some argue, values always creep into the diagnostic categories, we have a strong example of how the dimension of meaning infiltrates our understanding of psychiatric entities. Fulford (1989) has raised the same issue regarding our basic notions of mental illness, arguing that current values always enter into our definitions.

The issue of values raises the understanding/explanation discussion to another level. We are now not talking about the networks of meaning we understand and interpret in the patient, and we are not talking about the balance of meaning and cause in our comprehension of the patient. Rather, we are discussing the meanings that we, the clinicians, bring to the patient and the field. There is no stronger argument for the enduring usefulness of understanding in psychiatry than this need to apply it to ourselves in our work and in our theorizing. It is appropriate, then, to conclude this chapter by invoking the work of Hans-Georg Gadamer (1975 [1960]), the century's preeminent theoretician of hermeneutics, who argues that we always interpret from a perspective—a horizon of understanding, in his language—and that the most we can do is to be as aware as possible of the perspective from which we are understanding and interpreting. We would do well to heed his words as we concoct our diagnoses, our treatments, and our theories.

NOTES

1. The terms had, in fact, been introduced earlier by the historian Johann Droysen (Mackkreel 1975: 36), but it was Dilthey who developed and generalized the concepts. These concepts also have ancient antecedents dating from classical times. Aristotle distinguished practical knowledge, *phronēsis*, from technical knowledge, *technē*. In a rough way his distinction corresponds to that between understanding and explanation. With the revolution in science in the seventeenth century, Aristotle's technical (and theoretical) knowledge was transformed into the scientific method, and his notion of practical knowledge was relegated to the diminished category of secondary qualities. This transformation has been studied by Toulmin (2001), and Gadamer (1975) has specifically spelled out the way in which Aristotelian practical knowledge has been revived in hermeneutic understanding. (See also Dunne 1993; Phillips 2002a, 2002b.)

2. Dilthey recognized that explanation does have a place in psychology (Mackkreel 1975: 59) and that man is not only psychic life but also natural process. He wrote, for instance, that "the human studies embrace many physical facts and are based on knowledge of the physical world. . . . In fact, an individual like any other animal originates, survives and develops through the functioning of his body and its relation to his physical environment; his sense of life is, at least partly, based on this functioning" (Dilthey 1976: 163). He gave this little attention, however, in his effort to assert the independence of the human studies.

3. A dimension of hermeneutical understanding not addressed by Dilthey—but underscored by some of these authors, especially by Taylor with his notion of man as a "self-interpreting animal"—is that the human subject always comes pre-interpreted. That is, our

interpretation of another person involves an interpretation of the self-understanding that that person brings to the encounter. Giddens (1977) refers to this as a double hermeneutic, and Schafer in psychoanalysis (1992) refers to a retelling along psychoanalytic lines of the story that the patient brings to the treatment (for a review of hermeneutics, see Phillips 1996).

4. Jaspers distinguished between psychoses that have no meaningful connection to experience, and for which experience can at most serve as a trigger, and psychoses (reactive psychoses) that flow meaningfully from life experience. Of the latter he writes: "The psychosis has a meaning, either as a whole or in its individual details. It serves as a defence, an escape, as a wish-fulfillment. It springs from a conflict with reality which has become intolerable. But we should not over-rate the significance of such understanding" (1963 [1946]: 389). Although Jaspers would probably place Mrs. D in his class of reactive psychoses, it is not clear that his distinction adequately addresses the interpenetration of cause and meaning in a condition such as hers.

5. To his credit, Karl Jaspers recognized the hermeneutic dimension of psychoanalysis decades earlier: "With regard to psychopathology, psychoanalysis has the merit of having intensified *the observation of meaningful connections*. The attention that was paid to small and minute signs and to phenomena which hitherto had been unnoticed or thought unimportant, taught our consciousness to apprehend countless expressive phenomena. Such apprehension expressed itself as interpretation. Gestures, actions, mistakes, modes of speech, forgetting, as well as neurotic symptoms, dream-contents and delusions, all came to mean something other than what they appeared to do at first or what was at first intended"(Jaspers 1963 [1946]: 360). Jaspers also recognized the limits of psychoanalysis as an interpretative discipline: "The *limits* of every psychology of meaningful connections must necessarily remain the same for psychoanalysis in so far as the latter is meaningful. . . . Psychoanalysis has always *shut its eyes* to these limitations and has *wanted to understand everything*" (363).

6. For a review of the issue of hermeneutics in psychoanalysis, see Phillips 1991.

REFERENCES

Apel, K.-O. (1967) *Analytic Philosophy of Language and the* Geisteswissenschaften. Dordrecht: D. Reidel.

Apel, K.-O. (1984) *Understanding and Explanation: A Transcendental-Pragmatic Perspective.* Translated by G. Warnke. Cambridge, MA: MIT Press.

Diggins, J. P. (1996) *Max Weber: Politics and the Spirit of Tragedy.* New York: Basic Books.

Dilthey, W. (1924 [1894]) "Ideen über eine beschreibende und zergliedernde Psychologie." In Georg Misch (ed.), *Gesammelte Schriften.* Vol. 5: *Die geistige Welt: Einleitung in die Philosophie des Lebens. Erste Hälfte: Abhandllungen zur Grundlegung der Geisteswissenschaften.* Göttingen: Vandenhoeck and Ruprecht.

Dilthey, W. (1976) *W. Dilthey: Selected Writings.* Edited, translated, and introduced by H. P. Rickman. Cambridge: Cambridge University Press.

Dilthey, W. (1989 [1883]) *Introduction to the Human Sciences. Selected Works.* Vol. 1. Princeton: Princeton University Press.

Droysen, J. G. (1943) *Historik,* 2nd ed. Edited by Rudolf Hübner. Munich: Verlag von R Oldenbourg.

Dunne, J. (1993) *Back to the Rough Ground: "Phronesis" and "Techne" in Modern Philosophy and in Aristotle.* Notre Dame: University of Notre Dame Press.

Engel, G. (1977) "The Need for a New Medical Model: A Challenge for Biomedicine." *Science* 196: 129–36.

Engel, G. (1980) "The Clinical Application of the Biopsychosocial Model." *American Journal of Psychiatry* 137: 5535–44.

Fulford, K. W. M. (1989) *Moral Theory and Medical Practice*. Cambridge: Cambridge University Press.

Gadamer, H.-G. (1975) *Truth and Method*. New York: Continuum Press.

Giddens, A. (1977) *Studies in Social and Political Theory*. New York: Basic Books.

Gill, M. (1976). "Metapsychology Is Not Psychology." In M. Gill and P. Holzman (eds.), *Psychology versus Metapsychology: Psychoanalytic Essays in Memory of George S. Klein*. Psychological Issues, vol. 9. Monograph no. 36. New York: International Universities Press, pp. 71–105.

Habermas, J. (1971 [1968]) *Knowledge and Human Interests*. Translated by J. Shapiro. Boston: Beacon Press.

Jaspers, K. (1963 [1946]) *General Psychopathology*. Translated by J. Hoenig and M. Hamilton. Manchester: Manchester University Press.

Klein, G. (1976) *Psychoanalytic Theory*. New York: International Universities Press.

Kuhn, T. (1970) *The Structure of Scientific Revolutions*, 2nd ed. Chicago: University of Chicago Press.

Kuhn, T. (1977) *The Essential Tension: Selected Studies in Scientific Tradition and Change*. Chicago: University of Chicago Press.

Mackkreel, R. (1975) *Dilthey: Philosopher of the Human Studies*. Princeton: Princeton University Press.

McHugh, P., and Slavney, P. (1998) *The Perspectives of Psychiatry*, 2nd ed. Baltimore: Johns Hopkins University Press.

Phillips, J. (1991) "Hermeneutics in Psychoanalysis: Review and Reconsideration." *Psychoanalysis and Contemporary Thought* 14: 371–424.

Phillips, J. (1996) "Key Concepts: Hermeneutics." *Philosophy, Psychiatry, and Psychology* 3: 61–69.

Phillips, J. (2002a) "Technical Reason in the DSM-IV: An Unacknowledged Value." In John Z. Sadler (ed.), *Descriptions and Prescriptions: Values, Mental Disorders, and the DSMs*. Baltimore: Johns Hopkins University Press, pp. 76–95.

Phillips, J. (2002b). "Managed Care's Reconstruction of Human Existence: The Triumph of Technical Reason." *Theoretical Medicine* 23: 339–58.

Ricoeur, P. (1970 [1965]) *Freud and Philosophy*. Translated by D. Savage. New Haven: Yale University Press.

Ricoeur, P. (1974 [1969]) "The Conflict of Interpretations." In D. Ihde (ed.), *Essays in Hermeneutics*. Evanston, IL: Northwestern University Press.

Ricoeur, P. (1981) *Hermeneutics and the Human Sciences: Essays on Language, Action, and Interpretation*. Translated by E. Thompson. Cambridge: Cambridge University Press.

Rorty, R. (1979) *Philosophy and the Mirror of Nature*. Princeton: Princeton University Press.

Sadler, J., and Hulgus, Y. (1991) "Clinical Controversy and the Domains of Scientific Evidence." *Family Process* 30: 21–36.

Sadler, J., Wiggins, O., and Schwartz, M. (eds.) (1994) *Philosophical Perspectives on Psychiatric Classification*. Baltimore: Johns Hopkins University Press.

Schafer, R. (1983) *The Analytic Attitude*. New York: Basic Books.

Schafer, R. (1992) *Retelling a Life: Narration and Dialogue in Psychoanalysis*. New York: Basic Books.

Schwartz, M., and Wiggins, O. (1987) "Diagnosis and Ideal Types: A Contribution to Psychiatric Classification." *Comprehensive Psychiatry* 28: 277–91.

Schwartz, M., Wiggins, O., et al. (1989) "Prototypes, Ideal Types, and Personality Disorders." *Journal of Personality Disorders* 3: 1–9.

Taylor, C. (1985) "Self-interpreting Animals." In C. Taylor (ed.), *Human Agency and Language: Philosophical Papers*, vol. 1. Cambridge: Cambridge University Press.

Toulmin, S. (2001) *Return to Reason.* Cambridge, MA: Harvard University Press.

Tuckett, D. E. (1994) "The Conceptualization and Communication of Clinical Facts in Psychoanalysis." *International Journal of Psycho-Analysis* 75: 865–1297.

von Wright, G. (1971) *Explanation and Understanding.* Ithaca, NY: Cornell University Press.

Winch, P. (1990) *The Idea of a Social Science and Its Relation to Philosophy*, 2nd ed. London: Routledge.

CHAPTER 13

REDUCTIONISM/ ANTIREDUCTIONISM

TIM THORNTON

SCIENTIFIC reductionism is the view that higher-level theories can be reduced to lower-level theories. In psychiatry it underpins the claims to preeminence of biological psychiatry and the assumption that brain imaging techniques are ipso facto ways of seeing the mind (Posner 1993). But while there have been important advances in both these areas, there are reasons to be skeptical that psychiatry might be reduced without remainder to a fully biological or neurophysiological science.

One area of difficulty is the fact that psychiatry trades in reasons as well as (other sorts of) causes. Jaspers (1974) gives a clear expression of this distinction in his "Causal and 'Meaningful' Connections." Psychiatry aims to make behavior intelligible within the "space of reasons" as well as the "realm of (natural) law" (to use the terminology of Wilfred Sellars, repopularized by John McDowell). Can its methods and its subject matter be unified in order to reduce it to lower-level scientific description?

Another area concerns the central concept of disorder. Can disorder be reduced to more basic scientific terms, or does it presuppose a special kind of intelligibility?

In this chapter I outline the origins of reductionism and its connection to the unity of science and to philosophical naturalism, explore its motivation for philosophers of mind and of mental disorder, and sketch out the backlash against it that emerges from a reappropriation of a prescientific revolution worldview.

REDUCTIONISM, THE UNITY OF SCIENCE, AND PHILOSOPHICAL NATURALISM

In the early part of the twentieth century, reductionism was construed not merely as an expression of the view that "the physical is all there is" but as an aspect of the broader thesis that the sciences could, ultimately, be unified. The logical positivists construed reductionism as a logical or semantic thesis about the relation between theories. Broadly, one theory could be reduced to another if its terms could be defined using the terms of the reducing theory and its laws could be explained by the laws of the reducing theory. "Bridge laws" would connect higher-level types to lower-level types. Scientific progress would reduce "higher-level" theories to lower-level ones.

The assumption is still widespread that psychiatry and psychology will eventually be reduced to biology (which might be construed as physiology or evolutionary biology), biology to chemistry, and chemistry to physics. Oppenheim and Putnam expressed this view in their classic 1958 paper "Unity of Science as Working Hypothesis":

> It is not absurd to suppose that psychological laws may eventually be explained in terms of the behavior of individual neurons in the brain; that the behavior of individual cells—including neurons—may eventually be explained in terms of their biochemical constitutuion; and that the behavior of molecules—including the macromolecules that make up living cells—may eventually be explained in terms of atomic physics. If this is achieved, then psychological laws will have, *in principle*, been reduced to laws of atomic physics. (Oppenheim and Putnam 1991: 407)

Oppenheim and Putnam go on to argue that the only method seriously available for the unity of science is "microreduction." These are reductions in which "the objects in the universe of discourse of [the reduced science or theory] are wholes which possess a decomposition into proper parts all of which belong to the universe of discourse of [the reducing science or theory] (Oppenheim and Putnam 1991: 407). If microreduction is possible, a number of conditions must obtain. Oppenheim and Putnam's list begins:

1. There must be several levels.
2. The number of levels must be finite.
3. There must be a unique lowest level.
4. Any thing of any level except the lowest must possess a decomposition into things belonging to the next lowest level. (409)

For Oppenheim and Putnam, the world is made up of basic building blocks or atoms which display regularities that can be described in the law statements of the most basic science. The basic atoms also combine to constitute larger structures that display characteristic regularities of their own. In turn, these can be codified in the law statements of higher-level sciences. But the higher-level regularities do not emerge out of nothing. They can be explained as the consequences of the more basic patterns of the behavior of atoms.

With this picture in place, it is easy to see how the most basic level can assume a metaphysical role. Because it appears to describe everything, to be complete, it can assume the status of a touchstone for what is *really real*. Thus, only what can be reduced can be real. In the rest of this section I outline how just such an assumption has had a role in an important recent philosophical project, "philosophical naturalism."

A major influence on the recent development of naturalism in philosophy was the late American philosopher V. W. O. Quine (1908–2000). In his hands naturalism was primarily an approach to philosophical method: namely, it was in continuity with science. But implicit in Quinean philosophy is a metaphysical view that has become explicit in contemporary philosophical naturalism. Nature is identified with the subject matter of physics. Philosophical naturalism is thus construed as a project of showing how features of the world can be related to physics.

The central assumption of the equivalence of nature and the physical is made explicit by Jerry Fodor (1987). Fodor's project is to naturalize intentionality. Naturalism and reductionism go hand in hand. In a revealing passage he says:

> I suppose that sooner or later the physicists will complete the catalogue they've been compiling of the ultimate and irreducible properties of things. When they do, the likes of *spin, charm* and *charge* will perhaps appear upon their list. But *aboutness* surely won't; intentionality simply doesn't go that deep. It's hard to see, in face of this consideration, how one can be a Realist about intentionality without also being, to some extent or other, a Reductionist. If the semantic and intentional are real properties of things, it must be in virtue of their identity with . . . properties that are *neither* intentional *nor* semantic. If aboutness is real, it must be really something else. (Fodor 1987: 97)

This passage clearly summarizes the motivation for reductionism in the philosophy of mental content but applies more generally. If the full extent of what exists in nature is describable by physics (by a future complete physics, that is), then it should be possible in principle to show how any genuine feature or property can be reduced to that underlying physical description.

Assumptions of this sort play a role in thinking about psychiatry. A reductionist naturalism in psychiatry assumes that unless its basic categories can be systematically related to more basic scientific categories, then it has no right to think that it "cuts nature at the joints." In the next two sections I examine the challenge that a reductionist view of psychiatry faces in two areas: both the concept of disorder and the meaning, content, or intentionality of mental states.

REDUCTIONISM AND MENTAL DISORDER

Bill Fulford has argued that debate about the nature of mental illness and disorder centrally concerns whether values are "in" or "out" of their analysis (1999: 412). But this debate can also be seen as being about the prospects of reductionist naturalism in the philosophy of psychiatry. Can the concept of disorder be fleshed out in more basic, nonevaluative terms?

Adopting this interpretation of the debate about mental illness suggests that the following assumption may be at work. If the diagnostic judgment of mental illness is an *evaluation*—an expression of our values—rather than simply a *description* of the facts, then mental illness cannot be an objective matter; it cannot be a feature of the fabric of the world, independent of our own perspective. Thus, the aim of a descriptive account of illness, generally via the notion of function, can be seen as establishing its naturalistic status through reduction eventually to the austere language of physics. And, by contrast, if value theorists can establish that illness presupposes irreducible values, such reductionism will fail.

The conditional assumption motivated by naturalism seems to underpin much work here. It operates, for example, within Szasz's influential attack on the status of psychiatry (e.g., Szasz 1960). It is because judgments of mental illness are evaluative that they lack the objectivity of judgments of physical disease. Szasz goes on to argue that because diagnosis of mental illness is evaluative, psychiatry—the discipline that charts mental illness—cannot be a science.

An alternative, reductionist response is to argue that the antecedent of the conditional—the claim that diagnostic judgments are evaluations—is false. If an austere descriptive account can be given of mental illness, then the status of psychiatry as a discipline that at least aspires to be a descriptive science of objective and worldly phenomena can be preserved. This is the aim of accounts by Kendell (1975), Boorse (1975), and, to a first approximation, Wakefield (1999).

Wakefield attempts to characterize disorder through the notion of failures of function. The hope is that talk of "failure of function" can itself be explained in purely descriptive terms using the idea, gleaned from the evolutionary theory, of *natural*, *biological*, or *proper* functions (these different terms are used by different philosophers of biology). I said "to a first approximation" because Wakefield adds to this descriptive account of function a second, explicitly evaluative element: illnesses are *harmful* failures of function. There is a rationale for this, however, which in no sense undermines the basic naturalistic aim. This is that medical science not only aims at an understanding of the functioning (and failures of functioning) of the body and mind; it also aims to intervene to cure those failures that are harmful.

I have suggested that the debate about whether values are "in" or "out" of the analysis of illness, disease, or disorder can be seen as an argument about the prospects of reductionism in this area and that that, in turn, can be seen as motivated by a conception of nature. Everyone appears to agree that values are not part of the nature of the world. The prospects for reductionist naturalism thus turn on whether a descriptive nonevaluative account of a failure of function can be given. I briefly suggest why I think that one cannot.

The most promising attempt to reduce the concept of disorder is using biological function. Wakefield's account of function is spelled out in the following way:

> A natural function of a biological mechanism is an effect of the mechanism that explains the existence, maintenance or nature of the mechanism via the same essential process (whatever it is) by which prototypical non-accidental beneficial effects . . . explain the mechanism which cause them. . . .
>
> It turns out that the process that explains the prototypical non-accidental benefits is natural selection acting to increase inclusive fitness of the organism. (Wakefield 1999: 471–72)

There is some debate among philosophers about how precisely to define a biological function, but Wakefield's account captures the central idea. A biological function (exemplified by a particular trait of an organism) is a function that explains the evolutionary success and survival value of that trait (see Millikan 1995). Crucially, biological functions are distinct from dispositions. Engineering limitations might cause the actual behavioral dispositions of a trait to diverge from the biological function it thus only partially exemplifies. The divergences might themselves be life threatening and play no positive part in explaining the value of the trait. The best explanation of the survival of that organism and those like it cites the function that helped propagation or predator evasion, for example, and not those aspects of its behavioral dispositions that diverged from it.

This point is sometimes made by saying that what matters is not what traits or dispositions are selected but what function they are selected *for*. The distinction between "selection of" and "selection for" can be illustrated by the example of a child's toy (Millikan 1995; Sober 1984). A box allows objects of different shapes to be inserted into it through differently shaped slots in the lid. The round slot thus allows the insertion of balls, for example. It may be that the actual balls allowed through or "selected" in one case are all green. But they are selected *for* their round cross-section and not their green color. Millikan stresses the fact that the biological function of a trait may be displayed in only a minority of actual cases. It is the function of sperm to fertilize an egg, but the great majority of sperm fails in this regard.

To see how invoking biological function works in the project of a devising reductionist account of disorder, consider a criticism voiced by Megone:

> According to Wakefield, on this model, "the heart exists for the purpose of pumping the blood in the sense that past hearts having this effect causally explains how hearts came to exist and be maintained in the species and the genesis of the heart's detailed structure" (Wakefield 2000: 28). The most basic difficulty here is that past hearts' pumping the blood figure in all sorts of causal stories, stories in which agents die young, or agents do not reproduce, or agents reproduce but defectively, and so on. It is not the case that hearts pumping the blood have simply caused hearts to exist. So hearts pumping the blood does not causally explain how

hearts came to exist. This cannot therefore be the sense in which the pumping of the blood is a functionally explicable activity of the heart. (Megone 2000: 60–61)

But Megone here illicitly runs together causal explanation and "simple" causal relations. By contrast, Wakefield, like Millikan (see discussion later in this chapter), relies on specifying the function of systems through what best explains their continued existence. Thus, he can reply that the divergent causal relations do not explain the heart's existence. Its dispositions are also genuine causal consequences of the system's nature but do not explain its existence.

Wakefield's approach faces two difficulties. I outline the first here and return to it in the context of Millikan's reductionist account of meaning in the next section.

The first difficulty is this. For a successful reduction of disorder to biological functions, such functions have to be cashed out in terms of a more basic vocabulary. Psychiatry is to be explained in terms of biology. But, if it is so explained, the biological account has to be able to justify the invocation of a pattern of explanation that mirrors a pattern in the "space of reasons" but that is built "bottom up" from biological happenings. My concern is that the kind of explanations given in evolutionary biology presuppose rather than explain space-of-reason explanations.

Recall that what singles out a proper function is what *best explains* the continued existence of biological trait. But the best explanation turns on seeing an explanatory pattern in the myriad causal relations that goes beyond the resources of simple descriptive causal language, beyond the data of evolutionary success.

One might try to extend this point by saying that although the function that the behavioral dispositions of a biological system partially exemplify has to be consistent with that behavior, it is not determined by it. In fact, the function does not have to be consistent with the behavior, because the behavior only partially exemplifies the function. But, although the causal transactions of evolutionary history provide some constraint in the ascription of function, there are still an infinite number of different functions that meet that constraint. These include, for example, all the functions that diverge only at a still future date; systems with those functions would have been just as successful in the past. Thus, the data themselves do not determine a particular function even if we find it natural to interpret the data in particular ways. I return to develop this objection a little further at the end of the next section.

The second objection is more straightforward. If disorder is explained as failure of function, then the problem is that there are far too many such failures. Recall the case of sperm. Most sperm fail in their biological function. Their function is that property of them that best explains their evolutionary success. But this does not require that nature is an efficient engineer. In other words, there is no general reason that most traits should behave according to their function. So, to identify disorder with such failures is to see them widespread in nature. This is implausible.

This outline of the prospects of reductionist naturalism has aimed to place the "values in, values out" debate in a broader philosophical context. Now, one argument against the possibility of naturalizing disorder is that it contains an ineliminable evaluative element (see Fulford 1999). I have not followed that line of argument directly

REDUCTIONISM/ANTIREDUCTIONISM 197

because it is open to a reductionist naturalist to argue that there are no values present, that there merely *seem* to be because there are biological functions implicit. Furthermore, a naturalist may continue that it was the great virtue of Darwin's work to show how nature can appear to contain genuine purposes or values when, in fact, it does not. Even with that argument in play, however, reductionism still faces a problem: the explanatory power of proper functions presupposes, rather than explains, a higher-level structure of intelligibility. As I outline in the next section, this same objection applies to a second feature of psychiatric concern: the meaning, content, or intentionality of mental states.

Reductionism in Philosophy of Mental Content

In sketching out the motivation for a reductionist form of naturalism, I quoted from Jerry Fodor's (1987) influential book *Psychosemantics*. Fodor's work is of particular relevance to psychology and psychiatry because it complements cognitivist approaches in these disciplines. Both Fodor and cognitivist psychology and psychiatry discuss the mind in terms of information processing; both populate the brain and nervous system with internal representations that encode meanings. But Fodor also accepts the challenge that cognitivism in psychiatry and psychology often ducks: he attempts to explain just how internal states of the body can encode meanings (see Thornton 2002). If he were successful in explaining this encoding, Fodor would provide a way of mapping the structure of intelligibility of the space of reasons onto the realm of law and thus could unify two key sets of psychiatric concepts. Thus, assessing Fodor provides a way of assessing the cognitivist assumption that meaning must be reducible to neurological processes.

That there are genuine difficulties in naturalizing meaning can be brought out by considering a familiar example. If someone understands a directional signpost, then they understand which way it points (toward, rather than away from, the arrowhead). We might attempt to give a broadly cognitivist account or explanation of this by saying that there must be an inner state that represents or encodes that meaning. We might think of this as a kind of inner signpost with an arrow pointing in the same direction as the outer signpost. But, of course, that representation will represent pointing in the direction of the arrowhead only to someone who already understands how to interpret it. And the problem is that specifying the correct interpretation of the inner representation would generate a vicious regress. What encodes that representation? A third arrow on a second inner signpost pointing in the same direction?

This point is familiar from Wittgenstein and his interpreters (e.g., Wittgenstein

1953). If meaning depends on interpretation, then it appears that a question is begged. Fodor is well aware of this line of thought and attempts to sidestep it by eschewing an interpretational theory altogether. His explanation of the intentionality, meaning, or content of mental states is based instead on a causal theory of meaning or reference. The underlying motivation for a causal theory is the fact that effects can sometimes carry information about their causes. One can say "those spots mean measles" or "smoke means fire." Grice (1957) called examples like these cases of "natural meaning." Fodor deploys this same idea to argue that states of mind, or, rather, the brain, mean or refer to what they do because they are caused by their subject matter. Thus, a particular type of neurological state might encode the meaning or content "Cow!" because it is caused (or "caused to be tokened") by the presence of cows.

However, this kind of simple causal theory cannot account for a key feature of mental content: its normativity. It cannot account for those occasions where having a mental representation corresponds to a false belief. In such cases, representations are caused by states of affairs that they do not depict or to which they do not refer. Nevertheless, a simple causal theory will include *all* these causes as parts of the content which a mental representation encodes. The mental representation will stand for a disjunction of all its possible causes, and misrepresentation will be impossible. Hence the label "disjunction problem." Thus, one condition of adequacy of causal theories is that they are able to discriminate between two kinds of circumstance in which a mental representation is produced in the mind. There must be occasions where the cause and the content coincide and occasions of "deviant" causation where the mental representation is caused by something from outside its extension. A number of attempts have been made to solve the disjunction problem as part of a piece of reductionist naturalism. I mention two here: Fodor's asymmetric dependence theory and Ruth Garrett Millikan's evolutionary biological theory.

Pure Descriptive Theories of Mental Content

Fodor's preferred solution to the disjunction problem is elegant and minimal. It is to distinguish between causal connections that are constitutive of content and those that are not, in terms of asymmetric dependence (Fodor 1987). A type of mental representation has the content "horse" if horses cause it to be tokened in the "belief box" of a thinker and if those occasions on which it is caused by nonhorses depend asymmetrically on the connection to horses. (Thus, if the former connection had not existed, then the latter would not have existed either, but not vice versa). Occasions when nonhorses cause the "horse" mental representation to be tokened can now be counted as errors.

Fodor's proposal has received much critical attention. Many published articles attempt to show that Fodor's theory gives the wrong result in particular circumstances (Loewer and Rey 1991). Godfrey-Smith (1989) highlights another more general problem: he asks what resources a purely causal theory has for distinguishing between the independent causal relation that determines the content of a mental representation and those dependent causal relations that correspond to error.

Consider a mental representation that is caused by normal-looking horses, athletic cows, muddy zebras, and so forth. One obvious interpretation of this is that the representation encodes horse-thoughts and that the connections between it and some cows and zebras asymmetrically depends on the connection to horses. But, given only the facts about causal connections, another interpretation is equally plausible: that is that the mental representation encodes a disjunctive content including normal-looking horses, and some cows and zebras. There is, after all, a reliable causal connection between those animals and the representation. It is only given the content of the mental representation that one can determine which connections are fundamental and which are dependent; which would hold in nearby possible worlds, and which would not. What this suggests is not just that there is a problem with Fodor's particular solution but that there is something generally wrong with attempts to reduce intentional notions to purely causal ones. Something is omitted by the causal account: it cannot determine which one is the *correct* interpretation of the mental representation.

Biological Teleological Theories of Mental Content

The other major approach to reductionist naturalism in the philosophy of content invokes evolutionary theory. So-called teleological theories of content appear to have an important extra resource for explaining the normativity of content over and above those available to pure descriptive theories because they employ the notion of a natural, proper, or biological function (see Millikan 1995). The distinction between correctness and incorrectness in the tokening of a mental representation can be defined by reference to its functioning in accord with its biological function.

It is worth noting just how ambitious this version of the reductionist project is. It is not merely the claim that a general evolutionary theoretical explanation can be given of the possession of intentional mental states (i.e., of why it is advantageous to be able to represent the world). It is, rather, that each particular type of content can be explained in this way. Furthermore, the explanations cannot be question-begging: the selective advantages conferred must be characterizable in nonintentional terms. The meaning must drop out of the evolutionary theory.

A teleological account of function is a form of interpretational theory (in the sense mentioned earlier) because the characterization of the function that explains the survival of a trait is, in effect, an interpretation of the past behavior. Past behavior replaces inner states as the set of signs that have to be interpreted. But there is no limit to the different ways past behavior can be interpreted. Like the interpretation of signs, such behavior is consistent with an unlimited number of possible functions or rules. What ensures the determinacy of biological function—what selects just one of the rules—is an explanation of the presence of a trait couched in intentional terms that interprets what the trait is for. But finite past behavior can be explained as exemplifying many different or "bent" functions or rules, all of which would have been equally successful in the past but which diverge in the future. (For the terminology "bent rule" see Blackburn 1984.)

Millikan dismisses these possible alternatives by claiming that the explanation of a trait turns on what caused it to survive *in the past*. She considers the case of the rules that govern a hoverfly's mating behavior. Such flies are disposed to take flight in a particular direction, depending on the angle at which a potential mate is observed. Engineering limitations mean that if the mate arrives in the blind spot of the fly, it takes no action. Nevertheless, the biological function of the (relevant trait of the) fly is to take off at an angle that is a regular trigonometric function of the observed mate's initial position. Proper function and disposition do not coincide, but the correct function can nevertheless be identified. She argues:

> [The "bent" rule] is not a rule the hoverfly has a biological purpose to follow. For it is not because their behavior coincided with *that* rule that the hoverfly's ancestors managed to catch females, and hence to proliferate. In saying that, I don't have any particular theory of the nature of explanation up my sleeve. But surely, on any reasonable account, a complexity that can simply be dropped from the explanans without affecting the tightness of the relation of explanans to explanandum is not a *functioning* part of the explanation. (Millikan 1993: 221)

The claim is that "bent" rules introduce additional and unnecessary complexities that can be dispensed with without damaging the explanation of the success of a biological trait. But the problem with this reply is that it works only in the context in which the simplicity of an explanation can be assessed in a non-question-begging way. The problem is that the explanation of the survival value of the trait corresponding to a particular mental content has to be given without presupposing its content. Recall that the articulation of a proper function is not a matter of looking to behavioral dispositions but selecting from that causal history a function that best explains it. And now the question is what governs the pattern of this kind of explanation.

My concern is that that pattern is visible only to someone sensitive to the structure of the space of reasons, not just the realm of natural law. The latter might be able in principle to explain the detailed history of a trait but not identify its function and thus its successes and failures. Such a determination, however, is an exemplification of the structure of the space of reasons, not an independent explanation of it.

Fodor's pure causal theory and Millikan's biological theory of mental content demonstrate the problem with reductionist naturalism in this area. Biologically minded and cognitivist psychiatrists may simply assume that some such reduction must be possible. Surely, they might argue, meaning must be encoded in the head. But more careful examination of what would have to be achieved makes that assumption problematic. In light of the scale of the problem, it is worth revisiting the underlying motivation for the approach.

PSYCHIATRY WITHOUT REDUCTIONIST NATURALISM

The two preceding sections have highlighted the difficulty of giving a reductionist account of two ingredients of psychiatry: the content of reasons and the concept of disorder. They have not undermined the argument from Fodor that I cited to explain the felt need for such a reduction, however. Fodor's argument seems to establish that unless a reduction of problematic concepts is possible, then these concepts cannot label real properties in nature. Fodor's argument depends on an assumption about the completeness of physical explanation, but this assumption can be questioned.

Drawing on a range of sources that includes Aristotle's ethics, Wittgenstein's account of rules and normativity, and a post-Kantian picture of experience, John McDowell has recently challenged just this assumption in his influential lectures *Mind and World* (1994). In a central passage in which he attempts to diagnose the source of the assumption, he says:

> What is at work here is a conception of nature that can seem sheer common
> sense, though it was not always so; the conception I mean was made available only
> by a hard-won achievement of human thought at a specific time, the time of the
> rise of modern science. Modern science understands its subject matter in a way
> that threatens, at least, to leave it disenchanted. . . . The image marks a contrast
> between two kinds of intelligibility: the kind that is sought by (as we call it) natu-
> ral science, and the kind we find in something when we place it in relation to
> other occupations of "the logical space of reasons," to repeat a suggested phrase
> from Wilfred Sellars. If we identify nature with what natural science aims to make
> comprehensible, we threaten, at least, to empty it of meaning. By way of compen-
> sation, so to speak, we see it as the home of a perhaps inexhaustible supply of
> intelligibility of the other kind, the kind we find in a phenomenon when we see it
> as governed by natural law. It was an achievement of modern thought when this
> second kind of intelligibility was clearly marked off from the first. (70–71)

McDowell commends a different response to the prospects of a failure of a reduction of nonphysical to physical concepts. Rather than regarding this as impugning the reality or worldliness of the properties or concepts concerned, it may merely show that reductionists have started with an impoverished conception of what is real or part of nature. To mark the contrast, McDowell suggests that the natural is not restricted to what fits within the "realm of law" articulated by the physical sciences but also includes those patterns and properties that have to be fitted within a different pattern of intelligibility: the "space of reasons." This phrase marks the rational pattern of intentional states. But an analogous notion might be used to mark nonintentional concepts that naturalists have attempted to reduce (e.g., necessity, causality, disorder). (This might address the criticism that there are not just two sorts of space: the sciences contain a variety of methods, narratives as well as laws (Rorty 1998: 143–46).)

By suggesting that nature includes more than just the realm of law, McDowell does not aim to slight the success of science. Nor does he suggest that there should be no place for a "disenchanted" view of nature within a scientific worldview:

> But it is one thing to recognise that the impersonal stance of scientific investigation is a methodological necessity for the achievement of a valuable mode of understanding reality; it is quite another thing to take the dawning grasp of this, in the modern era, for a metaphysical insight into the notion of objectivity as such, so that objective correctness in any mode of thought must be anchored in this kind of access to the real. . . . [It] is not the educated common sense it represents itself as being; it is shallow metaphysics. (McDowell 1998: 182)

The alternative view, he suggests, is one in which the space of reasons is a genuinely autonomous structure of intelligibility. (In fact, he argues for the inverse of the normal priority by suggesting that it underpins the realm of law.) There is no need to connect its method of accessing truths about human thought and subjectivity with the kind of nomological explanation aspired to in biological psychiatry. The psychiatry of reasons and the psychiatry of causes stand on equal footing.

The idea that psychiatry might consist of two distinct and equally well grounded approaches might still seem implausible because of the grip of the hierachical picture of nature I described at the start. It is that which makes it seem that physics must be uniquely complete in describing the basic atoms of the world. But even this assumption can be questioned. Nancy Cartwright, a philosopher of science, suggests an alternative view:

> The laws that describe this world are a patchwork, not a pyramid. They do not take after the simple, elegant and abstract structure of a system of axioms and theorems. Rather they look like—and steadfastly stick to looking like—science as we know it: apportioned into disciplines, apparently arbitrarily grown up; governing different sets of properties at different levels of abstraction; pockets of great precision; large parcels of qualitative maxims resisting precise formulation; erratic overlaps; here and there, once in a while, corners that line up, but mostly ragged edges; and always the cover of law just loosely attached to the jumbled world of material things. For all we know, most of what happens in nature occurs by hap, subject to no law at all. What happens is more like an outcome of negotiation between domains than the logical consequence of a system of order. (1999: 1)

Elsewhere she writes:

> I imagine that natural objects are much like people in societies. Their behavior is constrained by some specific laws and by a handful of general principles, but it is not determined in detail even statistically. What happens on most occasions is dictated by no law at all. This is not a metaphysical picture that I urge. My claim is that this picture is as plausible as the alternative. God may have written just a few laws and grown tired. (Cartwright 1983: 49)

Cartwright's position is radical and contested. But merely as a sketch of an alternative to the usual assumption of the completeness of physics, it shows that the thesis needs some argument or support. Clearly, it is not analytically true. Cartwright adds to that the observation that the empirical evidence falls very far short of establishing it.

None of this is to say that reductions cannot take place within science. Oppenheim and Putnam's hypothesis that at least some branches of science can be unified can continue to play a methodological role. But by reminding us of the differences between the space of reasons and realm of law—such as the different pattern of explanation, attitude to exceptions, and so on—McDowell also suggests a picture of nature much more like Cartwright's than the logical positivists' hierachy. From the perspective of tidy intellectual housekeeping, it is psychiatry's misfortune, but also its great practical strength, that it straddles this divide.

REFERENCES

Blackburn, S. (1984) *Spreading the Word*. Oxford: Oxford University Press.

Boorse, C. (1975) "On the Distinction between Disease and Illness." *Philosophy and Public Affairs* 5: 49–68.

Cartwright, N. (1983) *How the Laws of Physics Lie*. Oxford: Oxford University Press.

Cartwright, N. (1999) *The Dappled World: A Study of the Boundaries of Science*. Cambridge: Cambridge University Press.

Dennett, D. (1987) *The Intentional Stance*. Cambridge, MA.: MIT Press.

Fodor, J. A. (1987) *Psychosemantics: The Problem of Meaning in the Philosophy of Mind*. Cambridge, MA: MIT Press.

Fulford, K. W. M. (1990) *Moral Theory and Medical Practice*. Cambridge: Cambridge University Press.

Fulford, K. W. M. (1999) "Nine Variations and a Coda on the Theme of an Evolutionary Definition of Dysfunction." *Journal of Abnormal Psychology* 108(3): 412–20.

Godfrey-Smith, P. (1989) "Misinformation." *Canadian Journal of Philosophy* 19: 533–50

Grice, H. P. (1957) "Meaning." *Philosophical Review* 66: 377–88.

Jaspers, K. T. (1974) "Causal and 'Meaningful' Connections between Life History and Psychosis." Translated by J. Hoenig. In S. R. Hirsch and M. Shepherd (eds.), *Themes and Variations in European Psychiatry*. Bristol: Wright.

Kendell, R. E. (1975) "The Concept of Disease and Its Implications for Psychiatry." *British Journal of Psychiatry* 127: 305–15

Loewer, B., and Rey, G. (eds.) (1991) *Meaning in Mind*. Oxford: Blackwell.

McDowell, J. (1994) *Mind and World*. Cambridge, MA: Harvard University Press.

McDowell, J. (1998) *Mind Value and Reality*. Cambridge, MA: Harvard University Press.

Megone, C. (2000) "Mental Illness, Human Function, and Values." *Philosophy, Psychiatry and Psychology* 7: 45–65.

Millikan, R. G. (1984) *Language, Thought and Other Biological Categories*. Cambridge, MA: MIT Press.

Millikan, R. G. (1993) *White Queen Psychology*. Cambridge, MA: MIT Press.

Millikan, R. G. (1995) "A Bet with Peacocke." In C. Macdonald and G. Macdonald (eds.), *Philosophy of Psychology*. Oxford: Blackwell.

Oppenheim, P., and Putnam, H. (1991) "Unity of Science as a Working Hypothesis." In R. Boyd, P. Gasper, and J. D. Trout (eds.), *Philosophy of Science*. Cambridge, MA: MIT Press.

Papineau, D. (1993) *Philosophical Naturalism*. Oxford: Blackwell.

Posner, M. I. (1993) "Seeing the Mind." *Science* 262: 673–79.

Rorty, R. (1998) "The Very Idea of Human Answerability to the World: John McDowell's Version of Empiricism." *Truth and Progress*. Cambridge: Cambridge University Press.

Sober, E. (1984) *The Nature of Selection*. Cambridge, MA: MIT Press.

Szasz, T. (1960) "The Myth of Mental Illness." *American Psychologist* 15: 113–18.

Thornton, T. (1998) *Wittgenstein on Language and Thought*. Edinburgh: Edinburgh University Press.

Thornton, T. (2000) "Mental Illness and Reductionism: Can Functions Be Naturalized?" *Philosophy, Psychiatry and Psychology* 7: 67–76.

Thornton, T. (2002) "Thought Insertion, Cognitivism and Inner Space." *Cognitive Neuropsychiatry* 7: 237–49.

Thornton, T. (forthcoming) *John McDowell*. Chesham: Acumen.

Thornton, T. (2002) "Reliability and Validity in Psychiatric Classification: Values and Neo-Humeanism." *Philosophy, Psychiatry and Psychology* 9: 229–35.

Wakefield, J. C. (1999) "Mental Disorder as a Black Box Essentialist Concept." *Journal of Abnormal Psychology* 108(3): 465–72.

Wakefield, J. C. (2000) "Aristotle as Sociobiologist: The 'Function of a Human Being' Argument, Black Box Essentialism, and the Concept of Mental Disorder." *Philosophy, Psychiatry and Psychology* 7: 17–44.

Wittgenstein, L. (1953) *Philosophical Investigations*. Oxford: Blackwell.

CHAPTER 14

FACTS/VALUES

Ten Principles of Values-Based Medicine

K. W. M. (BILL) FULFORD

VALUES-BASED MEDICINE (VBM) is the theory and practice of effective health-care decision making for situations in which legitimately different (and hence potentially conflicting) value perspectives are in play.

As a theory, VBM is the values counterpart of Evidence-Based Medicine, or EBM. VBM and EBM are both responses to the growing complexity of decision making in health care: EBM is a response to the growing complexity of the relevant *facts*; VBM is a response to the growing complexity of the relevant *values* (see Principles 1–5 in table 14.1 and table 14.2). As a practice, VBM is a skills-based counterpart of the currently dominant quasi-legal form of clinical bioethics. Quasi-legal ethics prescribes good *outcomes* in the form of increasingly complex ethical rules and regulations. VBM emphasizes the importance of good *process* in the form particularly of improved clinical practice skills (see Principles 6–10 in table 14.1 and table 14.3).

Table 14.1. Ten Principles of Values-Based Medicine (VBM)

The Theory

1st principle of VBM

All decisions stand on two feet, on values as well as on facts, including decisions about diagnosis (the "two-feet" principle)

2nd principle of VBM

We tend to notice values only when they are diverse or conflicting and hence are likely to be problematic (the "squeaky wheel" principle)

3rd principle of VBM

Scientific progress, in opening up choices, is increasingly bringing the full diversity of human values into play in all areas of health care (the "science-driven" principle)

4th principle of VBM

VBM's "first call" for information is the perspective of the patient or patient group concerned in a given decision (the "patient-perspective" principle)

5th principle of VBM

In VBM, conflicts of values are resolved primarily, not by reference to a rule prescribing a "right" outcome but by processes designed to support a balance of legitimately different perspectives (the "multiperspective" principle)

The Practice

6th principle of VBM

Careful attention to language use in a given context is one of a range of powerful methods for raising awareness of values (the "values-blindness" principle)

7th principle of VBM

A rich resource of both empirical and philosophical methods is available for improving our knowledge of other people's values (the "values-myopia" principle)

8th principle of VBM

Ethical reasoning is employed in VBM primarily to explore differences of values, not, as in quasi-legal bioethics, to determine "what is right" (the "space of values" principle)

9th principle of VBM

In VBM, communication skills have a substantive rather than (as in quasi-legal ethics) a merely executive role in clinical decision making (the "how it's done" principle)

10th principle of VBM

VBM, although involving a partnership with ethicists and lawyers (equivalent to the partnership with scientists and statisticians in EBM), puts decision making back where it belongs, with users and providers at the clinical coal-face (the "who decides" principle)

Adapted from K. W. M. Fulford (forthcoming), *Values-Based Medicine: Effective Healthcare Decision Making in the Context of Value Diversity* (Cambridge: Cambridge University Press).

PHILOSOPHY AND VALUES-BASED MEDICINE

VBM is derived primarily from philosophical value theory—that part of ethics (and of aesthetics) that is concerned with the logic, with the meanings and implications, of value terms (paradigmatically, good, bad, right, and so on; and, in aesthetics, beauty). VBM draws on philosophical value theory particularly as developed through careful attention to language use.[1]

Being an analytic rather than substantive branch of philosophy,[2] philosophical value theory has in recent years been largely neglected in favor of ethical theories that seek to establish what for want of a better word might be called moral "facts."[3] The charge against philosophical value theory has been that, if not actually incoherent, it has little relevance to practical issues (Williams (1985).[4] Bioethics, similarly, while drawing extensively on substantive ethical theories such as deontology (in rights-based codes connecting ethics with law), consequentialism (as in health economics [Williams 1995], and virtue theory (in professional education [e.g., May 1994]), has made little use of philosophical value theory. Yet it is precisely in being an *analytic* discipline that philosophical value theory is a potentially rich resource for an *empirical* discipline like health care.[5] In my *Moral Theory and Medical Practice* (1989) I showed how ideas derived from philosophical value theory help transform the traditional fact-centered "medical" model of the conceptual structure of health care into a more balanced fact + value model. VBM is the practitioner's "cut" of this fact + value model of health care.[6]

VBM: THE THEORY (PRINCIPLES 1–5)

As noted, VBM stands to the values bearing on clinical decision making much as Evidence-Based Medicine (EBM) stands to the facts (see table 14.2). There is of course considerable debate, not least among those concerned with the development of EBM (Eddy 1991; Hudson Jones 1999), as to whether, in its current form, EBM is a sufficient response to the "fact" side of health-care decision making. A fact + value model, nonetheless, suggests that in the increasingly complex environment of modern health care, to the extent that we need EBM (albeit an enlightened EBM), so, too, do we need VBM.

Principles 1–5 of VBM thus define the theory of VBM as a values counterpart of EBM. For Principles 1–3, as we will see, VBM and EBM run closely parallel. For Principles 4 and 5, VBM and EBM are antiparallel, though still complementary (see table 14.2).

Table 14.2. Comparison of VBM and EBM

Principles of VBM	VBM (Values-Based Medicine)	EBM (Evidence-Based Medicine)
Similarities		
1. The "two-feet" principle	Has a key role in clinical decision making (the values input)	Has a key role in clinical decision making (the fact input)
2. The "squeaky wheel" principle	Is a response to the growing complexity of values	Is a response to the growing complexity of facts
3. The "science-driven" principle	Complexity (of values) generated primarily by scientific progress	Complexity (of facts) generated primarily by scientific progress
Differences		
4. The "patient-perspective" principle	At the top of the "values hierarchy" are the value perspectives or individual patients of patient groups	At the top of the "evidence hierarchy" are facts that are as perspective-free as possible
5. The "multiperspective" principle	Disagreements over values are resolved primarily by processes that seek to balance legitimately different value perspectives	Disagreements over facts are resolved primarily by research methods aimed at establishing perspective-free facts

Values and Clinical Decision Making

1st Principle of VBM: All decisions stand on two feet, on values as well as on facts, including decisions about diagnosis (the "two-feet" principle).

The origins of VBM, then, are in the growing complexity of the values involved in all areas of health-care decision making. The most obvious evidence of this growing complexity is the recent explosion of ethical issues. But values come in many varieties—epistemic, aesthetic, and prudential, for example, as well as moral and ethical; they also take different logical forms (e.g., needs, wishes, desires); they have many origins (e.g., personal, professional, cultural); and they have a rich grammar (encompassing nouns, verbs, adverbs and so on). Matters are further complicated by the fact that the very word "value," besides its central use of judgments of good and bad, has a number of other meanings.[7]

VBM is concerned with values in health care in the central sense of the term, as covering any judgment of good and bad. A unifying feature of such judgments, as a former White's Professor of Moral Philosophy in Oxford, R. M. Hare, pointed out, is that they are prescriptive or *action-guiding* (Hare 1952).

It is this action-guiding property of values that explains why values are one of

---

Box 1 Diane Abbot's (overtly evidence-based) decision to start on lithium

Diane Abbot, a 64-year-old artist and art historian, was referred by her family doctor to a psychiatrist, Dr. Kirk.* She had a history of occasional but increasingly disruptive episodes of hypomania. One of her academic colleagues had been successfully treated for a similar condition with lithium. She wanted to discuss the latest evidence on efficacy, on possible adverse side effects, and so on, before deciding whether to start on lithium herself. The resources of EBM were essential to this process. Combined with Dr. Kirk's individual expertise, and Diane Abbot's understanding of her colleagues' experience, the resources of EBM allowed everyone concerned to be satisfied that her eventual decision to start on lithium was securely evidence based. But values, too, although not explicitly part of the decision-making process, were also essential. For without values, those concerned would have had no basis on which to make a decision "on the evidence." In any decision about treatment, then, EBM is an increasingly essential resource. But it is the *values*, implicit or explicit, attaching respectively to clinical *effectiveness*, to *cost*, to *adverse* side effects, and so forth, that have to be balanced in coming to a decision in a given case.

*Diane Abbot's story is described in Fulford (forthcoming), "Evidence-Based Medicine: Thomas Szasz' Legacy to Twenty-first Century Psychiatry," in J. A. Schaler (ed.), *Szasz under Fire: Thomas Szasz Faces His Critics* (Chicago: Open Court).

---

the two feet on which all decisions in health care (and, indeed, in any other context) stand. All our decisions, conscious or unconscious, deliberative or reflective, are guided in part by matters of fact. EBM, as I noted a moment ago, is a response to the growing complexity of the facts that guide clinical decision making. But values, too, are essential. We need facts to guide our decisions; but we also need values. This is illustrated by the relatively straightforward decision about prescribing lithium presented in Box 1.

The importance of values in treatment decisions is relatively self-evident. The fact + value model of VBM, though, suggests that values are important also in areas of health-care decision making that, in the traditional fact-centered medical model, have been assumed to be exclusively matters for science, notably diagnosis. Principle 2 of VBM explains why this is so.

Values Visible and Invisible

2nd Principle of VBM: We tend to notice values only when they are diverse or conflicting and hence are likely to be problematic (the "squeaky wheel" principle).

Values are sometimes more and sometimes less visible in relation to health-care decision making. For example, values are highly visible in the current furor over whether cheap anti-AIDS drugs should be made available for developing countries. By contrast, values are more or less invisible in a crash team's decision over what drugs to use in a cardiac emergency.

The fact that values fall on a scale, from implicit to explicit, from invisible to visible, has led many to think of decisions in medicine as being divided into two distinct types, scientific and ethical. On this view, the anti-AIDS drug manufacturer's decision is a matter for ethics, while the crash team's decision is a matter for science. It is on this view, too, that, as noted at the end of the preceding section, treatment in general is considered a matter inter alia for ethics, while diagnosis is considered a matter exclusively for science.

A different way of interpreting the visible/invisible scale of values, which again we owe to R. M. Hare and others in the "Oxford school," is that it is a function of *diversity*. Hare pointed out that where values are uniform, where they are largely shared, they tend to be implicit. It is only where values are *not* shared, where *different* values are operative in a given context, that they tend to become visible (Hare 1952, 1963). Thus, the crash team's decisions are driven by the shared value of saving the life of their patient. The furor over anti-AIDS drugs, by contrast, directly reflects a clash of clinical and commercial values. This is a case of what is sometimes said to be "the squeaky wheel getting the grease"! As Box 2 illustrates, it is only when values cause trouble, it is only when there is conflict or disagreement over them, that we notice they are there.

Hare's interpretation of the visible/invisible scale of values can now be applied to the relative visibility of values in relation to treatment decisions compared with decisions about diagnosis. In the traditional fact-centered model of medicine, as noted, diagnosis is assumed to be essentially a matter for medical science. This is because in most of medicine diagnosis does indeed appear to be value free. But this in turn, according to Hare's interpretation, is because in the acute, life-threatening, and often painful conditions with which medicine has traditionally been concerned, the operative values are largely shared. A heart attack (myocardial infarction), for example, involving as it does severe physical pain and imminent death, is, in and of itself, a bad condition by anyone's standards. Over such conditions, that is to say, our values are largely shared; hence they tend not to be problematic; hence, consistently with Hare's interpretation of the visible/invisible scale, the values involved in taking a heart attack to be a *bad* condition (and, hence, to this extent a disease),[8] go largely unnoticed. Yet the values are there, nonetheless.

The values involved in diagnosis come close to being fully visible in psychiatry.[9] Indeed, psychiatric diagnostic classification is more overtly value laden than its counterparts in other areas of medicine in no less than four respects: (1) the language of psychiatry's official classifications, such as the American *Diagnostic and Statistical Manual*, is value laden, (2) some of the specific categories are defined in part by value judgments (e.g., personality disorders and the paraphilias), (3) the differential diagnosis of many psychiatric disorders includes moral categories (e.g., alcoholism vs.

Box 2 Diane Abbot's (overtly values-based) decision to stop lithium

A few months after starting on lithium, Diane Abbot returned to Dr. Kirk with a letter from her family doctor explaining that she had decided to stop taking lithium. He, the family doctor, was concerned about this because her mood had been well stabilized and she had had no significant side effects "medically speaking." The implication was, could Dr. Kirk make her see sense? Diane Abbot explained that although she had had no "real" problem with the lithium, and that although her mood had indeed been more stable, she could no longer "see colors." No, she did not mean that she had become color-blind! But colors had lost their emotional intensity, which, for her as an artist, was a disaster. She recognized her doctor's concerns, which were indeed shared by her colleagues—that in her hypomanic episodes she risked embarrassing and potentially costly consequences of her disinhibited behavior. But, from her point of view, what mattered above all was her work as an artist. This was why she had decided to stop taking lithium.*

Whereas, therefore, Diane Abbot's decision to start lithium (described in Box 1) was overtly evidence based, her decision to stop lithium was overtly values based. On closer inspection, of course, both decisions are seen to be based on facts (evidence), as well as on values. In the present case, the relevant fact was that lithium was blunting Diane Abbot's appreciation of color. There is evidence, from personal narratives (Jamison 1994) as well as from wider field trials (Keller et al. 1992), that a degree of blunting of normal mood is a common side effect of lithium. It is a side effect to which little attention has been paid because, to most people, it is relatively unimportant. Hence, it did not figure in the evidence-based discussions that led to Diane Abbot's decision to start on lithium. Had Diane Abbot appreciated the extent to which lithium might impair her ability to "really see" colors, her values as an artist might have surfaced more explicitly at that stage. In the event, it was only when her values led to her decision to stop treatment, it was only when her values thus became discrepant with those of her doctor and her colleagues, that they became fully visible. The same principle, that values tend to become visible only when they are discrepant, explains the overtly value-laden nature of psychiatric diagnosis compared with diagnosis in most areas of physical medicine (see text).

*She was reluctant to experiment with lower doses of lithium (she had started at the bottom of the normal "therapeutic" range). Instead, she worked out with Dr. Kirk and her family doctor an advance directive for early intervention in further hypomanic episodes (see Box 3).

---

drunkenness, psychopathy vs. delinquency, hysteria vs. malingering), and (4) Criterion B (social/occupational dysfunction) for schizophrenia, and corresponding criteria for other conditions, are overtly evaluative in form.

The diagnosis of functional psychotic disorders makes fully explicit the need for a fact + value conceptual framework for diagnosis. What is required for a diagnosis of schizophrenia, say, is *both* the presence of certain specific experiences and/or behaviors (defined descriptively and listed under Criterion A) *and* a change in social and/or occupational functioning which is a change for the worse (defined by one or more of the negative value judgments specified by Criterion B). The same fact + value framework is implicit in all areas of medicine. In other areas, though, the evaluative element remains implicit because the operative values are largely shared. There is no "Criterion B" for a heart attack, not because the diagnosis of a heart attack is *more scientific* than that of schizophrenia but because a heart attack is *less complex evaluatively*. A heart attack, as noted, is a bad condition by anyone's standards. Hence the evaluative part of the diagnosis is unproblematic. Hence it can be (and properly is) ignored in practice.

In the traditional fact-centered medical model, the more value-laden nature of psychiatric diagnosis is taken to be a mark of the (supposedly) primitive state of psychiatric science (Boorse 1975, 1976; Phillips 2000). In the fact + value model that supports VBM, it is a mark of the evaluatively (as well as scientifically) more complex nature of psychiatry. Psychiatry, that is to say, and consistently with Hare's interpretation of the visible/invisible scale of values, is concerned with areas of human experience and behavior, such as emotion, desire, volition, and belief, over which human values vary widely and legitimately. This is why we need a Criterion B for the diagnosis of schizophrenia but not for a heart attack. Schizophrenia is evaluatively (as well as descriptively) complex. A heart attack is not.

More Science Equals More Values, Not Less

> *3rd Principle of VBM:* Scientific progress, in opening up choices, is increasingly bringing the full diversity of human values into play in all areas of health care (the "science-driven" principle).

The "squeaky wheel" principle, however, raises a question: human values, we must assume, have always been diverse. So why should it be only recently, in the closing years of the twentieth century, that values have become so visible in medicine? From the perspective of the traditional fact-centered medical model, this is counterintuitive. According to the traditional model, as science progresses the importance of values in health care will become less, not more. The fact + value model of VBM, by contrast, as we will see in this section, anticipates that, as science progresses, so the importance of values in health care should become, as thus far they have become, more, not less.

The increasing visibility of values in health care at this time is capable of different interpretations. Some ethicists and lawyers see it as a case of medicine finally waking up, or finally being woken up, to ethical issues: and about time too, is the implication! Hare's interpretation of the visible/invisible scale of values, however—that the degree to which values are visible is a function of diversity—suggests, rather, that medicine has been moving from a time when the operative values were shared to a time in which they are increasingly divergent. The growing visibility of values in medicine, Hare's interpretation suggests, reflects a growing diversity of the values that guide decision making in health care.

So where has this growing diversity come from? We do not have to look far for possible candidates. First, there is the diversity of values themselves, as noted earlier. Needs, wishes, interests, and so on may all be relevant to, and yet all pull in different directions in, medicine. Then again, there is the variety of origins of values: individual, cultural, professional. Again, these may pull in different directions. A third source of diversity, less well recognized but no less important, is the diversity of our values as individual human beings. For human values differ widely and legitimately, from person to person, for the same person in different contexts or at different times, from culture to culture, and at different historical periods (Fulford et al. 2002a).

These sources of diversity of values are all largely static, however. Hence, there must have been some other factor or factors involved in opening the stopcock, as it were, in letting the diversity of human values through into medicine at the present time. Again, we do not have to look far for likely candidates, some external and others internal to medicine. Externally, there is our increasing individualism (we are less inclined to take our values from each other) and our rejection of authority (of handed-down values). There is also global travel and communication (which expose us to a wider range of values) and our increasingly cosmopolitan society (which brings different people with different cultural values into direct contact).

In addition to these external factors, however, significant as they have been, there is a factor of even greater importance that is internal to medicine: scientific progress. On the traditional fact-centered medical model, it may sound a bit farfetched to claim that scientific progress, rather than increasingly eliminating values from medicine, is actually letting them in. But the link between scientific progress and the growing visibility of values in medicine is, in fact, entirely straightforward: it is that scientific progress increasingly *opens up choices*, and with choices go *values*. As long as I have no choice in a given situation, my values are irrelevant. It is only when I have a choice that my values become relevant to guiding the choice I make. This is illustrated for psychiatry by the story of Diane Abbot, in Box 3. But in all areas of health care, technological and scientific advances are increasingly giving us an ever wider range of choices over an ever wider range of aspects of our lives.[10]

Patient-Centered Practice

4th Principle of VBM: VBM's "first call" for information is the perspective of the patient or patient group concerned in a given decision (the "patient-perspective" principle).

Thus far, we have seen that values guide all decisions (Principle 1), that values become visible where they are diverse rather than shared (Principle 2), and that they

---

Box 3 Science gives Diane Abbot choices

Diane Abbot's decisions were made possible by advances in the medical sciences that underpin psychiatry. Without the Australian psychiatrist John Cade's original observation of the mood-stabilizing properties of lithium, and subsequent studies that clarified its effects and side effects, Diane Abbot would not have been in a position to start on lithium. Equally important, though, without the availability of other options for managing her hypomanic mood swings, she might not have been in a position to stop taking lithium. Had her options been either to take lithium and to continue working, albeit with less emotional intensity, or to stop lithium and risk potentially damaging periods of hypomania, she might well have opted for lithium. As it was, she worked out with Dr. Kirk, her psychiatrist, an "advance directive," in which she agreed with her family doctor and her colleagues that they could insist on early treatment with neuroleptics, if necessary as an involuntary inpatient, when she showed warning signs of a relapse. This was a feasible strategy in Diane Abbot's case because her warning signs were clear-cut—notably that she stopped sleeping and that she consistently misinterpreted these signs, at the time, as "entering a productive phase." But Diane Abbot's decision to stop lithium, nonetheless, was made possible, ultimately, by science. It was science that made lithium available and it was science that made the alternatives to lithium available.

The sciences, particularly the "brain" sciences, have had a bad press recently. For many in the user movement, indeed, there has been something of a moral imperative to refuse treatments, such as ECT (electroconvulsive therapy), even when an individual has found such treatments helpful (Perkins 2001). But, as Peter Campbell, a user advocate who writes about his own experience of manic-depressive illness, has pointed out, what matters is not that a particular treatment is or is not used. What matters is that the use or otherwise of a given treatment is guided primarily by the values of the person receiving it (Campbell 1996). In psychiatry, as described in the text, the values that guide treatment decisions are inherently diverse (i.e., because human values are inherently diverse in the areas of experience and behavior with which psychiatry is concerned). But scientific progress, in opening up an ever-wider range of choices, is increasingly allowing the full diversity of human values to come through into clinical decision making in all areas of medicine.*

*The effect of scientific progress in opening up choices, and hence bringing the full diversity of human values into other areas of medicine, is illustrated by a number of articles in Fulford et al. 2002b: see, e.g., J. Raphael-Leff on gamete donation (Leff 2002) and Paul Cain on cardiopulmonary resuscitation (Cain 2002).

---

are becoming increasingly visible in medicine because scientific progress, by opening up choices, is allowing the full diversity of human values into play in health-care decision making (Principle 3). In these three respects, as anticipated, VBM runs parallel with EBM (see table 14.2). We now come to two respects in which EBM and VBM, although still complementary, run antiparallel.

**Box 4 Diane Abbot's values as the "first call" in her decision to
start on lithium**

Given the prominence afforded autonomy of patient choice in medicine, at least
in industrialized countries (Okasha 2000), it may seem self-evident that when it
came to stopping lithium, Diane Abbot's values should have taken precedence over
those of her colleagues and her doctor. Importantly, though, her values were also
the "first call" in her original decision to start treatment. Yet that decision, with
hindsight, turned out to have been wrong—"wrong," that is, as judged by her values
as an artist. Had her need to be able to "really see" colors been more apparent at
the time, then the evidence of lithium's "emotional blunting" effects would probably have been discussed at that stage. Diane Abbot might still have decided to
start on lithium, but with her eyes open to the possibility of this side effect and
with her doctor also aware that this was a concern.

   The skills that would have allowed Diane Abbot's values to have been more
accurately weighed in the decision to start on lithium are discussed later (under
Principles 6–9). It is worth noting, though, that Diane Abbot herself was guided to
a significant extent by the positive experiences of her colleague on lithium. So this
is not a case of a patient's being misled by a naive use of EBM. Narrative, as well
as meta-analytic, sources of evidence were in play. Yet, still the wrong decision was
made.* Things worked out well. But this was a result of the way in which the
subsequent decision to stop lithium was handled (see Box 5).

* Or, more accurately, the right decision (to have a *trial* of lithium) on the wrong or incomplete grounds (because the possibility of emotional blunting had not been discussed).

The first antiparallel between VBM and EBM is in their respective "first calls"
for information. In EBM, our first call is objective information: information that is
as free as possible from the particular subjective perspective of this or that individual
or group. The aim of science, classically conceived, is what the American philosopher
Thomas Nagel (1986) has called the "view from nowhere." This is why, in EBM, the
information derived from meta-analyses of high-quality research is at the top of the
"evidence hierarchy" (Sackett et al. 2000). Such information is as perspective-free as
it is possible to get.

   In VBM, by contrast, as Box 4 illustrates, our "first call" is the perspective of the
particular patient (or group of patients) concerned in a given decision. This follows
from the diversity of human values noted earlier. The point is that human values are
not, merely, different but *legitimately* different.[11] Hence, in a given clinical situation,
while we may have a great deal of general information about the values that are likely
to be operative, and while such information is indeed an important part of the knowledge base of VBM (see Principle 7), it can never be a substitute for the *actual* values
of the *particular* individuals concerned.

Resolving Differences

> *5th Principle of VBM*: In VBM, conflicts of values are resolved primarily, not
> by reference to a rule that prescribes a "right" outcome, but by processes de-
> signed to support a balance of legitimately different perspectives (the "multi-
> perspective" principle).

Principle 4, in centering VBM firmly on the values of the person (or group) concerned in a particular decision, is, in this rather precise sense, "patient-centered"
(Fulford 1995). The diversity of human values, however, has a second and in a sense
opposite corollary: namely, disagreements are *inevitable*. The given diversity of human values makes it inevitable that the values of a particular patient may well be
different from those of their doctor; and both may be different from those of a nurse
or social worker, or from those of the informal caregivers concerned, and so forth.

How, then, to resolve such differences? This brings us to the second antiparallel
between VBM and EBM. In EBM, differences of view about the facts are resolved,
in principle, by consensus: more facts (more data) are accumulated, crucial experiments are carried out, or a wider evidence base is accessed, all with the aim of
deciding which view is right. But when it comes to values, there may be no uniquely
right view. And if Principles 2 and 3 of VBM are right, value diversity, rather than
uniquely right values, will become increasingly the norm in health care. Values-
Based Medicine, then, aims to resolve differences, not by consensus but by what I
have called elsewhere "dissensus" (Fulford 1998)—that is, by *processes that support
effective action through a balance of legitimately different value perspectives*.

It is worth looking at this notion of dissensus in a little more detail, since it is at
the heart of the practice of VBM. Thus, in the quasi-legal model of bioethics, differences of values are resolved, in principle, by reference to a rule (embodied in a
code or guideline and often supported by law), which has been settled in advance
by consensus. Differences of interpretation may arise, of course. But these are settled,
again in principle, by reference to a regulatory body with executive decision-making
powers.[12] Quasi-legal bioethics is thus outcome focused. It seeks to determine the
outcome of decisions by reference to rules that express particular values. In this
respect, quasi-legal bioethics is like EBM. Both are outcome focused. Both, that is
to say, aim to provide rules (or guidelines) on what to do in a given situation. These
rules are based on consensus, respectively on the facts (EBM) and the values (quasi-
legal bioethics) that guide clinical decision making. VBM, as Box 5 illustrates for the
case of Diane Abbot, shifts the emphasis from outcome to process. In VBM there is
a clear place for rules and regulation in providing a framework for practice. Such a
framework, as we will see at the start of the next section, is essential. In VBM, though,
the framework of rules and regulation is limited to those values that for a given
community are largely shared and hence over which consensus (agreement on a
particular value) is appropriate. A key insight of VBM, furthermore, summarized in

Box 5 Diane Abbot's values and the "dissensual" basis of her decision to stop lithium

As noted in Box 2 and described in the text (under Principle 2), Diane Abbot's decision to stop lithium was overtly values based because the operative values were contested. When she started on lithium, her values were concordant with those of her family doctor and her colleagues. But when it came to stopping lithium, what mattered to Diane Abbot was her ability to "really see" colors, while what mattered to her doctor and her colleagues was the potentially damaging effects of a further episode of hypomania. And her doctor and her colleagues had a point! Diane Abbot, when hypomanic, was a considerable liability to herself and to everyone else. Moreover, whatever her subjective impression, objectively her output as an artist had been enhanced rather than restricted while on lithium. Stabilizing her mood may have taken some of the excitement out of her work; but this, in the view of her colleagues, was more than compensated for by her greater consistency. Even in her own terms, then, it seemed (to everyone else) imprudent, to say the least, that she should come off lithium.

Quasi-legal ethics and VBM, in these circumstances, lead to the same outcome: that Diane Abbot should stop taking lithium. But, whereas in quasi-legal ethics stopping lithium is an outcome prescribed by a rule expressing a "right" value (patient autonomy), in VBM stopping lithium is the product of a process aimed at achieving a balance of different, and legitimately different, values. As described in the text, the quasi-legal rule is justified by a (supposed) consensus (on the value of autonomy), whereas the VBM process, of balancing legitimately different value perspectives, starts from the premise that there is often no one right perspective—hence the neologistic "dissensus." The shift in VBM from outcome to process, from *what* is done to *how* it is done, depends critically on the skills summarized under Principles 6–9.

Principle 3, is that, as scientific advances open up choices, so diversity, rather than shared values, will increasingly become the norm in health-care decision making. Increasingly, then, dissensual, as well as consensual, approaches to clinical decision making will be needed. Increasingly, that is to say, instead of relying solely or even primarily on rules and regulation to prescribe outcomes, we will need to develop processes that allow effective decision making through a balance of legitimately different value perspectives.

This "multiperspective" approach, in the context of health-care decision making, depends critically on a number of key clinical skills. This is one specific sense in which VBM is process rather than outcome focused. In VBM, good clinical decision making, in the increasingly values-diverse context of modern health care depends, in the well-worn phrase, not just on *what* is done but on *how* it is done. It is to the skills base of VBM that we turn in the next section.

VBM: THE PRACTICE (PRINCIPLES 6–10)

As a strategy for resolving differences, dissensus, in VBM is antiparallel not only with EBM but also with bioethics. As a theoretical discipline, bioethics is a rich and varied discipline fully cognizant of the diversity of human values. In its connections with practice, however, it has taken a predominantly quasi-legal form premised on the (generally unacknowledged) assumption of "right values." The growing mountain of ever more complex rules and regulations governing all areas of health care aim to give effect to these right values: the rules tell us what the values are; regulatory bodies have executive authority to interpret the rules in equivocal cases.[13]

It is no part of VBM to suggest that we can do without rules and regulation altogether (Fulford and Bloch 2000). To the contrary, as already noted, VBM incorporates rules and regulation but as a framework for practice defined by the values shared within a given community.[14] Such values, then, set benchmark outcomes against which decisions taken within the relevant community can be measured. By the same token, though, quasi-legal ethics is *in*appropriate in situations in which legitimately *different* values are in play.[15] In such situations, we should rely not on "good outcomes" but on "good process," not, as I put it a moment ago, on *what* is done but on *how* it is done. The "how" of VBM depends on four key areas of clinical skill and an important shift in the locus of clinical decision-making (see table 14.3).

Skills Area 1: Awareness of Values

> *6th Principle of VBM:* Careful attention to language use in a given context is one of a range of powerful methods for raising awareness of values (the "values blindness" principle).

At the heart of many of the problems with values in health care is what might be called "values blindness." That is to say, problems arise in practice not so much from direct conflicts of values as from a failure to recognize values for what they are. In multidisciplinary teamwork, for example, a recent empirical study has shown that deep but largely unrecognized differences of values among psychiatrists, social workers, community nurses, patients, and informal caregivers may be a key factor behind failures of collaborative decision making (Colombo et al. 2003; Fulford 2001).

This "values blindness" has many sources: the tendency of values to become invisible when shared (see Principle 2); the development of professional identity (which includes a shared value system; Fulford 1994c); and the success of science (tending to eclipse values and other humanities-related aspects of medicine, for example in medical education; Hope and Fulford 1993).

Table 14.3. Comparison of VBM and Quasi-Legal Ethics

Principles of VBM	VBM (Values-Based Medicine)	Quasi-Legal Ethics
6. The "values-blindness" principle	Values are important in all areas of health care	Values are concerned with ethical issues
7. The "values-myopia" principle	A full range of empirical methods is used for increasing knowledge of values	Empirical methods are subject to prior values
8. The "space of values" principle	Ethical reasoning is used to explore differences (the space of values)	Ethical reasoning is used to decide "what is right"
9. The "how it's done" principle	Communication skills have a substantive role	Communication skills have a merely executive role
10. The "who decides" principle	Primarily patients and practitioners	Primarily ethicists and lawyers

A key skill underpinning VBM, then, is greater awareness of where, what, and how values come into health care. Improved knowledge of values, and the reasoning and communication skills described later in this chapter, all contribute to this. A distinct skill, however, is greater alertness to language use, to the words and phrases actually used in a given context. This approach is based on the work of the Oxford philosopher J. L. Austin (1956–57). Austin argued for what he called "philosophical field work"; that is, rather than just thinking about meanings in the abstract, Austin said that we should examine the language people actually use as a guide to understanding. This approach, which is illustrated for the case of Diane Abbot in Box 6, has been applied as a method of inquiry across a range of issues in the philosophy of psychiatry (Fulford 1990; Fulford et al., forthcoming) and, combined with empirical social science methods, in research (Fulford 2001). Recently, the approach has been developed as the basis of new training programs in values-based practice for health-care professionals (e.g., nurses, social workers, psychologists) working in such areas as assertive outreach, community care, and acute inpatient care. In this context, in particular, Austin's methodology has turned out to be a particularly powerful method for raising awareness of the often very wide differences in values between different team members, and between providers and users of services (Fulford et al. 2002).

Having raised awareness of the extent to which values and differences in values permeate health care, however, we must consider what the next step is. Where do we go from there?

Box 6 Awareness of the values operative in Diane Abbot's case

As described in the text, a first, and essential, skill for VBM is raised awareness of values. The effectiveness of linguistic analysis, of careful attention to language use, as a method for raising awareness of values is illustrated by the account of the opening stage in Diane Abbot's story in Box 1. In the first part of this box, Diane Abbot's overtly evidence-based decision to start on lithium was described in the language of a clinical case history. Here we were concentrating on the message — that is, the importance of EBM, combined with Dr. Kirk's clinical experience and Diane Abbot's legal colleague's positive personal experience, as the basis of her decision. In the second part of the box, by contrast, we were made aware of the significance of values, alongside evidence, in her decision. This was done by standing back for a moment from the message (the importance of EBM) and looking at the actual words in which the message (as a standard clinical case history) was delivered. The key words, italicized in Box 1, were *value* words — "effectiveness," "cost," and "adverse." The values-awareness workshop and other new training initiatives, described in the text, are based on this linguistic-analytic approach.

Skills Area 2: Knowledge of Values

7th Principle of VBM: A rich resource of both empirical and philosophical methods is available for improving our knowledge of other people's values (the "values-myopia" principle).

Where Principle 6 is concerned with values blindness, Principle 7 is concerned with "values myopia" — with our tendency, even when aware of values, to assume that other people's values are the same as our own. Within health care, this tendency is evident, for example, both in clinical interactions and, on a larger scale, in needs assessment (Marshall 1994) and service planning (Campbell 1996). But values myopia, as Box 7 illustrates, may have subtle and complex interactions with the evidence base of practice.

A second skill that underpins VBM is thus, straightforwardly, knowledge of the values bearing, or likely to bear, on a given decision in a given context. Our resources in this respect are partly empirical, partly philosophical. Empirical methods for gaining better understanding of other people's values include firsthand narratives (the growing "user literature," for example), the use of poetry and other literary sources, anthropological methods (such as ethnography), psychological techniques (cognitive-behavioral; psychoanalysis), and surveys. Among philosophical methods, Continental philosophy, which is more text-based than Anglo-American analytic philosophy, is a rich resource. This includes phenomenology (concerned with the structure and content of experience) and hermeneutics (concerned with revealing meanings).[16]

Box 7 Knowledge of the values operative in Diane Abbot's case

Knowledge of values in VBM includes knowledge both of the extent of the *differences* between people in their values and of the extent to which people *underestimate* these differences: we all tend to assume that other people's values are similar to our own. In Diane Abbot's case this "values myopia" (see text) led to one of the fault lines in her original decision to start lithium. The evidence base for this decision, insofar as it was derived from EBM, was the effects and side effects of lithium as characterized by the results of meta-analyses of high-quality research. But the effects and side effects described in such studies are picked out by reference to values that are widely shared: an "effect" of a drug is one that is positively valued by most people in most contexts, a side effect one that is negatively valued by most people in most contexts.

There is nothing wrong with this as such. To the contrary, such values, positive and negative, are essential: they pick out, severally, variables (the effects and side effects) relevant to a given research paradigm; taken together, they determine whether the research is "worth" doing in the first place. But a failure to recognize the (inevitable and appropriate) skewing of research toward values that are largely shared can lead to decisions that fail to reflect the sometimes very different values of a given individual in a particular context. The emotional blunting side effect of lithium was known. But, being a side effect of relative unimportance to most people, it had not figured prominently in EBM analyses of lithium or, indeed, in Dr. Kirk's clinical experience. Hence, although emotional blunting turned out to be a key side effect from Diane Abbot's perspective as an artist, it was not on Dr. Kirk's agenda in his initial discussion with her. Again, this is not a fault with EBM as such. Diane Abbot was equally misled by the narrative information from her colleague. The fault line runs rather from a "values-myopic" use of evidence, whether meta-analytic, clinical, or experiential, in clinical decision making.

There is no shortage of methods, then—empirical, literary, philosophical, and so forth—for building up our knowledge of the values likely to be operative in a given case. In some instances this may be enough to resolve difficulties; greater knowledge of the values in play in a given clinical context may help to remove misunderstandings, to increase mutual respect, and so forth. To understand all is to forgive all! Sometimes, though, conflicts and difficulties will remain. It is here that reasoning skills may be helpful.

Skills Area 3: Reasoning about Values

8th Principle of VBM: Ethical reasoning is employed in VBM primarily to explore *differences* of values, rather than, as in quasi-legal bioethics, to determine "what is right" (the "space of values" principle).

Methods for reasoning about values can be derived from any area of ethics (Dickenson and Fulford 2000: ch. 2). Methods commonly used in health care include consequentialism (e.g., the utilitarian basis of much health economics) and deontology (e.g., rights-based documents and standards). In the clinical context, two methods have gained wide currency:

- Principles: "top down" reasoning from general principles
- Casuistry: "bottom up" reasoning, direct from cases

All of these methods may be helpful in VBM. The aim of ethical reasoning in VBM, however, is radically different from its aim in the quasi-legal form of bioethics (Fulford et al. 2002a). In quasi-legal ethics, as in legal reasoning itself, the aim is to decide "what is right." As noted earlier, this is appropriate where values are more or less shared. In VBM, by contrast, in the context of value diversity, the aim is rather to explore the nature and extent of *differences* of values. There are limits, of course, and these are reflected in the framework for practice provided by quasi-legal bioethics and law (limited to situations where values are shared; see earlier discussion). But in situations of value diversity, the first aim of ethical reasoning is to explore the "space of values" (Fulford and Bloch 2000).

The radically different aim of ethical reasoning in VBM, to explore differences of values, has important implications for practice. These are illustrated by the case of Diane Abbot in Box 8. But it also carries with it a radically different way of thinking about differences of values themselves in health care. In quasi-legal bioethics, the assumption of uniquely "right" values has the implication that differences of values are a problem to be "solved" (by consensus, by dictat, or whatever means). The assumption in quasi-legal bioethics is that differences of values are a barrier to effective clinical decision making. In VBM, by contrast, differences of values, while indeed sometimes requiring resolution, may also be a *resource* for clinical decision making. For, as management theorists rather than ethicists have recognized (Heifetz 1994),[17] we are all better at understanding other people's values when they are similar to our own. In VBM, then, different value perspectives, as represented by different members of a multidisciplinary team, for example (see later discussion), operate as a series of lenses or filters for highlighting the often very different value perspectives of individual clients or patients. Different value perspectives within the clinical team, on this VBM model, far from being an impediment to effective clinical decision making, offer a positive resource for matching decisions as closely as possible to the values of those concerned.

There will be situations, though, in which, despite our being fully aware of the origin of a problem in differences of values (Principle 6), and despite our having fully explored the values concerned (Principles 7 and 8), conflicts remain. This is inevitable (and indeed to be welcomed!) if, as VBM suggests, *legitimately* different value perspectives are the norm in health care. In health care, moreover, matters can never be left in the air (Fulford 1994). Practical situations demand practical action, even if this means "leaving well enough alone." It is here that communication skills become important in VBM.

Box 8 Reasoning about the values operative in Diane Abbot's case

The fault line in Diane Abbot's original decision, noted in Box 7—a values-myopic use of evidence—illustrates the key difference between quasi-legal ethics and VBM in their approaches to reasoning about values. The quasi-legal aim of coming to an agreement on the "right" outcome (consensus), inevitably leads to a focus on shared values. This is especially true of casuistry, or case-based reasoning, the very justification of which is that agreement on actual cases reflects shared values (Fulford and Bloch 2000). Diane Abbot was, in a sense, guided in her decision to start lithium by casuistic reasoning: by the case of her colleague on lithium and his positive experience of that treatment.

The aim of ethical reasoning in VBM, by contrast, is to explore *differences* of values. In Diane Abbot's case, such reasoning might have alerted her, and Dr. Kirk, to a key difference between herself and her colleague—that, whereas she was a creative artist, he was a lawyer. Both were successful academics whose work required high levels of sustained attention. For both, therefore, the attention disrupting effects of hypomania were highly negatively evaluated. But whereas for the lawyer emotional blunting was unimportant (it was not indeed a side effect of which he had even been aware), for the artist it was of the essence. Casuistic reasoning, it is important to add, is not the only way in which this difference of values might have been anticipated. Principles reasoning, although much criticized in bioethics, offers a powerful tool for exploring differences of values.*

*Tom Beauchamp and Richard Childress (1989), in their original description of the role of principles reasoning in medicine, are much closer to VBM than to quasi-legal ethics. Their "prima facie" principles are, in effect, dimensions along which the values operative in a given case can be explored (Fulford et al. 2002a).

Skills Area 4: Communication Skills

9th Principle of VBM: In VBM, communication skills have a substantive rather than (as in quasi-legal ethics) a merely executive role in clinical decision making (the "how it's done" principle).

In VBM, awareness, knowledge, and ethical reasoning are combined with communication skills to effect action. Educationally, this is an extension of a model of "ethics training" for medical students developed in Oxford, in which traditional ethics and law are fully integrated with communication skills in a clinical problem-solving approach to ethical reasoning (Hope et al. 1996).

A wide range of communication skills is important in VBM. Two particular kinds of skill stand out, though, as being essential:

- *Patient-perspective skills.* These are the skills of listening to and exploring the values of a client or patient. They are the basis of the patient-centered principle of VBM (Principle 4). Raised awareness (Principle 6), improved knowledge (Principle 7), and ethical reasoning (Principle 8) may all be helpful in this respect, particularly where there are difficulties of communication. But, as Principle 4 emphasizes, the values of the particular individual concerned are irreducible.

- *Multiperspective skills.* These are the skills involved in coming to a balance of values in situations of conflict and disagreement. They are the basis of the multiperspective principle of VBM (Principle 5), the principle that replaces consensus with dissensus — that is, with effective action in the context of legitimately different value perspectives. Relevant perspectives in health care include those of other colleagues (medical and nonmedical), of informal caregivers, of managers, and so forth. Mutual understanding and respect are fundamental in this respect. But specific skills, such as negotiation and conflict resolution, are also essential.

Communication skills, although of course important also in quasi-legal ethics, have a deeper importance in VBM. In quasi-legal ethics, communication skills are *executive*, their role being primarily to help in implementing the rules (which, in turn, are taken to express "right" values; see earlier discussion). In VBM, by contrast, as Box 9 illustrates for the case of Diane Abbot, communication skills have a *substantive* role. In VBM, communication skills are central (1) to establishing the different value perspectives bearing on a given situation (complementing, at an interpersonal level, the philosophical and empirical methods outlined under Principles 6–8), and (2) to resolving a course of action where the operative value perspectives are genuinely in conflict. This is why, as noted under Principle 5, in VBM good practice depends not just on *what* is done but on *how* it is done.[18]

Taking Back the Territory

10th Principle of VBM: VBM, although involving a partnership with ethicists and lawyers (equivalent to the partnership with scientists and statisticians in EBM), puts decision making back where it belongs, with users and providers at the clinical coal-face (the "who decides?" principle).

Where Principles 6–9 of VBM are concerned with the skills base of decision making in the context of value diversity, Principle 10 is concerned with "who decides?"

In quasi-legal ethics, the assumption of "right" values, and its consequent proliferation of rules and regulatory authorities, inevitably leads to a model of the ethicist as an expert. And ethicists, like scientists, may indeed bring a range of relevant expertise to policy, practice, education, and research in health care. As we saw earlier, however, where legitimately different values are in play, the particular value pre-

---

Box 9 Communication skills and the values operative in Diane Abbot's case

Both patient-perspective and multiperspective communication skills, as described in the text, were important to securing the good outcome achieved in Diane Abbott's case. These skills were especially important at the apparently unproblematic initial stage, when everyone agreed with her decision to start on lithium. A quasi-legal approach would have endorsed Diane Abbot's choice on grounds of the "right" value of autonomy. As such, there would have been a risk of alienating her colleagues and her family doctor when her decision to stop lithium ran counter to their concerns for her welfare: such concerns, expressed in terms of beneficence in Beauchamp and Childress's *Four Principles*, tend to be relabeled pejoratively in quasi-legal bioethics as "paternalistic."

In VBM, by contrast, the dissensual nature of decision making starts from (the meta-value of) respect for differences of values. A precondition of such respect is that the voices of those concerned, of *all* those concerned, are listened to. This is not as easy as it sounds! First, it is time consuming, although the time spent in coming to an understanding of the relevant perspectives tends to pay off in the longer term because those concerned, as in Diane Abbot's case, feel understood and fully engaged (see Principle 10). Second, it is not always easy to understand other people's values where they are different from one's own. As noted in the text, this is one reason (among many others) why the different value perspectives represented by a well-functioning multidisciplinary team may be crucial to good clinical care. These perspectives operate as a series of "lenses" sensitive to the different values operative in a given case. A further and increasingly important series of such lenses is provided by support groups and networks of those with firsthand experience of the situation in question. Talking with people who have "been through it" provides invaluable experiential information. Diane Abbot's lawyer colleague was helpful to her not just in starting lithium but also in her decision to stop it. Given the differences in their values, though, it might have been helpful, too, if Diane Abbot had been able to talk to someone from the creative arts with personal experience of lithium therapy. A key role of advocacy groups in VBM is to support decision making by helping to put service users with similar backgrounds and experience in touch with each other.

---

scribed by a quasi-legal ethical rule, however enlightened, will necessarily conflict with the very different values of many of those to whom the rule is intended to apply.

The complaint of ethicists against the medical culture has been that "doctor knows best." Bioethics has thus rightly emphasized the importance of patient autonomy in health-care decision making. Quasi-legal bioethics, however, if extended from areas of value uniformity to areas of value diversity, risks a new culture of "ethicist knows best" (Fulford et al. 2002a). VBM, in starting from the legitimately different value perspectives that are increasingly in play in all areas of health care, puts ethical decision making back where it belongs—with those concerned, as users and provid-

---

Box 10 "Who decides?" and the outcome in Diane Abbot's case

The shift in the locus of decision making in VBM from ethicists and lawyers to patients and professionals carries with it a shift from rights to responsibilities. The "right values" of quasi-legal ethics creates a culture of legal rights. The meta-value of respect for differences in VBM creates a culture of mutual responsibility. In Diane Abbot's case, Dr. Kirk's failure to mention emotional blunting as a potential side effect of lithium might have led a rights-minded lawyer to consider an action for breach of duty of care. The action would probably not be pursued because the damages, in this case, were negligible. But an increasingly defensive approach to practice is the result of an overreliance on such rights-based approaches. In Diane Abbot's case, the defensive strategy would have been to give her a checklist of potential side effects of lithium and to ask her to sign a consent form, or something similar. Instead, a positive relationship of trust was built up among all those concerned such that Diane Abbot, her colleagues, and her family doctor all felt engaged in, and hence had a sense of ownership of, the decisions made.

This had a number of positive therapeutic effects. First, the experience of emotional blunting helped Diane Abbot to appreciate that her mood swings were not, as such, pathological but (within limits) a positive aspect of her work as an artist. Second, it allowed her to take responsibility (with help from others) for managing future overswings. As noted in the text, her positive decision to stop lithium was combined with an advance directive for early intervention in a future hypomanic episode. This was felt to be important (by Diane Abbot as well as by her doctor and her colleagues) because of her lack of insight in the past into the warning signs of a relapse. In the event when these signs eventually recurred it was Diane Abbot herself who initiated contact with her doctor. Somehow, her engagement in the process of managing her condition had given her improved insight at this crucial early stage. We can only speculate on the mechanisms involved here: some combination, perhaps, of her improved understanding of her condition; of her new trust in her family doctor, Dr. Kirk, and her colleagues; and of her confidence that she would be treated with due regard to her values. This improved insight may not prove to be a permanent change, of course. But her recognition of the positive as well as negative aspects of her mood swings and her ability to take responsibility as well as to receive help are consistent with the improved prognosis associated with recovery approaches to the functional psychoses (Mueser et al. 2002).

---

ers, as patients, professionals, and as managers, at the clinical coal face. As the outcome of Diane Abbot's story (described in Box 10) illustrates, this re-engagement of those concerned with the decisions they make is the basis of a close connection between VBM and the emphasis on agency that is at the heart of the recovery model of mental health practice (Mueser et al. 2002).

CONCLUSIONS: PSYCHIATRY FIRST

Although this chapter has been about Values-Based *Medicine*, the main driver for the development of the ten principles outlined here has been psychiatry. In one sense, this is how it should be. Psychiatry, as noted under Principle 2, is more value laden than any other branch of medicine essentially because it is concerned with areas of human experience and behavior in which human values are particularly diverse. Hence, it would seem, it is natural that it is here, in psychiatry, that VBM should be developed first.

In the traditional fact-centered model of medicine, however, the development of VBM in psychiatry would be interpreted very differently—namely, as an apology or as a substitute for its (supposed) lack of a mature underpinning scientific theory. According to this model, as also noted under Principle 2, psychiatry's more overtly value-laden nature is a mark of scientific deficiency. Correspondingly, therefore, according to the fact-centered traditional medical model, psychiatry needs VBM because it lacks science. Philosophical value theory, by contrast, suggests that the more value-laden nature of psychiatry is a mark not of scientific inadequacy but of values complexity. Psychiatry is more value laden than other areas of medicine because it is concerned with areas of human experience and behavior, such as emotion, desire, volition, and belief, in which human values are highly (and legitimately) diverse (Fulford 1989: ch. 5).

It is as a response to value complexity, then, not as a substitute for scientific sophistication, that VBM has developed first in psychiatry. Principle 3 of VBM, furthermore, the "science-driven" principle, shows that, with future progress in medical science and technology, similar value complexity will increasingly become the norm in *all* areas of medicine. Far from lagging behind medical science, therefore, psychiatry, in developing the theory and practice of VBM, is providing a lead that other areas of medicine, under the pressure of scientific progress, will eventually be obliged to follow. VBM, then, is indeed a first for psychiatry. And given its origins in philosophical value theory, the extent of the penetration of VBM already into policy and practice in mental health makes it also a first for the *philosophy* of psychiatry.

ACKNOWLEDGMENTS

I am grateful to the many colleagues who have contributed, with suggestions, examples, and case studies, to the development of the ideas set out in this chapter. My particular thanks go to Gillian Bendelow, Jeremy Dale, Melissa and Paul Falzer, John Geddes, Christa Kruger, Eric Matthews, Sarah Matthews, John Sadler, Giovanni Stonghellini, Werdie van Staden, and the members of the Values Project Group of the National Institutes of Mental Health in England (NIMHE): Piers Allott (chair), Simon Allard, Catherine Laurence, Liz Mayne, David Morris, Albert Persaud, Anthony Sheehan, and Kim Woodbridge.

NOTES

....

1. This approach, associated particularly with Oxford analytic philosophy, is sometimes called the "Oxford school." Exemplars include Philippa Foot (1958–59); R. M. Hare (1952, 1963), J. O. Urmson (1950), and G. J. Warnock (1971). Although it focuses particularly on moral values, philosophical value theory seeks to characterize the logical properties of value terms of all kinds. Von Wright (1963) defined several hundred kinds of values in his compendious *The Varieties of Goodness*. In the current pandemic of ethical issues in medicine, we tend to forget that many other kinds of value bear on decision making at all levels in health care—policy, managerial, and clinical—and indeed in research (see Sadler 1996; also Sadler, chapter 11 in this volume. See also Principle 1).

2. E.g., a branch of philosophy that is concerned with clarifying meanings rather than (directly) producing "answers."

3. See, e.g., A. MacIntyre (1985) and J. Dancy (1993).

4. I return to the practical importance of analytic ethical theory later; see especially note 11.

5. Compare the contribution of mathematics to the physical sciences.

6. The ten principles of VBM outlined in this chapter are based on Fulford, *Values-Based Medicine* (forthcoming) (Cambridge: Cambridge University Press).

7. As when mathematicians speak of evaluating an equation, for example.

8. The value judgments involved in taking a condition to be a disease/illness, for example, express not just negative value but a particular *kind* of negative value: that is, disease is different from ugliness (negative aesthetic value), delinquency (negative moral value), foolishness (negative prudential value), and so on. The characterization of the particular kind of negative value expressed by disease, illness, and the like is an important task for philosophy, particularly in relation to psychiatry; see my *Moral Theory and Medical Practice* (1989: chs. 6–10), and work by the Swedish philosopher Lennart Nordenfelt (1987), for one approach to this via agency. VBM, as presented here, however, does not depend on this further characterization. A negative value judgment, according to this approach, is at least a necessary, albeit not sufficient, prerequisite for a condition to be a disease/illness; and VBM is based primarily on the generic properties shared by all value terms, rather than the properties that mark out "medical" value judgments from value judgments of other kinds.

9. See Fulford 1989: chs. 8 and 9; also Fulford 1994a. For an account of Criterion B for schizophrenia and the dependence of the differential diagnosis between psychosis and religious experience on value judgments, see Jackson and Fulford (1997). Values in the diagnosis of manic-depressive disorder are discussed in Moore et al. (1994). For recent work on values in psychiatric diagnosis, see the edited collection by John Sadler, *Descriptions and Prescriptions: Values, Mental Disorders, and the DSMs* (2002), and his forthcoming monograph, *Values and Psychiatric Diagnosis*.

10. Reproductive medicine is a case in point. Even a few years ago, reproductive medicine was concerned mainly with major pathology, like "impacted fetus" or infertility, over which people's values are largely shared (like a heart attack, these are *bad* conditions, in themselves, for anyone). But now a series of remarkable advances in "assisted reproduction"

are giving us choices in areas that until recently were the stuff of science fiction: we can reverse the menopause, we can select fetuses, we are close to "designer" babies. Small wonder, then, that the full diversity of human values has been brought into play in this area of medicine!

11. The central importance of individual perspectives as our "first call" in VBM is sufficiently grounded on the given diversity of human values in health care (illustrated by the edited collection Fulford et al. 2002a). That our values are not only different but *legitimately* different also follows analytically from the logical separation of fact and value (or, more exactly, of description and evaluation) insisted on by "nondescriptivism" in philosophical value theory. The eighteenth-century British empirist philosopher David Hume is generally credited with the first explicit account of the claim that no description of a state of affairs in the world can ever, in itself, add up to a value judgment of that state of affairs: "no ought from an is" is how Hume's "law" is often summarized. Hare (1952) is perhaps the clearest exponent of this position among twentieth-century philosophers. The opposing school, descriptivism, points to situations in which we feel compelled to make a given value judgment on the basis of a given description (e.g., Warnock 1971). Exponents of the Hume-Hare version of nondescriptivism argue that in such cases the "compulsion" to make a given value judgment is only a psychological, not a logical, compulsion. The compulsion, that is to say, arises from the fact that in response to the situation in question, human values being what they are, most or even all people would make the same value judgment. But this leaves the analytic separation (the separation of *meaning*) intact.

In *Moral Theory and Medical Practice* (1989), and in two subsequent articles, "Nine Variations and a Coda on the Theme of an Evolutionary Definition of Dysfunction" (1999) and "Teleology without Tears: Naturalism, Neo-Naturalism and Evaluationism in the Analysis of Function Statements in Biology (and a Bet on the Twenty-first Century)" (2000), I have argued that the Hume-Hare separation of fact and value applied to concepts of disease and illness has a rich crop of implications for practice in psychiatry and medicine. The phenomenology specifically of delusion, furthermore, has interesting implications for the debate about fact and value in philosophical value theory. (The traditional debate has been in "horizontal" terms: that is, directly between fact and value; the phenomenology of delusion, however—in particular that delusions may take the form of value judgments, as well as of factual beliefs—points to a "vertical" connection between fact and value. That is, both depend on, and hence are (logically) related through, a background structure of practical reasoning; see Fulford 1989: ch. 10). Many of the practical implications of philosophical value theory, however, can be derived equally from descriptivist theory, to the extent that health care is concerned with areas in which human values are largely shared (Fulford 1991). The practical dangers of descriptivism arise from the temptation to extend the claimed derivation of "values" from "facts" to areas in which human values are legitimately different. In such areas—that is, in areas in which people's values are *not* shared—descriptivism is at risk of abusive consequences by imposing the values of one group or individual on those whose values are different.

This risk is greatly increased because of our tendency to underestimate the extent of the differences of values between us (see Principle 7). And it is a risk to which psychiatry, as an area of particular diversity of human values (Principle 3), has been peculiarly vulnerable in practice (Fulford 1998). In psychiatry, through much of the twentieth century, abusive practices arose, not primarily from malicious intent but because one person's or group's beliefs about "best" practice were allowed to exclude all other views (Fulford 2000a, 2000b). In psychiatry, then, a nondescriptivist rather than descriptivist basis for VBM is required. Furthermore, VBM's Principle 3 suggests that scientific progress is driving all areas of medicine increasingly into areas of value diversity. A nondescriptivist rather than descriptivist basis for VBM is thus likely to be increasingly important in all areas of medicine if we are to avoid the abusive imposition of one person's or group's values on others. See also Principle 10.

12. In the United Kingdom, for example, the Human Fertilisation and Embryology Authority has such powers.

13. It is no coincidence that the form of ethical regulatory codes is similar to that of practice guidelines derived from EBM. Both assume a unique "right" answer (in principle) for every situation; both assume that we approximate to the right answer by consensus. Quasi-legal bioethics, I have argued elsewhere, has indeed adopted this model (unwittingly) from scientific medicine (Fulford 2000b). In this respect, then, although developed originally as a guardian against the misuse of medical technology, bioethics has taken on the colors of its enemy!

14. VBM, in emphasizing value diversity, might be thought to risk ethical relativism and, hence, ethical chaos! There are several reasons why this is not so: (1) Human values, if more diverse than has generally been recognized, at least in health care, are not chaotic (if they were, law, which is self-evidently values based, would be chaotic!). (2) The shared values that, in VBM, are the proper remit of the rules and regulation of quasi-legal ethics provide, for a given group, a framework for decision making. (3) Where values are not shared, VBM starts not from the postmodern "anything goes" but from a principle of *mutual* respect with a range of clear and definite implications for policy and practice (mutual respect, for example, precludes racism because racism is incompatible with respect for differences (see the NIMHE Values Framework described in note 18). Far from being a recipe for ethical chaos, then, VBM is more like the values equivalent of a political democracy. Like a political democracy, VBM might be thought to be weaker than an authoritarian autocracy, such as a monarchy or a totalitarian regime. And in situations of extreme danger (e.g., war or famine), an autocracy may be more effective (indeed, we declare "marshal law" when a single shared value of survival is at stake). But the lesson of the twentieth century is that totalitarian solutions, in our civilization, however well intentioned, collapse into abusive ideology and that democracy, is, in practice, the stronger system (see also Principle 10).

15. That is, because the "right" values expressed in the rules and regulations governing the decision in question will necessarily be in conflict with the necessarily different values of many of those to whom the rules and regulations are intended to apply. See also Principle 10.

16. Illustrations of each of these resources, empirical and philosophical, with practical relevance for health care, and drawing on a rich international literature, are given in an anthology combining firsthand narratives from patients and caregivers with academic articles, poetry, and other literary sources (Fulford et al. 2002b). The aim of this anthology is twofold: first, to illustrate the remarkable diversity of human values relevant to every aspect of health-care decision making (from first contact through diagnosis to treatment and outcome); second, to build up a picture of the extent of the arsenal of methods available for improving our knowledge of values in relation to health-care decision making.

17. Heifetz was a psychiatrist before he moved into management and leadership studies. His book *Leadership without Easy Answers* (1994) develops a theory of "adaptive work" supported by a series of clear practical strategies for effective decision making in contexts of conflicting values.

18. Exploring values may sound like a tall order (a luxury perhaps?) in the contingencies of day-to-day practice. But the practical importance of values in modern health care has been recognized in the United Kingdom by the priority afforded values in the work of the National Institute for Mental Health (England). The NIMHE is a department of the Modernization Agency in the U.K.'s National Health Service (NHS) with responsibility for im-

plementing the U.K. government's key strategy for mental health, the National Service Framework for Mental Health. The first action of the NIMHE was to establish a Values Project Group to develop a framework of values and, importantly, a "process for implementation" (Ministerial Announcement 2001), for all stakeholders, both users and providers, in mental health. The Values Project Group worked in partnership with each of the other NIMHE programs, including such key areas as recovery practice, equality, inclusion, and "users as experts," to produce a framework for Values-Based Practice. This has now been formally adopted and is published at www.connects.org.uk/conferences. The framework will be developed further in conjunction with other training and policy initiatives within the NHS Modernisation Agency, such as the black and ethnic minority mental health strategy (Department of Health 2003). NIMHE thus recognizes that understanding patients' values and the values of colleagues is an *investment* in time. It is an up-front cost that could pay huge dividends in terms of the quality of the patient's experience, the job satisfaction of providers, compliance, responsiveness to change, and so forth.

REFERENCES

Austin, J. L. (1956–57) "A Plea for Excuses." *Proceedings of the Aristotelian Society* 57: 1–30. Reprinted in A. R. White (ed.) (1968) *The Philosophy of Action* (New York: Oxford University Press).

Beauchamp, T. L., and Childress, J. F. (1989; 4th ed. 1994) *Principles of Biomedical Ethics.* New York: Oxford University Press.

Boorse, C. (1975) "On the Distinction between Disease and Illness." *Philosophy and Public Affairs* 5: 49–68.

Boorse, C. (1976) "What a Theory of Mental Health Should Be." *Journal for the Theory of Social Behaviour* 6: 61–84.

Cain, P. (2002) " 'Partnership' Is Not Enough: Professional-Client Relations Revisited." Pages 278–81 in K. W. M. Fulford, D. Dickenson, and T. H. Murray (eds.), *Healthcare Ethics and Human Values: An Introductory Text with Readings and Case Studies.* Oxford: Blackwell.

Campbell, P. (1996) "What We Want from Crisis Services." In J. Read and J. Reynolds (eds.), *Speaking Our Minds: An Anthology.* Basingstoke, England: Macmillan Press for The Open University, pp. 180–83.

Colombo, A., Bendelow, G., Fulford, K. W. M., and Williams, S. (2003) "Evaluating the Influence of Implicit Models of Mental Disorder on Processes of Shared Decision Making within Community-Based Multi-disciplinary Teams." *Social Science and Medicine* 56: 1557–1570.

Dancy, J. (1993) *Moral Reasons.* Oxford: Blackwell.

Department of Health (2003) *Inside Outside: Improving Mental Health Services for Black and Minority Ethnic Communities in England.* London: Department of Health.

Dickenson, D., and Fulford, K. W. M. (2000) *In Two Minds: A Casebook of Psychiatric Ethics.* Oxford: Oxford University Press.

Eddy, D. M. (1991) "Clinical Decision Making: From Theory to Practice. Rationing by Patient Choice." *JAMA* 265: 105–8.

Foot, P. (1958–59) "Moral Beliefs." *Proceedings of the Aristotelian Society* 59: 83–104. Reprinted in Foot, P. (ed.) (1967) *Theories of Ethics.* Oxford: Oxford University Press.

Fulford, K. W. M. (1989) *Moral Theory and Medical Practice*. Cambridge: Cambridge University Press. Reprinted 1995 and 1999.

Fulford, K. W. M. (1990) "Philosophy and Medicine: The Oxford Connection." *British Journal of Psychiatry* 157: 111–15.

Fulford, K. W. M. (1991) "The Concept of Disease." In Sidney Bloch and Paul Chodoff (eds.), *Psychiatric Ethics*, 2nd ed. Oxford: Oxford University Press, pp. 77–99.

Fulford, K. W. M. (1994a) "Closet Logics: Hidden Conceptual Elements in the DSM and ICD Classifications of Mental Disorders." In J. Z. Sadler, O. P. Wiggins, and M. A. Schwartz (eds.), *Philosophical Perspectives on Psychiatric Diagnostic Classification*. Baltimore: Johns Hopkins University Press.

Fulford, K. W. M. (1994b) "Not More Medical Ethics." In K. W. M. Fulford, G. R. Gillett, and J. M. Soskice (eds.), *Medicine and Moral Reasoning*. Cambridge: Cambridge University Press.

Fulford, K. W. M. (1994c) "Medical Education: Knowledge and Know-how." In R. Chadwick (ed.), *Ethics and the Professions*. Aldershot, England: Avebury Press.

Fulford K. W. M. (1995) "The Concept of Patient-Centred Care." In K. W. M. Fulford, S. Ersser, and T. Hope (eds.), *Essential Practice in Patient-Centred Care*. Oxford: Blackwell Science.

Fulford, K. W. M. (1998) "Dissent and Dissensus: The Limits of Consensus Formation in Psychiatry." In H.A.M.J. ten Have and H-M. Saas (eds.), *Consensus Formation in Health Care Ethics*. Philosophy and Medicine Series. Dordrecht: Kluwer Academic, pp. 175–92.

Fulford, K. W. M. (1999) "Nine Variations and a Coda on the Theme of an Evolutionary Definition of Dysfunction." *Journal of Abnormal Psychology* 108(3): 412–20.

Fulford, K. W. M. (2000a) "Teleology without Tears: Naturalism, Neo-Naturalism and Evaluationism in the Analysis of Function Statements in Biology (and a Bet on the Twenty-first Century)." *Philosophy, Psychiatry, and Psychology* 7(1): 77–94.

Fulford, K. W. M. (2000b) "Philosophy Meets Psychiatry in the Twentieth Century: Four Looks Back and a Brief Look Forward." In P. Louhiala and S. Stenman (eds.), *Philosophy Meets Medicine*. Helsinki: Helsinki University Press, pp. 114–31.

Fulford, K. W. M. (2001) "Philosophy into Practice: The Case for Ordinary Language Philosophy." In L. Nordenfelt (ed.), *Health, Science and Ordinary Language*. Amsterdam: Rodopi.

Fulford, K. W. M. (forthcoming) "Values-Based Medicine: Thomas Szasz' Legacy to Twenty-first Century Psychiatry." In J. A. Schaler (ed.), *Szasz under Fire: Thomas Szasz Faces His Critics*. Chicago: Open Court.

Fulford, K. W. M., and Bloch, S. (2000) "Psychiatric Ethics: Codes, Concepts, and Clinical Practice Skills." In M. Gelder, J. J. Lopez-Ibor, and N. Andreasen (eds.), *New Oxford Textbook of Psychiatry*. Oxford: Oxford University Press, pp. 27–32.

Fulford, K. W. M., Dickenson, D., and Murray, T. H. (2002a) "Introduction: Many Voices: Human Values in Healthcare Ethics." Pages 1–19 in K. W. M. Fulford, D. Dickenson, and T. H. Murray (eds.), *Healthcare Ethics and Human Values: An Introductory Text with Readings and Case Studies*. Oxford: Blackwell.

Fulford, K. W. M., Dickenson, D., and Murray, T. H. (eds.) (2002b) *Healthcare Ethics and Human Values: An Introductory Text with Readings and Case Studies*. Oxford: Blackwell.

Fulford, K. W. M., Williamson, T., and Woodbridge, K. (2002) "Values-Added Practice." *Mental Health Today* (October), pp. 25–27.

Fulford, K. W. M., Thornton, T., and Graham, G. (forthcoming) "Introduction: Origins,

Outcomes and How to Use This Book." In K. W. M. Fulford, T. Thornton, and G. Graham, *The Shorter Oxford Textbook of Philosophy and Psychiatry*. Oxford: Oxford University Press.

Hare, R. M. (1952) *The Language of Morals*. Oxford: Oxford University Press.

Hare, R. M. (1963) Descriptivism. *Proceedings of the British Academy* 49: 115–34. Reprinted in Hare, R. M. (1972) *Essays on the Moral Concepts*. London: Macmillan.

Heifetz, R. (1994) *Leadership without Easy Answers*. Cambridge, MA: Harvard University Press.

Hope, R. A., and Fulford, K. W. M. (1993) "Medical Education: Patients, Principles and Practice Skills." In R. Gillon (ed.), *Principles of Health Care Ethics*. Chichester, England: Wiley.

Hope, T., Fulford, K. W. M., and Yates, A. (1996) *The Oxford Practice Skills Course: Ethics, Law and Communication Skills in Health Care Education*. Oxford: Oxford University Press.

Hudson Jones, A. (1999) "Narrative in Medical Ethics." *British Medical Journal* 318: 253–56.

Jackson, M., and Fulford, K. W. M. (1997) "Spiritual Experience and Psychopathology." *Philosophy, Psychiatry, and Psychology* 4(1): 41–66. Commentaries by R. Littlewood, F. G. Lu et al., A. Sims, and A. Storr and response by authors, pp. 67–90.

Jamison, K. R. (1994) *Touched with Fire: Manic Depressive Illness and the Artistic Temperament*. New York: Free Press.

Keller, M. B., Lavori, P. W., Kane, J. M. Gelenberg, A. J., Rosenbaum, J. F., Walzer, E. A., and Baker, L. A. (1992) "Subsyndromal Symptoms in Bipolar Disorder: A Comparison of Standard and Low Serum Levels of Lithium." *Archives of General Psychiatry* 49(5): 371–76.

MacIntyre, A. (1985) *After Virtue: A Study in Moral Theory*. London: Duckworth.

Marshall, M. (1994) "How Should We Measure Need? Concept and Practice in the Development of a Standardized Assessment Schedule." *Philosophy, Psychiatry, and Psychology* 1(1): 27–36.

May, W. F. (1994) "The Virtues in a Professional Setting." In K. W. M. Fulford, G. R. Gillett, and J. M. Soskice (eds.), *Medicine and Moral Reasoning*. Cambridge: Cambridge University Press.

Ministerial Announcement (2001) Made at launch of the National Institutes for Mental Health in England (NIMHE).

Moore, A., Hope, T., and Fulford, K. W. M. (1994) "Mild Mania and Well-Being." *Philosophy, Psychiatry, and Psychology* 1(3): 165–78.

Mueser, K. T., Corrigan, P. W., Hilton, D. W., Tanzman, B., Schaub, A., Gingerich, S., Essock, S. M., Tarrier, N., Morey, B., Vogel-Scibilia, S., and Herz, M. I. (2002) "Illness Management and Recovery: A Review of the Research." *Psychiatric Services* 53(10): 1272–84.

Nagel, T. (1986) *The View from Nowhere*. New York: Oxford University Press.

Nordenfelt, L. (1987) *On the Nature of Health: An Action-Theoretic Approach*. Dordrecht: D. Reidel.

Okasha, A. (2000) "Ethics of Psychiatric Practice: Consent, Compulsion and Confidentiality." *Current Opinion in Psychiatry* 13: 693–98.

Perkins, R. (2001) "What Constitutes Success? The Relative Priority of Service Users' and Clinicians' Views of Mental Health Services." *British Journal of Psychiatry* 179: 9–10.

Phillips, J. (2000) "Conceptual Models for Psychiatry." *Current Opinion in Psychiatry* 13: 683–88.

Raphael-Leff, J. (2002) "The 'Kinder Egg': Some Intrapsychic, Interpersonal, and Ethical Implications of Infertility Treatment and Gamete Donation." In K. W. M. Fulford, D. Dickenson, and T. H. Murray (eds.), *Healthcare Ethics and Human Values: An Introductory Text with Readings and Case Studies*. Oxford: Blackwell, pp. 201–5.

Sackett, D. L., Straus, S. E., Scott Richardson, W., Rosenberg, W., and Haynes, R. B. (2000) *Evidence-Based Medicine: How to Practice and Teach EBM*, 2nd ed. Edinburgh: Churchill Livingstone.

Sadler, J. Z. (1996) "Epistemic Value Commitments in the Debate over Categorical vs. Dimensional Personality Diagnosis." *Philosophy, Psychiatry, and Psychology* 3(3): 203–22.

Sadler, J. Z. (ed.) (2002) *Descriptions and Prescriptions: Values, Mental Disorders, and the DSMs*. Baltimore: Johns Hopkins University Press.

Sadler, J. Z. (forthcoming) *Values and Psychiatric Diagnosis*. Oxford: Oxford University Press.

Straus, S. E. (2002) "Individualizing Treatment Decisions: The Likelihood of Being Helped or Harmed." *Evaluation and the Health Professions* 25(2): 210–24.

Urmson, J. O. (1950) "On Grading." *Mind* 59: 145–69.

von Wright, H. G. (1963) *The Varieties of Goodness*. London: Routledge and Kegan Paul and New York: Humanities Press.

Warnock, G. J. (1971) *The Object of Morality*. London: Methuen.

Williams, B. (1985) *Ethics and the Limits of Philosophy*. London: Fontana.

Williams, A. (1995) "Economics, QALYs and Medical Ethics: A Health Economist's Perspective." *Health Care Analysis* 3(3): 221–26.

PART III

NORMS, VALUES, AND ETHICS

CHAPTER 15

GENDER

NANCY POTTER

GENDER is an analytical category that refers to the social organization of the relation between the sexes. The term "gender" is used to designate psychological, social, and cultural aspects of maleness and femaleness. It includes gender attribution, gender assignment, gender role, and gender identity. *Gender attribution* is a complex, interactive process of inferring and then attributing the gender of someone on the basis of what we take to be "cues"—various body features, dress, behavior, mannerisms, and so on, that function as signifiers—of a particular gender. *Gender assignment* is a special case of gender attribution that (usually) occurs once, at birth. Usually, assignment is made after inspection of the infant's genitals, which are categorized according to presence of either vagina or penis; gender is announced on the basis of that inspection. *Gender role* is a set of prescriptions and expectations about what behaviors are appropriate for people of one gender. Gender roles include interests, activities, dress, skills, and sexual partner choice. For each of these components, there are clear, and different, expectations for those who occupy the male role and those who occupy the female role, although expectations and norms vary somewhat, depending on culture. *Gender identity* is the self-attribution of gender: how one considers oneself in relation to the categories of gender. Rules for self-attribution are not necessarily the same as rules for attributing gender to others. One's gender identity can be relatively independent of the gender attributions made by others.

Although many people assume that a healthy individual will have a stable and unified gender that correlates with his or her biological sex, these aspects of gender frequently do not line up in a neat package. In much of the Western world, the gender attribution process is the method by which people construct a world of two genders. However, although secondary gender characteristics and genitals are important cues, they are never sufficient for making a gender attribution. Nor is knowing the relationship among the gender components sufficient for making a correct gender attribution. Experiences and expressions of gender are more fluid, flexible, and dynamic than the social organization of gender indicates. For example, fantasy (which plays an important role in identity formation and transformation, assertion of agency, and experiences of autonomy) may circulate around culturally proscribed or transgressive domains of behavior. Both sexual fantasies and role fantasies may be at odds with gender attribution and may complicate or disrupt a person's gender identity.

The social organization of gender is identified as a *sex/gender system*, which is a set of arrangements by which a society transforms biological sexuality into gendered beings whose activities and interests are expected to contribute to a productive and generative society in culturally specified ways. The sex/gender system in Western industrialized societies follows a dichotomized system of human sexual difference. In most of the Western world, male biology is expected to correlate with masculine gender attribution, role, and identity, and male sexual desire is supposed to be desire for its "counterpart," the female. Similarly, female biology is expected to correlate with feminine gender attribution, role, and identity, and female sexual desire is supposed to have males as its object. Men and women who physically deviate from biological expectations have historically been medicalized and treated for genital anomalies (e.g., morphology and reproductivity are "fixed" to correlate with the more likely gender attribution, and gender is assigned accordingly). But different cultures form different sex/gender systems and, thus, view gender differently. Not all sex/gender systems are dichotomous. For the past 100 years, ethnologists have been reporting findings of a category of people among some aboriginal societies who receive social sanction to become a gender other than that to which they had originally been assigned. This category, usually called *berdache*, appears to be a "third gender" in that it is not simply an oppositional identity and role, or a form of homosexuality or cross-dressing. Although both the findings and interpretations are disputed, many ethnologists report that berdache is an accepted, and even honored, category in many aboriginal cultures and is not viewed as a deviance or pathology.

Within the dichotomous sex/gender system that most readers will be familiar with, gender is one axis of power, together with race and class. Gender, race, and class are axes of power in that they not only mark difference as binary oppositions (male/female, white/nonwhite, middle class/poor) but express those differences as inequality, inferiority, or pathology. Since the time of Pythagoras and Aristotle's "Table of Opposites," maleness has been associated with rationality, abstract thinking, impartiality, unity, and goodness, and femaleness has been viewed as derivative or deformed and associated with emotionality, particularist thinking, plurality, and evil. Not surprisingly, "light" is on the side of goodness and maleness, while "dark" is located in the column along with "female" and "evil." With the modern period and the Enlightenment, mind and body were added to the oppositional view of metaphysics. Such associations have justified the exclusion of women from public life and civic action and the outsider status of girlchildren and women when it comes to laws against assault for domestic, sexual, and workplace violence. Men have also suffered under this asymmetrical value system for gender through a socialization process where boys and men are turned away from emotionality and attachment, through assumptions that the primary emotion acceptable in males is anger, and through the repudiation of femaleness in their lives. But the racial axis of power complicates this analysis, because people of color—both men and women—are often characterized in ways similar to the qualities associated with femaleness (e.g., emotionality, particularist reasoning, or evil, especially sexual evils). Any thoroughgoing understanding of gender as a contributor to mental ease or distress must include considerations of racialization processes and experiences of being raced.

The legacy of gender inferiority for females, and gender superiority for males, cannot be underestimated. Gender is one of the central ways by which we come to form and express identity and selfhood, and thus an understanding of gender as a concept and an experience is crucial to a commitment to foster healthy, flourishing individuals or to minimize psychosocial anguish and difficulty.

Cultural influences combine with biological ones to affect both behavior and interpretation of behavior. Research indicates that interpretations of male and female behavior contain biases in diagnosis and treatment. An examination of the history of madness in the Western world reveals that women more frequently have been viewed as mad and are more likely to be treated with medications. Although readers might think that such biases are a thing of the past, they would be mistaken. During the period from 1960 to 1994, new diagnostic categories were introduced that indicate that the values upholding traditional gender roles are still entrenched in psychiatric fields. Hysteria, the paradigm case of a "female disorder," did not disappear but, instead, resurfaced as a personality disorder marked by an exaggerated feminine response that included manipulativity and excessive sexuality. Promiscuity, viewed as "natural" in men but as a potential symptom in women, is liable to gender bias either way. The equation of sexual prowess with natural maleness turns against men whose interest in sexual activity is minimal, rendering a diagnosis of sexual dysphoria that, for women, would not arise under an assumption of women's lesser interest in sexual matters. Women who are sexually active in unconventional ways (e.g., with many partners or with relative strangers), alternatively, tend to be viewed as symptomatic of problem sexuality and may be assessed for borderline personality disorder, which is diagnosed in women far more than in men. Homosexuality, too, is linked to a dichotomous and asymmetrical sex/gender value system in which males, whose biology is supposed to line up with masculine behavior and female object-choice of desire, have been diagnosed as sexually deviant and exposed to treatments, cures, and confinement. This diagnosis has been challenged, as has the diagnosis of masochism, a disorder thought to be typically female. Masochism was rejected as a mental illness when its gender biases were uncovered; homosexuality was removed from the *Diagnostic and Statistical Manual* when assumptions about gender, including an assumption that heterosexuality is the natural entailment of biological sex, were called into question. Nevertheless, many unfounded and potentially damaging biases remain.

This is not to suggest that gender is wholly cultural or social. I discuss one way in which biological influences are gender-related. Development of females in adolescence is affected by physiological features such as internal sex organs, the onset of menarche, and breast development. Because of their differing sexual anatomy and function, adolescent girls are likely to experience their bodies as ambiguous, paradoxical, and discontinuous. Female body image tends to be fragmented or even ego-alien, and teenage females describe their bodies primarily in terms of appearance and attractiveness rather than, as teenage boys do, in terms of strength, virility, and effectiveness. Self-descriptions do not, themselves, show a patterned difference in attitude toward male or female embodiedness, but eating disorders are far more common among females than males: behavior suggests that the contours and shifting of muscle-to-fat ratio that occurs in female adolescence combines with a cultural over-valuation of thin, attractive females that prompts deep concern and loathing for the female body. Negative or shaming cultural attitudes toward menstruation combine with physical discomfort, so that many young girls experience their bodies as having betrayed them by menstruation. Finally, differences between male and female genitalia should be considered when understanding physiological gender differences. The penis is external, and its workings and pleasures during adolescence are readily discoverable. Not so for girls, whose clitoris may be stimulated without being discovered, or discovered through indirect stimulation but not seen, or perhaps not discovered by themselves but through stimulation by another. Adolescent girls often grow up unaware or unclear about the workings of their own bodies, especially where sexual pleasure is concerned. Research also indicates that female adolescents masturbate far less than do young males—a finding that is related, at least in part, to their differing anatomies. This finding matters because masturbation is a way toward autonomy through self-soothing and through an increased understanding of one's body and how to meet its needs. Masturbation, for both males and females, is an important activity that promotes healthy development—contrary to the historical view of masturbation as deeply disturbing to one's mental health—yet physical and attitudinal differences about masturbation may inhibit this activity for many females. Female physiology is no more or less likely to produce psychiatric problems than is male physiology, historic theories of female biology notwithstanding. Still, it is important to appreciate the kinds of physiological differences in male and female biology and to understand that female physiology, when combined with denigrating attitudes toward things female, can hinder healthy psychological development and can give rise to mental distress in women's lives.

Research into gender differences and gender-specific problems in mental health needs to address biases both in assumptions about femininity and womanliness and in subject matter. Norms for mental health have historically been masculinist. For example, the association of reason with maleness has led to a persistent devaluation of emotionality such that the "overemotional" person is liable to be viewed as problematic and, when appearing with other behaviors, symptomatic of pathology. The charge of manipulativity, a characteristic of borderline personality disorder, is much more often given to women, but without an understanding of how representations of manipulativity are filtered through the ideology of gender and without an understanding of how restricted access to power may affect a person's ability to be directly effective in the world. Research into topics such as possible gendered interpretations of manipulativity would be useful to the field. But research into women as a class has been too often overlooked in the medical fields, and when it is undertaken, it is sometimes infused with a priori assumptions about female inferiority. In other words, research into "women's issues" does not necessarily correct for gender biases. For example, Gilligan's seminal work (*In a Different Voice*, 1982) on the different moral reasoning of women has been criticized for entrenching, rather than debunking, cultural stereotypes that women are more caring, more oriented toward relationships, and more particularist than are men. This characterization has a long history not only of stereotyping women in ways that legitimize exclusion from participation in the public domain but also of functioning as a norm by which women who deviate from or repudiate those characteristics are assessed as less womanly, not fully female, or "not real women." Thus, while Gilligan argued that her research shows that women's moral voices are different, but not inferior, to men's moral voices, critics worry that her conclusions may reflect assumptions about the gender dichotomy that hark back to the oppositional thinking of ancient times. Herman's (1992) research into etiology, symptoms, and treatment of posttraumatic stress disorder is a better example of work that is focused on experiences that are primarily female — namely, child sexual abuse — while avoiding gender stereotypes. A central way she accomplishes this task is by offering a rich and nuanced analysis of child sexual abuse that pays attention to patterns but does not fall prey to generalizations. Women, who as a class are potentially victimized as children, are nevertheless treated as particular individuals whose experiences and responses vary.

Psychiatrists in clinical practice and in the academy may perpetuate gender stereotypes that ultimately undermine psychiatrists' own attempts to facilitate psychological health. In addition to the issues already discussed, psychiatrists need to attend to language and dialogue in a number of ways. I mention two of them.

Gender differences are marked and constituted, in part, by the words we utter and the kinds of speech acts we engage in. Gender-neutral language is now the norm in most scholarly journals because it is recognized that terms such as "man" and "mankind" are ambiguous: sometimes they refer to all humans, but at other times they refer only to males. There are other ways in which gender bias shows up in language. A classic example is the ways in which sexual acts were talked about at least up through the 1980s: men were the actors, women the acted-upon (men "screwed" and women "got screwed," and so on). This formation of gender through subject/object positions in grammar can be even more subtle. Irigaray (1985), for example, argues that the structure and the components of language as we know it today are male, in that the dominant order is symbolically structured around and through males and masculinity. This line of reasoning leads some mental health theorists and practitioners to search for another language — a feminine one — that will allow for women to situate themselves as subjects, not in dominant discourse but in an alternative discourse of their own making.

Psychiatrists may not know where to begin assisting female patients in the formation of alternative liberatory discourses. But a first step, it seems to me, would be to understand that language can work to dominate and subjugate in far more complex ways than we might think, and that we may inadvertently participate in others' subjugation by the ways we speak.

A related way that language can subjugate is through our styles of engagement in dialogue. Naming is an activity that historically has been denied to women, and this is particularly true when it comes to women's experiences and their interpretations of them. If psychiatrists wish to understand the ways gender differences may give rise to mental distress, they would do well to attend to the subtle ways that individual women's struggles to communicate and to be heard are overridden. An offer of an interpretation, on the part of a psychiatrist, may arise out of a desire to relieve distress, to point out what the patient is failing to notice, or to move the patient along toward a more flourishing path. But even an unintentional imposition of interpretation can deprive a female patient of meaning-making, undermining her attempts at autonomy.

A final consideration for practice is that of building trust. Whether the psychiatrist is male or female, and whether the patient is male or female, trust is likely to be a salient issue for the patient. This is not simply a function of the doctor/patient relation but a matter of gender and power. Gender, as a lived analytic category and a cultural construct, is a signifier for both psychiatrist and patient, and the patient may implicitly base his or her trust (or distrust) on indications of the psychiatrist's apparent attitudes and values with respect to the medical establishment and cultural norms. Being a trustworthy psychiatrist involves understanding ways in which the position one holds vis-à-vis each particular patient can impede or enhance that patient's trust in one, and issues of gender can never be entirely independent of either party's situatedness.

REFERENCES

Baker, Robert (1975) "Pricks and Chicks: A Plea for Persons." In Robert Baker and Frederick Elliston (eds.), *Philosophy and Sex*. Buffalo, NY: Prometheus Books, pp. 45–64.

Bayer, Ronald (1987) *Homosexuality and American Psychiatry*. Princeton, NJ: Princeton University Press.

Butler, Judith (1990) *Gender Trouble: Feminism and the Subversion of Identity*. New York: Routledge.

Caplan, Paula (1987) *The Myth of Women's Masochism*. New York: E. P. Dutton.

Chessler, Phyllis (1997) *Women and Madness*, 25th anniversary ed. New York: Four Walls Eight Windows.

Cross, Lisa (1993) "Body and Self in Feminine Development: Implications for Eating Disorders and Delicate Self-Mutilation." *Bulletin of the Menninger Clinic* 57(1): 41–69.

Friedman, Marilyn (1994) "Beyond Caring: The De-moralization of Gender." In Larry May and Shari Collins Sharratt (eds.), *Applied Ethics: A Multicultural Approach*. Englewood Cliffs, NJ: Prentice Hall.

Fulton, Robert, and Anderson, Steven (1992) "The Amerindian 'Man-Woman': Gender, Liminality, and Cultural Continuity." *Current Anthropology* 33(5): 603–10.

GAP Report (Group for the Advancement of Psychiatry) (2000) *Homosexuality and the Mental Health Professions: The Impact of Bias.* Hillsdale, NJ: Analytic Press.

Gilligan, Carol (1982) *In a Different Voice: Psychological Theory and Women's Development.* Cambridge, MA: Harvard University Press.

Gilman, Sander (1985) *Difference and Pathology: Stereotypes of Sexuality, Race, and Madness.* Ithaca, NY: Cornell University Press.

Goulet, Jean-Guy (2001) "The 'Berdache'/'Two-Spirit': A Comparison of Anthropological and Native Constructions of Gendered Identities among the Northern Athapaskans." *Journal of the Royal Anthropological Institute* 2: 683–701.

Herman, Judith Lewis (1992) *Trauma and Recovery.* New York: Basic Books.

Irigaray, Luce (1985) *This Sex Which Is Not One.* Translated by Catherine Porter. Ithaca, NY: Cornell University Press.

Jimenez, Mary Ann (1997) "Gender and Psychiatry: Psychiatric Conceptions of Mental Disorders in Women, 1960–1994." *Affilia: Journal of Women and Social Work* 12(2): 154–76.

Kessler, Suzanne, and McKenna, Wendy (1978) *Gender: An Ethnomethodological Approach.* Chicago: University of Chicago Press.

Lloyd, Genevieve (1993) *The Man of Reason: "Male" and "Female" in Western Philosophy.* Minneapolis: University of Minnesota Press.

Martin, Norah (2001) "Feminist Bioethics and Psychiatry." *Journal of Medicine and Philosophy* 26(4): 431–41.

Murray, Stephen (1994) "On Subordinating Native American Cosmologies to the Empire of Gender." *Current Anthropology* 35(1): 59–61.

Showalter, Elaine (1985) *The Female Malady: Women, Madness, and English Culture, 1830–1980.* New York: Penguin Books.

Trexler, Richard (2002) "Making the American Berdache: Choice or Constraint?" *Journal of Social History* 35(3): 213–36.

Walton, Jean (2001) *Fair Sex, Savage Dreams: Race, Psychoanalysis, Sexual Difference.* Durham, NC, and London: Duke University Press.

Whitbeck, Caroline (1973) "Theories of Sex Difference." *Philosophical Forum* 5(1–2): 54–80.

CHAPTER 16

RACE AND CULTURE

MARILYN NISSIM-SABAT

THIS chapter deals with issues that warrant interdisciplinary work; the relevant disciplines are philosophy, psychiatry, theory of culture,[1] and critical race theory.[2]

Conjoining race and culture signifies both linkage and separateness of these concepts and the existential phenomena they denote. That "race" is a cultural construct is now widely acknowledged, not only in critical race theory (Zack 1977: 98–99) but in medicine as well (*Nature/Genetics* 2001; R. S. Schwartz 2001). As such, "race" is not the same phenomenon as biological diversity within the species; therefore, it is not an aspect of the biological substrate of human cultures. Rather, race exists by virtue of "raciation,"[3] a process of cultural production. Moreover, raciation is racism: cultures constitute groups as raced others, and thereby as deficient in some alleged essential characteristics of humanness. Thus, race and culture are linked in and through the historical and material character of race as a cultural construct.

Given this, why is race not subsumed within culture as one of many culturally constituted phenomena? Why race *and* culture? The separation entails an assumption: while it may be that human existence is necessarily enculturated, it is not inevitable that human cultures engender raciation. Thus, we are here concerned with culture insofar as racialized oppression exists within it, and insofar as it may be possible to reconstitute some institutions—for example, psychiatry—as relatively non-racist.

We can now formulate an organizing thread in the form of a question: How can the psychosocial situatedness of persons who are oppressed, yet inherently free, be understood and changed? This question pertains to the etiology, diagnosis, and treatment of mental disorders in that such disorders reflect, on the one hand, inner compulsions (that is, modes of self-oppression) and, on the other hand, oppression originating outside, both in the family and in broader cultural institutions and practices. The values in play here are mental health and empowerment of patients and practitioners. Actualizing these values requires a critical examination of the relation between inner (psychic) and outer (cultural) oppression in the etiology of mental disorders. The question we have posed can now be existentially contextualized: Why would individuals freely adopt modes of crippling inner oppression as a consequence of outer oppression? This brings to the fore the issue of victim status.

One of the most pervasive ways that collusion with oppression is enacted is victim blaming. Even when oppression is acknowledged, victim blaming (by victims, perpetrators, or society) denies any relation between, on the one hand, oppression originating in society, such as racism, and, on the other hand, inner oppression, such as self-blame or other psychic compulsions. As a result, the victim-blaming stance posits either a decontextualized, abstract, and thus dehumanized notion of human freedom — agency as atomized willing ("Just say no!") — or an insuperable determinism as denial of human freedom.[4] In psychiatry, some racialized victim blaming has taken the form of belief in putative biological racial characteristics that increase susceptibility to certain mental disorders, as well as the belief that racial characteristics preclude mature agency. Individuals and institutions that blame victims fail to acknowledge the existence of forces that originate externally in cultural institutions that induce inner, psychic self-oppression. Such collusion, in the form, for example, of identification with the oppressor, might be instituted to ward off psychic collapse or to avoid actions against oppression that could result in physical or psychic death. Thus, "collusion" is both a free act and a response to oppressive forces where no other option is, or is believed to be, available. What is necessary is to develop a stance on freedom or agency in relation to oppression that obviates victim blaming and thus enables resistance and change.

I discuss three attempts to theorize the philosophical and cultural issues relevant to raciation in psychiatry: the work of Michel Foucault, the work of Frantz Fanon, and psychoanalytic Marxism. In the conclusion, I discuss the development of a view that can build on the strengths of previous work and enable forward movement.

RACIATION IN PSYCHIATRY

Two examples of racist practices in psychiatry are (1) the racialized attempt to exterminate the Jews of Europe by the Nazis and their collaborators, including psychiatrists,[5] and (2) the continued institutionalization and practice of antiblack racism in psychiatry in the United States, Great Britain, and other European and non-European countries and cultures. The focus here is on antiblack racism.

Raciation generates social attitudes that institutionalize the victim-blaming stance, which holds that black people are the problem, rather than what is actually the case: that the problem is racism against blacks (Gordon 2000: 69–72).

Collusion of Psychiatry with Raciation

An important contribution is A. Thomas's and S. Sillen's *Racism and Psychiatry* (1972). Written to document how racism was institutionalized under the rubric of "scientific" psychiatry, the authors cite numerous works written by psychiatrists and social scientists. Myths of the inferiority of the brains of black people, myths of phylogenetic traits that allegedly reveal racial inferiority, and falsification and misuse of statistics "proving" much higher incidence of mental illness in blacks are all documented. For example, "a well-known physician ... had a psychiatric explanation for runaway slaves ... [–]*drapetomania*, literally the flight-from-home madness" (2). These 'diagnoses' coincided with the "view that psychological characteristics ... are determined by an inherited constitutional structure" (4). A more recent treatment is *Forensic Psychiatry, Race and Culture* by S. Fernando et al. (1998). The authors cite evidence to show that, "today in the UK, and very likely in most European countries ... the forensic thrust within general psychiatry confuse[s] questions of crime and illness, and ... allow[s] racism to become intimately involved in this amalgam" (119). Of particular interest is the discussion of racism in relation to schizophrenia. The authors conclude:

> Schizophrenia was associated at its birth ... with ideas of racial degeneration ... at a time when the dogma of skin-colour racism was being incorporated into European thinking. ... Europe ... has become multiracial. ... As stresses ... arising from ... racial interaction affect Europe, ... schizophrenia is again being implicated. ... And [it] ... is the diagnosis ... used to medicalise black protest, despair and anger. (66)

Cross Cultural Psychiatry (J. M. Herrera et al. 1999) contains articles on psychopharmacology and ethnicity. For example, W. B. Lawson states that

> African Americans ... are more likely ... to be involuntarily committed and to be placed in seclusion or restraints. ... African Americans ... are overdiagnosed with schizophrenia and consequently are more likely to receive antipsychotics when they are not needed. ... African American patients with clear cut bipolar affective disorder ... were often initially diagnosed with schizophrenia. (67–68)

In *Fair Sex, Savage Dreams: Race, Psychoanalysis, Sexual Difference* (2001), Jean Walton discusses, for example, Joan Riviere's influential essay, "Womanliness as Masquerade." Riviere analyzes a woman's dream and ignores the fact that the threatening male in the dream is black (18–24). Walton shows that psychoanalysis has colluded with racism from its inception.

Impact of Racism on Victims

A classic treatment is W. H. Grier and P. M. Cobbs's *Black Rage* (1968). The authors, both psychiatrists, present case histories that illustrate the inseparability of racism and mental disorder. They discuss, for example, a black woman who "thought it a fundamental truth that black women . . . were ugly . . . she was ugly" (9). A recent treatment is C. J. P. Harrell's (1999) *Manichean Psychology: Racism and the Minds of People of African Descent*. Harrell details the devastating physiological, cognitive, developmental, and emotional consequences of racism, which he encapsulates as "Manichean psychology":

> The Manicheans conceived of blackness . . . as evil. Whiteness . . . became associated with good. . . . People of African descent become associated with evil and inferiority. We come to see Caucasians as superior and inherently good . . . [thus, racism] influences . . . beliefs about the efficacy and competence of human beings as a function of their race [and] racist information influences standards of beauty and body image. (15)

These works document the racism in psychiatry and provide rich resources for further study.

What are the causes of racism in psychiatry? Certainly, they are the same as the causes of racism in culture at large. However, there is no generally accepted explanation of the causes of racism. There is, however, a consensus that racism is a form of dehumanization, of denial of the humanity of a group of persons who are different in ways that are held to be "inferior—that is, nonhuman or inhuman. Denial of the role of external oppression in the formation of mental disorders is an enactment of dehumanization in that it is equivalently denial of sociality, of interdependency as a constitutive character of the human (Gordon 2000: 60–86).[6] It is, then, pertinent to inquire whether there are aspects of psychiatry that collude with dehumanization. An aspect of psychiatry that is often held to be dehumanizing is the "medical" or "biomedical" model.

The medical model entails a disease concept that somatizes symptoms and abstracts from socially constituted stressors. It abstracts from history, culture, and the person as subject; consequently, cultural and individual differences and their effect on etiology, diagnosis, and treatment are discounted. Moreover, the medical model is associated with the positing, and imposing, of ethnocentric cultural "universals" of normality that derive from a biomedical conceptualization of the person. Finally, the medical model incorrectly purports to be a value-free perspective on health and illness.[7]

No claim is made here that the medical model is the only factor that sustains racism. Nevertheless, as shown earlier and as is shown in the discussion that follows, those who have studied this issue extensively focus on the medical model as the central factor in and through which racism has been instituted and perpetuated in psychiatry.

THREE PERSPECTIVES ON RACIATION
IN PSYCHIATRY

....

These perspectives have been selected for discussion because in them the cultural production of race is a central feature of the perspective as a whole.

Michel Foucault

Michel Foucault, the French philosopher and cultural historian (1925–84), was influenced by Kant and Nietzsche. Foucault points out that, in his essay on the Enlightenment, Kant, for the first time, questioned the meaning of humanity in a particular historical situatedness (Foucault 1982: 216). But Foucault also saw the philosophical tradition as having failed to free itself from the binary of reason and unreason, sanity and madness, that is, two sides of the way in which state power, by creating internal warfare, institutes and sustains oppressive practices. The influence of Nietzsche is shown in Foucault's appropriation of Nietzsche's genealogical method, which allows for historical analysis without presupposing either an origin or ultimate foundation of the phenomena in question (Dreyfus and Rabinow 1982: 108–9).

Foucault's early work is an indictment of the medicalization of psychiatry as a process that has served not merely to rationalize existing forms of domination but to create them. For Foucault, the new form of political power that began developing in the seventeenth century, the state form, necessitated the development of techniques to control society and, as well, to regulate individuals. Consequently, psychiatry became a medical specialty whose discourse generated the socially operative concepts of normality and abnormality. These then led to practices of exclusion of the abnormal, the mad, from society (Foucault 1976: 64–75).

Foucault terms this historically evolved form of state power "biopower." This means that the state assumed power, not merely, as in previous periods, over life in that the sovereign power could let live or kill; now the bourgeois state assumed control over the conditions and qualities of human life. Once the bourgeoisie gained power, it became preoccupied with health and the transmission of heredity diseases and "degeneracy." For Foucault, sexuality and race are produced in this process. Given Foucault's nominalist philosophical stance, sexuality and race are social "objects" produced by discourse, with no extradiscursive reference. Thus, psychiatry participated in the creation and deployment of state biopower by providing a scientific rationale for discourses of sexual and racial purity (Foucault 1978: 135–59).

Foucault discusses race in several texts. The focus here is on his (1991) article, "Faire vivre et laisser mourir: la naissance du racisme" (as cited, translated, and discussed by Stoler 2000). Foucault wrote that "what inscribes racism in the mechanisms of the state is the emergence of biopower"; [it is a] "means of introducing . . .

a fundamental division between those who must live and those who must die" (84). For Stoler, interpreting Foucault, racism "fragments the biological field, it establishes a break . . . inside the biological continuum of human beings by defining a hierarchy of races, as a set of subdivisions in which certain races are classified as 'good,' fit, and superior" (84). And, "racism is the condition that makes it acceptable to put [people] to death in a society of normalization" (85, quoting Foucault). Thus, "races," for example, Africans, become abnormal by definition, and, as such, expendable.

Of particular interest is Foucault's (1982) view of the formation of the subject as a process of subjectification or subjugation: "This form of power . . . categorizes the individual, marks him by his own individuality, attaches him to his own identity. . . . It . . . makes individuals subjects . . . [i.e.,] subject to someone else by control and dependence. . . . Both meanings suggest a form of power which subjugates and makes subject to" (212).

Thus, Foucault engaged the issue of victim status in recognizing that oppression functions on the intrapsychic level and does so by constructing forms of subjectification that are forms of subjugation. He clarified the ways that oppressive state power, by imposing processes of normalization through the collusion of psychiatry, colonizes the individual who becomes an instrument for the enforcement of existing power relations, including racism.

Two problematic aspects of Foucault's thought are denial of agency (i.e., Foucault's antihumanist stance) and relativism. Freundlich (1994) shows that Foucault's "virtually complete neglect of human agency and of processes of reasoning does not allow him to account for historical change . . . other than in terms of the 'agency' of a system of anonymous rules and elements" (168). Freundlich also shows that "the epistemological role that the theoretical concept of a discourse as a historical a priori plays in Foucault . . . leads to a self-destructive relativism" (154). That is, Foucault accords a range of freedom to his own discourse that he denies to all other discourses. To these problems we can add that emphasized by Stoler: Foucault's elision of the phenomenon of colonialism.

Frantz Fanon

In contrast to Foucault, Frantz Fanon (1925–61) proclaimed his perspective to be that of a new humanism. From the beginning, Fanon criticized the dehumanizing practices of psychiatry. Fanon, born in Martinique, trained as a psychiatrist in France and then took a post in a hospital in Algeria.

Fanon was influenced by both Marxism and the existential phenomenology of Jean-Paul Sartre, as well as by psychoanalysis. His work is important because it shows that the Freudian register of psychosexual development in colonial societies must be subsumed within a sociogenesis of mental disorder (Gordon 1997: 144). Fanon stressed that the oppressor relied on the "epidermal" character of antiblack racism (38), and he discovered that the psyche of the colonized person is pervaded, consciously and unconsciously, by the belief structure of the colonists: that is, denial of the humanity of the colonized. Thus, Fanon found that the pathology of his psychiatric patients in Algeria was neither ontogenic nor phylogenic; rather, it was sociogenic—brought about by the totalistic oppressive system of the French in Martinique and Algeria (Fanon 1967: 11; 1963: 249–310).

Summarizing Fanon's work, Gordon writes: "Like Fanon, philosophy must de-center itself in the hope of radical theory and become, in its embodiment, a critically self-questioning practice" (1997: 45). Gordon alludes to Fanon's awareness that philosophy was not self-critical regarding race. Kant and Hegel, both of whom made extensive, explicitly racist remarks, are exemplary. Fanon wrote that "ontology, when it is admitted once and for all that it leaves existence by the wayside, does not permit us to understand the being of the black" (1967: 88). Fanon indicts Western philosophy for ontologizing the human essence as white so that whiteness became a criterion for humanness. This ontology does not permit us to understand the lived experience of the black, or, therefore, to empathize with the incalculable suffering this ontology has imposed. Fanon's aim in both *Black Skin/White Masks* and *The Wretched of the Earth* was to initiate a process of black disidentification with whiteness that would free blacks to re-create their own lived reality, the conditions of their actual existence. Thus, beliefs regarding who and what one ontologically, existentially is, must be bracketed, "left by the wayside." This process of decentering philosophy as lived in one's sense of one's own existence would lead, Fanon hoped, to overcoming any sociogenic identification with the oppressor and to a struggle for liberation in the name of all humanity.

Fanon did not reject psychiatry as such. Indeed, in *The Wretched of the Earth* (1963), he included numerous case histories showing that racism in psychiatry is caused sociogenically by the Eurocentric ontology of whiteness (Gordon 1997: 144) within a medical model that then legitimates it with the imprimatur of science. But, Fanon believed that there can be a non-Eurocentric psychiatry. Indeed, his support for revolution in Algeria was a psychiatric prescription for the restoration of mental health, not, as some have argued erroneously, through catharsis but rather through detoxification. Given the almost unimaginable brutality of French oppression in Algeria, Fanon believed that only confrontation with the oppressor offered the oppressed the possibility of detoxification—the possibility, that is, of claiming their lives as human beings (Bulhan 1985: 131–53).

Foucault praised psychoanalysis as liberating individuals from subjecthood. For Fanon, in sharp contrast to Foucault, it is not subjecthood that is dehumanizing; it is, rather, the denial of subjecthood, of humanness, that leads to pathological defenses like self-blame and identification with the aggressor. True to his Sartrean inspiration, Fanon posited freedom as the being of humanity; his views are thus incompatible with Foucault's denial of agency.

Critique of Fanon is through hindsight. Fanon died in 1961 at the age of 36, near the end of the Algerian revolution. From a Fanonian perspective, did the Algerian revolution succeed? Have Algerians disidentified with whiteness? These questions cannot be answered here. However, European and non-European cultures are still afflicted with racisms, including antiblack racism. Moreover, raciation in psychiatry is barely diminished. Following Fanon, I propose that psychiatry, including psychoanalysis, must revise itself to incorporate the sociogenic aspect of the etiology of mental disorder, including instances in which sociogenesis is the primary etiological factor. A relevant question is this: Isn't sociogenesis an etiologic factor in all mental disorders? And, if it is, what sort of theory can encompass this etiology? I argue not that Fanon would have disagreed regarding the ubiquity of sociogenesis but only that, in hindsight, we can see that the sociogenesis of raciation is, as Foucault maintained, a means of maintaining the status quo by constitution of society as riven by internal wars. Alternatively, cannot psychiatry in general, and psychoanalysis in particular, recognize the ubiquity of sociogenesis and see it as an etiological, diagnostic, and treatment factor, one that can function as a potential source, not only of genuinely ameliorative psychiatric therapy, but of liberatory practice as well, even in societies not on the brink of revolution? Can genuinely ameliorative therapy be anything but liberatory practice, if, that is, oppression is an etiological factor? These are the questions that psychiatry must ask if racism is to be addressed.

E. V. Wolfenstein

E. V. Wolfenstein's 1993 book, *Psychoanalytic Marxism*, is a remarkable compendium and analysis of the tradition of Freudian Marxism: a critique of the latter and its major figures, and a treatise that develops a unique perspective on Marxism, Hegel's dialectical philosophy, psychoanalysis, and critical race theory.

Freudian Marxism

As Wolfenstein points out, "classical Freudian-Marxism is primarily the work of three men: Wilhelm Reich, Erich Fromm, and Herbert Marcuse" (53). All three saw psychoanalysis as a supplement to Marxism. Reich, originator of "sexual politics," was a psychoanalyst and social theorist who fled "from the problematics of social life into sexual romanticism and a reduction of mind to body" (90) and eventually abandoned social theory. For Wolfenstein, Fromm's social psychology and effort to integrate psychoanalysis with "Marx's historical ontology" are valuable contributions; however, his "relational concept of selfhood" elides the individual and results in the "sacrifice of psychoanalysis at the Marxist altar" (73). Marcuse's contribution was to place repression (Freud) and alienation (Marx) within the same theoretical frame, and this helps us clarify the relationship between them. However, Marcuse's Hegelian-Marxism splits the "bad totality of the present" and "a purely Utopian future," leading Marcuse to declare that "the class struggle is over and we have lost" (87). For Marcuse, Freud's theories entail that the death drive and pleasure (absence of stimulation) are the same, and this ultimately determines human experience.

Psychoanalytic-Marxism

In his chapter 4, Wolfenstein discusses how psychoanalytic Marxism moves beyond Freudian-Marxism. Wolfenstein believes that Kleinian object relations theory's emphasis on the reparative capacity of the psyche is more attuned than is Freudian orthodoxy to the social aspects of human development. In addition, Wolfenstein advocates a renewal of Hegelian Marxism's emphasis on the dialectic of recognition. He further maintains that psychoanalytic Marxism goes beyond Freudian Marxism's focus on individuals and families on one extreme and political-economic structures on the other by recognizing that "the pluralization of emancipatory politics . . . generated other theoretical categories, most notably those of race and gender. Henceforward psychoanalytic-Marxism must also be a critical theory of patriarchy/phallocentrism and racism" (169).

Wolfenstein deals with the issue of race throughout the book, including a psychoanalytic-Marxist analysis of racism. In that section, he discusses Ralph Ellison's famous novel, *The Invisible Man* (1989). In his analysis, Wolfenstein touches on the issue of the sociogenesis of mental disorders. He provides a Kleinian psychoanalytic diagnosis of the protagonist as attempting a "schizoid solution to the problematics of the paranoid-schizoid position" in his efforts to "heal himself from the wounds of invisibility" (346) — that is, from the effects of a racist society. Citing Foucault and others, Wolfenstein remarks that "the paranoid-schizoid position is a social structure, a placement and deployment of power, a combination of real persecutory forces" (348). If the Invisible Man were not to advance beyond this point (as numerous actual invisible men do not), we would have an example of a person who internalized oppression by adopting a self-crippling psychic structure. The Invisible Man is attempting to cope with psychic extinction — the psychic consequences of his invisibility. At this point, his efforts to heal himself were self-defeating. Here Wolfenstein does touch on the phenomena that generate the question that is the organizing thread of this chapter: How could, and why would, a person freely assent to oppression and, in so doing, institute modes of self-oppression? Up to this point, Wolfenstein's analysis is sound. So on one hand Wolfenstein sees that the pathology of the Invisible Man cannot be understood apart from sociogenic etiological factors. On the other hand, significantly for Wolfenstein, the Invisible Man is not a patient in psychoanalysis.

Wolfenstein's psychoanalytic reading of Ellison's novel notwithstanding, we must raise this question: How is it that in his book Wolfenstein does not deal with racism *within* psychiatry and psychoanalysis? Though he sees psychoanalysis as a liberatory praxis on the individual level, and despite his awareness of sociogenesis, for example, in *The Invisible Man*, Wolfenstein separates this from liberatory praxis on the political level. Since he claims that psychoanalysis as therapy suspends all political phenomena, Wolfenstein does not see sociogenesis as an etiological factor to be dealt with in the consulting room. Describing the psychoanalytic dyad, he writes:

> Both patient and analyst are members of a given social order. They create a microcosm . . . in which, to a greater or lesser extent, interests and conflicts of interest of the macrocosm are suspended. Thus, they are able to give their full attention to

the project of individual self-liberation — but only to individual self-liberation. The freedom they create extends to but not beyond the point at which social reality has been bracketed. (387)

The Invisible Man was attempting to, and in the novel, does, cure himself; but he was not undergoing psychoanalysis as construed by Wolfenstein. Moreover, given the latter's view of psychoanalysis as therapy, psychoanalysts are not racists or, if they are, their racism will be suspended in the practice of psychoanalysis. But, we may ask, whose practice of psychoanalysis? Contemporary psychoanalysis has moved beyond the view that doing psychoanalysis exempts the analyst from acting out prejudices in the treatment. Moreover, contemporary psychoanalysis is much more explicit than was Freud in identifying parental failure as the primary etiological factor in mental disorder (see, e.g., Pizer 1998).

It is important to ask how it is that Wolfenstein fails to motivate self-investigation within psychoanalysis. The chief factor is his view that psychoanalytic Marxism is not, and should not be, a synthesis of psychoanalysis and Marxism (as both philosophy and emancipatory practice) and that such a synthesis will inevitably fail to do justice to either the individual or the collectivity. Wolfenstein's critique of both Fromm (for abandoning the intrasubjective dimension) and Marcuse (for abandoning the intersubjective dimension) alleges just such failures. What inhibits Wolfenstein from identifying racism within psychiatry itself and calling for psychiatry's self-investigation is, then, his repudiation of the possibility of a coincidence within psychoanalysis of the aims of praxis: that is, a coincidence between liberatory praxis in the consulting room, on the one hand, and the struggle to overcome oppression originating in society, on the other hand. However, unless such a coincidence of practical aims is established, thus motivating radical self-investigation, victim blaming cannot be transcended.

CONCLUSION

In examining the problematic of the relations among inner and outer oppression and victim status, we find that these phenomena cannot be understood unless the relation between individual and collectivity is encompassed within a perspective that is beyond psychoanalytic Marxism, for the latter construes individual and social praxis as two separate planes of liberatory praxis.[8] The desired philosophical stance would show that intersubjective life is constitutive for the individual subject at the same time that the subjects, as individuals, constitute intersubjective life. This is not unlike the Marxist idea that an authentically human society is one in which "the free development of each is the condition for the free development of all" (Marx and Engels 1988: 75). This means that human life is individual-psychic (intrasubjective) such that each individual is unique and, at the same time, intersubjective or collective. Thus, the relation between individual and society is mediated by processes of co-constitution.

Individuals, each with her or his own unique contribution, collectively co-constitute and are constituted historically and culturally by society. If sociality were not constitutive for human beings as nevertheless unique individuals, then the relation between inner (self) and outer (social) oppression could not be understood. Why would an individual consciously or unconsciously blame him- or herself for circumstances over which that individual either had or believed him-or herself to have no or little control? Thus, self-blame and identification with an oppressor, pervasive subjective features of mental disorders, suggest that the subject is threatened with actual, existential loss of intersubjective embeddedness and thus with psychic extinction. As we have seen, Wolfenstein's relegation of the intrapsychic and intersubjective dimensions of experience to separate planes of praxis cannot resolve the problem. These insights move us beyond psychoanalytic Marxism to a phenomenological psychoanalysis based on the transcendental phenomenology of Edmund Husserl and to a conception of a psychiatric practice that can dialectically sublate both the existential humanism of Fanon and Marx on one hand and psychoanalysis on the other hand. This would result in the transformation of psychiatry's self-understanding as a natural-medical science into a self-understanding as "the truly decisive field" (Husserl 1970: 208) of the humanistic disciplines.

The characteristics of transcendental phenomenology that render it the philosophical foundation for psychiatry are as follows:

1. Phenomenology begins with adoption of an attitude that is condition for the possibility of incorporating Fanon's methodological principle: "We must leave ontology by the wayside." The attitude of methodological suspension of all ontological commitments, and, equivalently, suspension of "the pregivenness of the world," or belief in the world's givenness prior to subjectivity, was called by Husserl the "transcendental reduction" (151–52).

2. Given the suspension of ontological commitments, phenomenology opens up the possibility of the most radical self-investigation possible for human beings.

3. For Husserl, each ego [self] constitutes itself uniquely within the stream of inner time. In this respect, Husserl speaks of "the primal 'I,' the ego of my epoche [transcendental reduction], which can never lose its uniqueness and personal indeclinability" (1970: 185). Moreover, "Only by starting from the ego and the system of its transcendental functions . . . can we. . . . exhibit . . . transcendental communalization, through which . . . the 'world for all' and for each subject *as* world for all is constituted" (185–86). Thus, transcendental phenomenology, by affirming the uniqueness of the individual in a manner that in no way rules out communal life, motivates the possibility of both psychogenesis and sociogenesis, as well as the interplay between them on all levels of human existence.

4. In this way, the standpoint of transcendental phenomenology instantiates hope: hope that in our freedom we can remake ourselves and our world so that there shall be no more victims (Nissim-Sabat 1998). Such a goal for a

humanistic psychiatry, a psychiatry premised on a methodology of radical self-examination, would enable psychiatry, perhaps for the first time, to actualize its core values of practitioner and patient empowerment.

NOTES

1. Though this chapter deals exclusively with psychiatry and culture with respect to issues of race, there is an important movement, generally referred to as "cultural psychiatry," that presents a broader critique of psychiatry. See, for example, Fabrega (1989) and Kleinman (1988). Fabrega's article provides a valuable history of cultural psychiatry, including R. J. Laing and the antipsychiatry movement. See also A. Kraus (2001).

2. The phrase "critical race theory" is used in its contemporary sense (beyond its origin in the Critical Legal Studies movement) to refer to interdisciplinary work in philosophy, psychology, literary studies, history, and other fields in which work raciation is studied from a liberatory perspective.

3. The term "raciation" is a less awkward equivalent of "racialization"; both terms refer to the cultural production of race and are so used by, for example, Walton (2001: 241).

4. For a thorough analysis of extant modalities of victim blaming in relation to oppression and psychology, see Nissim-Sabat (1998).

5. For extensive discussion and documentation of the role of German psychiatry in the Holocaust, see *Medical Murder* (2002). This document, published on the official web site of the city of Hamburg, begins with the following: "The participation of physicians, especially psychiatrists, in the Holocaust is unprecedented in history. The crimes of German Psychiatry are unique and unprecedented in the history of mankind." These statements are fully grounded in documented evidence.

6. Gordon here critiques psychology as naturalized, as psychologism, not psychology as construed within phenomenology itself. Phenomeology is discussed in the conclusion of this chapter.

7. For a thorough and incisive discussion of the strengths and weaknesses of the medical model in psychiatry, see Schwartz and Wiggins (1985).

8. In addition, understanding requires eschewing a stance like Heidegger's, for whom self and other are held to be unseparated (Zimmerman 1985: 25). The notion of the unmediated "We" that rules out mediation between individual and collectivity (Heidegger) does not enable a stance outside the ambit of potential victim blaming because it fails to motivate the free act of assent to oppression that the self as unique individual takes to be in his or her best interest.

REFERENCES

Bulhan, A. B. (1985) *Frantz Fanon and the Psychology of Oppression.* New York: Plenum.
Dreyfus, H. L., and Rabinow, P. (1982) *Michel Foucault: Beyond Structuralism and Hermeneutics.* Chicago: University of Chicago Press.

Ellison, Ralph (1947) *The Invisible Man.* New York: Vintage.

Fabrega Jr., Horacio (1989) "Cultural Relativism and Psychiatric Illness." *Journal of Nervous and Mental Disease* 177(7): 415–30.

Fanon, F. (1963) *The Wretched of the Earth.* Translated by Constance Parrington. New York: Grove Press. French version originally published in 1961.

Fanon, F. (1967) *Black Skin, White Masks.* Translated by Charles Lam Markman. New York: Grove Press. French version originally published in 1952.

Fernando, S., et al. (1998) *Forensic Psychiatry, Race and Culture.* London: Routledge.

Foucault, M. (1976) *Mental Illness and Psychology.* Translated by Alan Sheridan. New York: Harper and Row. French version originally published in 1954.

Foucault, M. (1978) *The History of Sexuality,* vol. 1. Translated by R. Hurly. New York: Pantheon. French version originally published in 1976.

Foucault, M. (1982) Afterward. In H. L. Dreyfus and P. Rabinow, *Michel Foucault.* Chicago: University of Chicago Press, pp. 208–26.

Freundlich, D. (1994) "Foucault's Theory of Discourse and Human Agency." In C. Jones and R. Porter (eds.), *Reassessing Foucault.* London: Routledge, pp. 152–80.

Gordon, L. R. (1997) "Fanon, Philosophy, and Racism." In Lewis R. Gordon, *Her Majesty's Other Children.* Lanham, MD: Rowman and Littlefield, pp. 25–50.

Gordon, L. R. (2000) *Existentia Africana.* New York: Routledge.

Grier, W. H., and Cobbs, P. M. (1968) *Black Rage.* New York: Bantam.

Harrell, C. J. P. (1999) *Manichean Psychology: Racism and the Minds of People of African Descent.* Washington, DC: Howard University Press.

Herrera, J. M., et al. (1989) *Cross Cultural Psychiatry.* New York: Wiley.

Husserl, E. (1970) *The Crisis of European Sciences and Transcendental Phenomenology.* Translated by David Carr. Evanston, IL: Northwestern University Press. German version originally published in 1954.

Kleinman, A. (1988) *Rethinking Psychiatry.* New York: Macmillan.

Kraus, A. (2001) "Phenomenological-Anthropological Psychiatry." Translated by O. Wiggins. In F. A. Henn et al. (eds.), *Contemporary Psychiatry.* New York: Springer-Verlag, pp. 339–55.

Lawson, W. B. (1999) "The Art and Science of Ethnopharmacotherapy." In John M. Herrera et al. (eds.), *Cross Cultural Psychiatry.* New York: Wiley, pp. 67–73.

Marx, K., and Engels, F. (1988). *The Communist Manifesto.* Norton Critical Edition. Edited by S. Bender; translated by S. Moore. Norton: New York. German version originally published in 1872.

Medical Murder (2002) Hamburg, Germany, pp. 1–9. Retrieved 3/15/02 from http://www.ITZ.uni-hamburg.de/rz3a035/psychiatry.html.

Nature/Genetics (2001) Editorial. 29(3): 239–40.

Nissim-Sabat, Marilyn (1998) "Victims No More." *Radical Philosophy Review* 1(1): 17–34.

Pizen, S. A. (1998) *Building Bridges: The Negotiation of Paradox in Psychoanalysis.* Hillsdale, NJ: Analytic Press.

Schwartz, M. A., and Wiggins, O. (1985) "Science, Humanism, and the Nature of Medical Practice: A Phenomenological View." *Perspectives in Biology and Medicine* 28: 231–61.

Schwartz, R. S. (2001) "Racial Profiling in Medical Research." *New England Journal of Medicine* 334(18): 1392–93.

Stoler, A. L. (2000) *Race and the Education of Desire: Foucault's History of Sexuality and the Colonial Order of Things.* Durham, NC: Duke University Press.

Thomas, A., and Sillen, S. (1972, 1991) *Racism and Psychiatry.* New York: Carol Publishing Group.

Walton, Jean (2001) *Fair Sex, Savage Dreams: Race, Psychoanalysis, Sexual Difference.* Durham, NC: Duke University Press.

Wolfenstein, E. V. (1993) *Psychoanalytic Marxism.* London: Free Association Books.

Zack, N. (1977) "Race, Life, Death, Identity, Tragedy and Good Faith." In Lewis R. Gordon (ed.), *Existence in Black.* New York: Routledge, pp. 99–109.

Zimmerman, Michael E. (1982) *Eclipse of the Self: The Development of Heidegger's Concept of Authenticity.* Athens: Ohio University Press.

CHAPTER 17

COMPETENCE

CHARLES M. CULVER
BERNARD GERT

"COMPETENCE" to consent to or to refuse treatment is a central concept in U.S. health law and bioethics. It is widely believed that a patient must be fully competent before his consent or refusal is valid. However, despite the wide acceptance of the central role that competence plays in the consent process, there is disagreement not only about how the term should be defined but also about its application to particular cases.

If a patient is judged to be competent to make health-care decisions, then, at least in general, her consent to or refusal of a suggested medical intervention is acceded to. If she has been given adequate information about the proposed intervention and no coercion has been employed during the consent process, her consent and refusal are judged to be valid and therefore determinative. It is regarded as legally sanctioned and ethically justified for the physician to proceed with a medical intervention in the presence of a valid consent. However, it is not regarded as legally sanctioned or ethically justified to carry out an intervention on a patient who has made a valid refusal. By contrast, if a patient is judged to be incompetent to consent, then, except in emergency situations, a physician should not carry out an intervention even if the patient has agreed to it, but rather some form of surrogate consent should be obtained. Similarly, if a patient who refuses an intervention is judged to be incompetent to refuse, then under some circumstances it is justified to carry out the intervention nonetheless.

Many definitions of competence have been proposed. Although there is a high degree of agreement among them on how they would classify a random sample of patients, there are some significant disagreements. Furthermore, these concordant classifications correlate strongly with most persons' intuitions about whether a particular patient's consent or refusal should be acceded to. The difficult philosophical problem is to provide an account of competence that accords with most people's considered judgments about when patients' consents or refusals should be accepted. In addition to providing a definition of competence, it is also important to provide the criteria by which, in particular cases, its relative presence or absence should be determined.[1]

LOGIC OF COMPETENCE

Before examining various definitions of competence, it is helpful to review some universally agreed-on features of how the term should be used. Persons are often referred to as "competent" or "incompetent," but this is a somewhat misleading shorthand locution. Competence is task-specific: a person is competent or incompetent to make a will, to perform a neurological examination, or to refuse a suggested medical intervention. It does not follow from the fact that a person is competent to do X that he is competent to do Y. For example, a somewhat confused man may be competent to eat his breakfast by himself or to tie his shoelaces but not competent to make a decision about having a radical prostatectomy. A person may even be competent to consent to a rather simple medical intervention (applying a Band-Aid to a cut finger) but not competent to consent to an intervention with a complex spectrum of risks and benefits (having a carotid endarterectomy for transient ischemic attacks). No one is competent to do everything, although some persons (the totally unconscious) are not competent to do anything. Saying that a person is "competent" is always shorthand for "competent to do X."

In discussing the competence that is a necessary requirement for valid consent or refusal, it is crucial to have a clear and precise account of the task that a patient must be competent to perform. The standard way of describing this task is to say that the patient must be competent to consent to or refuse a medical intervention. However, this way of describing the task is ambiguous in important ways. This ambiguity is responsible for the different definitions of competence that have been proposed. As we shall see later, specifying the task in an unambiguous way leads to a more adequate account of competence and also makes clear what criteria should be used to determine if the patient is competent to perform that task.

DEFINING COMPETENCE TO CONSENT OR REFUSE

The Understand and Appreciate (U+A) Definition

Various definitions of competence have much in common, but they differ in significant ways. Thus, it is possible, although it seldom happens, for a patient to be competent on one definition but incompetent on another. One thing all definitions have in common is the stipulation that the patient understands the factual information relevant to the decision she is being asked to make. Suppose a patient has been given adequate information in a language that she speaks and in terms that most speakers of that language would understand. However, she cannot understand what she has been told (because, for example, she is significantly retarded, or because she is suffering from cognitive confusion secondary to a moderate degree of delirium). Then, even if she does consent or refuse, she is not regarded as competent to make that decision. Valid consents or refusals require understanding, and if a patient does not adequately understand, then one necessary condition of competence has not been satisfied.

"Understanding" refers to whether a patient has adequately carried out a certain kind of mental process but says nothing about the content of the decision (that is, the consent or the refusal) that the patient actually goes on to make. What is at issue is limited to whether the patient has understood whatever (adequate) information he has been given.

"Appreciation" refers to whether a patient has adequately carried out another kind of mental process. It requires more than that the patient understand the information given to her; it requires that she appreciate that the information she has understood is indeed applicable to her at this given point in time. But, like understanding, appreciation says nothing about the content of the decision. One reason a criterion of appreciation has been invoked, in addition to a criterion of understanding, is that on rare occasions patients have delusions that impinge on the consent process and that affect a patient's appreciation but not her understanding. For example, a patient can fully understand the risks that a suggested intervention carries but also believe that he is Superman and that no harm can befall him. If he consents to a risky procedure with the false belief that he cannot be harmed by it because he is Superman, then it is plausible to say he is not competent to consent because, although he knows the risks, he falsely believes they do not apply to him. "Appreciation" could be regarded as a particular kind of understanding—one could say that "understand" means to understand the nature of an intervention's risks and benefits and also to understand that they do indeed apply to oneself in the current situation— but usually it is listed as a separate criterion.

Understanding and appreciating are frequently combined into a single understand-and-appreciate (U+A) criterion, and it is possible to define competence to consent or refuse using only these two measures. We call this a "pure U+A" definition. An important feature of defining competence in this way, which is seen by many as its particular strength, is that the patient's actual decision does not enter into the determination of competence. Competence, as defined by U+A criteria, can in theory, and frequently in practice, be determined before knowing whether the patient will consent to or refuse treatment. If the patient understands the (adequate) information she has been given and appreciates that indeed it applies to her in the current situation, then she is competent, and, absent coercion, whatever decision she makes is determinative and should be heeded.[2]

There are advantages to the pure U+A definition of competence that may in part explain its popularity. First, it fits well with the goal that many have of allowing competent patients to make any decision they want. Second, the determination of whether a patient understands and appreciates information is usually relatively easy to make (there are inevitable borderline cases) and can be investigated by briefly quizzing the patient about the content and the pertinence of what she has just been told. If the patient does U+A, then the physician can simply let the patient decide and behave accordingly. It seems far more difficult and less objective to determine whether a patient's decision is "autonomous" or "irrational" or "authentic" or to apply some other concept of that ilk (see later discussion).

Inadequacy of the Pure U+A Definition

The problem with the pure U+A definition is that it sometimes gives a result that is so counterintuitive that no responsible physician would act on it. Here is an example of such a case:

> Case #1. An elderly depressed woman is refractory to antidepressant drug treatment and has lost a significant amount of weight. She is very frightened about the prospect of having electroconvulsive treatment (ECT), and she cannot bring herself to consent to the procedure, either verbally or in writing. She does not disagree with her doctor's opinion that she may die without ECT, and she acknowledges that ECT would likely prevent her death, but she still cannot bring herself to consent. She did consent to have ECT when she was similarly depressed several years ago, and she remembers that ECT rather quickly alleviated her depression. She was similarly frightened of ECT on this earlier occasion, but her husband somehow pressured her to consent to the procedure. Her husband is no longer living, and her two grown sons, although they very much want their mother to have ECT, have been thoroughly unsuccessful in influencing her to consent. She understands and appreciates everything her doctor has told her and disagrees with none of it, but she has an irrational fear that prevents her from consenting to ECT.[3]

This patient clearly satisfies the U+A definition of competence.[4] Her refusal to consent is not based on any lack of ability to understand or appreciate information; it is based on the strong irrational fear that she has of the ECT procedure. And yet essentially everyone familiar with this case believes the patient should be given ECT.

Here is another example:

Case #2. A severely depressed man, weakened by a cardiac disorder, refuses life-saving treatment for his eminently treatable and potentially reversible cardiac condition. Unlike some depressed patients, he manifests no cognitive delusions or distortions: he understands the relevant information about the likely sequelae of treatment and nontreatment and appreciates that they apply to him. He refuses all treatments and also nutrition and hydration because he wants to die. He gives, and apparently has, no reason to refuse, other than his wish to die, and there is no reason to think his life would not be satisfactory and enjoyable to him if he were to recover from his current condition. The only explanation for his refusal is that he is severely depressed.[5]

This patient also satisfies the U+A definition of competence: he understands and appreciates all of the facts about his situation. His overwhelming desire is to die and all of his actions (refusing cardiac treatment and refusing nutrition and hydration) are logically consistent with his goal of satisfying his desire to die.

Irrationality of a Patient's Decision

The woman in Case #1 suffers from a seriously irrational fear of ECT treatment, and the man in Case #2 has a seriously irrational desire to die.[6] Most physicians believe that these patients' refusals should be overruled. However, if only incompetent patients' refusals can be overruled and if the formal U+A criteria are used strictly and exclusively to define competence, then both of these patients are competent to refuse, and the irrationality of their actual choices can have no role in determining their competence.

The U+A definition usually yields a result that coincides with physicians' judgments about which patients' refusals should be overruled, because people who make seriously irrational treatment refusals often do so because they do not adequately understand and appreciate the facts about their situation. However, sometimes refusals are made because of irrational fears or irrational desires. Patients like the two described can irrationally refuse treatment even though they do understand and appreciate all of the relevant information. Irrational fears (phobias) and irrational desires do not always cause the kinds of cognitive distortions that the U+A definition treats as the only features that make a person incompetent. If only the refusal of incompetent patients can be overruled, the U+A definition does not allow overruling the patients in Cases #1 and #2. Since the primary point of determining competence is to prevent others' overruling patients whose decisions should not be overruled but to allow them to overrule patients whose decisions should be overruled, it is not sufficient for the criteria defining competence to work just part of the time; they must work in every case.

Thus, a dilemma exists. If competent patients can make any treatment decision they want, no matter how irrational, without interference, then competence cannot be defined solely by the use of the formal criteria of U+A. Whatever formal criteria are invoked to define competence, so long as these do not specify anything about the content of the patient's actual decision, they will allow for cases in which the definition is satisfied but the patient makes such a seriously irrational decision that nearly everyone would favor overruling the patient.[7,8] It appears that both U+A criteria and the rationality/irrationality of the patient's decision play some part in judgments about competence and that these two criteria operate to some extent independently.

However, there is a justifiable concern about allowing the rationality/irrationality of the patient's decision to play any part in judgments about competence. Irrationality is often defined in such a way that any decision that deviates from the preferred decision of the doctor is labeled as irrational. When irrational is used in this way, the freedom of otherwise competent patients to make their own decisions about whether to accept or reject a proposed treatment is lost. However, if rational is used to mean "not irrational" and no decision is regarded as irrational unless (1) it would result in the patient's suffering significant harm for a reason that almost no one with similar knowledge and intelligence would regard as adequate for suffering that harm and (2) persisting in that decision would result in the person's satisfying the definition for having a mental disorder, then the freedom that would be lost is not a freedom that any rational person wants to have.[9]

Modifying the U+A Definition of Competence

There are at least three ways in which the criteria we have discussed can be combined to define an approach to competence. The first (A) has been discussed: competence can be defined exclusively by U+A (or other formal) criteria. However, within this first approach, there are two opposing views about the role of U+A competence in determining whether to overrule a patient's decision. The first (A1) is to claim that competence defined in this way is determinative: if the patient consents, proceed with the intervention; if the patient refuses, don't proceed with the intervention. Thus, according to this view the patients described in Cases #1 and #2 would both be regarded as competent and therefore would not be treated. Someone who held this view might acknowledge that most persons' intuitions would favor overruling the refusals in cases like these. However, the argument could be made by exponents of this view that it is better in the long run to give everyone unbridled freedom of choice, even if, as a result, some persons make seriously irrational decisions that cause them great harm.

The second position (A2) that can be taken is that although competence should be defined exclusively by U+A, and that a finding of competence generally justifies acceding to a patient's decision, the irrationality of the patient's decision should sometimes have an important role in determining whether to override that decision. The claim is that it is ethically justified to overrule the seriously irrational decision of a competent patient.[10] This approach has the advantage of being more congruent with persons' intuitions about whether to overrule in actual cases. For example, the patients in Cases #1 and #2 would be labeled as competent, but their refusals would be regarded as seriously irrational, and on the basis of that serious irrationality it would be ethically justified to overrule them.[11] The disadvantage of this approach is that the notion of sometimes overruling a competent patient is at variance with the U.S. legal tradition that competent patients' decisions should never be overruled.[12]

A different position (B) that can be taken is to change the definition of competence so that it is no longer defined exclusively in U+A terms. Several theorists have suggested that the definition of competence be plastic and shifting so that it varies with the kind of clinical situation the patient is in.[13] Thus, if a suggested intervention holds the promise of only limited benefit and limited risk (i.e., nothing of great moment is at stake), then a patient might be deemed competent to consent or refuse simply on the basis of expressing a choice (a formal criterion). The rationality of a refusal in this situation would not be a factor in determining competence. Even if a patient's refusal were thought to be mildly irrational—that is, only minor harm would be suffered—he would be deemed competent to refuse. In a clinical situation in which a patient was refusing life-sustaining treatment, however, it would be necessary for the patient's refusal to be rational for the patient to be deemed competent.

This shifting-definition approach has problems. It is odd to have a key central theoretical term change its very meaning from situation to situation. More important, it leads to strange results. For example, two doctors can disagree about the seriousness of a patient's condition because they have a reasonable disagreement about the patient's underlying diagnosis. The patient firmly refuses further diagnostic tests but refuses to discuss his reasons for doing so. One doctor believes the malady from which the patient is suffering is minor and that there is no urgency to conduct additional diagnostic tests unless the clinical situation changes. The other doctor believes it is more probable than not that the patient is suffering from a serious occult disorder and that further tests might be clarifying and even life saving. Under the shifting-definition approach, the first doctor could claim that the patient was competent to refuse and the second doctor could claim that the patient was not competent to refuse. The two doctors' disagreement about competence would stem from the differing diagnostic inferences they have made, based on the signs and symptoms they observe. But if "competence" is a mental attribute of persons, which most theorists believe, then changes in competence should vary only with changes in mental characteristics of the person, not with changes in his physical condition. The diagnostic disagreements between the two physicians should be irrelevant in determining the competence of the patient.[14]

Any account of irrationality to be incorporated into the concept of competence must be such that no decision is regarded as irrational if any significant number of persons would regard that decision as rational. All irrational decisions must be such that they would result in the patient's suffering significant harm for a reason that almost no one with similar knowledge and intelligence would regard as adequate for suffering that harm. This means that no decision based on religious beliefs that are held by any significant number of people will be irrational. The only irrational decisions are those that would be persisted in by people because of a mental disorder.

Symmetry and Asymmetry of Consents and Refusals

Suppose a patient at a given time consents to a suggested intervention. Using a particular definition of competence, she is judged to be competent to consent. Now suppose nothing about her situation is altered, but after further reflection she changes her mind and refuses the intervention. Is she, automatically, to be judged competent to refuse? Different definitions of competence yield different answers to that question. Under the strict U+A definition, there is a symmetry between consent and refusal. Since competence is judged on the basis of U+A, and not on the basis of the content of the patient's decision, if the patient is competent to decide in one way then, unless her U+A is somehow altered in the interim, she is competent to decide in the other. For example, on the strict U+A definition, the patients in Cases #1 and #2 would be judged competent in either case: whether they consented to or refused treatment. In contrast, with definition B, if these patients consented to treatment, they would be considered competent, but if they refused, they would be considered incompetent. Thus, there is an asymmetry between consent and refusal.

If a definition of competence makes it possible to always determine whether a patient is competent before the patient's actual decision to consent or refuse is known, then there is symmetry, and the definition is one where U+A are determinative. If a definition of competence allows the patient's actual decision to consent or refuse to sometimes determine whether a patient is competent, then there is asymmetry, and irrationality or some similar normative term is, one way or another, being included in the definition of competence.

Competence as the Ability to Make a Rational Decision

If the task that a patient must be competent to perform is described as consenting to or refusing a medical intervention—that is, deciding whether to consent or refuse— then it seems there should be symmetry. However, as pointed out, this way of describing the task is ambiguous in important ways. It is not clear what counts as competent to consent or refuse. People often decide to do something without having any information about the consequences of their decision, so it is not clear why everyone agrees that understanding and appreciating the relevant information is necessary for being competent to decide whether to consent to or refuse a medical intervention.

Reflecting on this fact makes it clear that the task that a patient must be competent to perform is that of making a rational decision about a proposed medical intervention. Thus, we define the competence required for valid consent or refusal as (C) *competence is the ability to make a rational decision.*[15] We noted earlier that competence was task-specific. This definition makes clear what the task is: to make a rational decision about the medical intervention being proposed. Thus, competence and rationality should not be defined independent of one another as has been done in the past; rather, they should be linked in the way the above definition indicates.

There are several conditions that can take away a person's ability to make a rational decision. Among them are the following:

a. A cognitive disability that prevents the person from understanding the information relevant to making a decision of a certain kind. In the case of medical treatment decisions, this would be the lack of ability to understand the "adequate information" given during the consent process.
b. A cognitive disability that prevents appreciating that the relevant information in (a) does indeed apply to one in one's current situation.
c. A cognitive disability that prevents coordinating the information in (a) with the patient's personal rational ranking of the various goods and harms associated with the various available options, insofar as these rankings are relevant.
d. The presence of a mental disorder such as a mood disorder or a volitional disability that causes one to make irrational decisions.[16]

[margin note: — can't associate it w/ their personal values]

If either (a), (b), (c), or (d) is present, then the person lacks the ability to make a rational decision of the particular kind involved, which is to say that she is not competent to make a rational decision of that kind. Thus, the ability to make a rational decision has intellectual, affective, and volitional components.

Each of the four factors listed may by itself take away a patient's ability to make a particular kind of rational decision. We think this list is exhaustive, and thus the absence of all four factors is sufficient to insure that the patient is competent to make a rational decision of the kind involved. However, more than one of the factors may be present. For example, a person may suffer from a delirium that renders him unable to understand the relevant information and also be sufficiently depressed that he would be unable to make a rational decision even if he were to understand the relevant information.

The vast majority of patients who make irrational treatment decisions are not competent to make rational decisions of the kind involved. Consider a middle-aged man who refuses to have an appendectomy for his acute appendicitis, even though it is in danger of rupturing and causing a possibly fatal peritonitis. It almost always is the case that patients of this kind (1) do not have the cognitive ability to understand the situation; or (2) do not have the volitional ability to consent because of, say, a fear of general anesthesia; or (3) are so depressed because of their situation that, despite their accurate cognitive understanding, they do not have the ability to make this kind of rational decision. Thus, this man will almost certainly be found, correctly, to be incompetent to refuse surgery. Seriously irrational decisions are seldom made by persons who have the ability to make rational decisions of the kind involved, and they are never persisted in unless the person is not competent to make that kind of decision.

Different definitions of competence vary in the way in which they articulate the concepts of "competence" and "rationality." The pure U+A definition of competence sharply distinguishes between competence to make a decision to consent or refuse a proposed intervention and the rationality or irrationality of the decision made. By contrast, definition B includes rationality/irrationality as a sometimes-important constituent of the definition of competence. Definition B specifies that treatment refusals in high-risk clinical situations must be rational before the person can be regarded as competent to make them, but the definition does not require rational decisions in less risky settings in order to classify patients as competent. Definition C specifies that a person is competent to make a particular medical decision if and only if she has the ability to make a rational decision of the particular kind involved. Being able to make a rational decision of a particular kind has constituent cognitive, volitional, and affective components.

Incorporating the rationality/irrationality of the patient's decision into the account of competence helps bridge the gap that has developed between the specified justifications for two morally similar procedures: overruling patient refusals of medical interventions, and involuntarily committing persons who are deemed dangerous to themselves or others. In most states, a person can be involuntarily committed if he is suffering from a mental illness that makes him dangerous to himself or to others. There is no mention of competence—defined as U+A or in any other way—in most states' statutory criteria for commitment. The concern is solely with the probability that the person will act dangerously because of a mental disorder. Acting in that way is exactly what we regard as acting in a seriously irrational way. A sufficient condition for incompetence should be the irrational refusal of a medical intervention because of a mental disorder.

Advantages of Definition (C)

Definition C has several advantages:

1. Everyone agrees that competence is task-specific, but definition C provides the first explicit statement of the kind of task that competent patients must be able to perform. Defining competence as the ability to make a rational decision explains the common intuition that a high degree of irrationality is a major factor in determining incompetence. By continuing to distinguish between the competence of the patient and the rationality of a particular decision, this definition makes clear that determining incompetence and justifying paternalistic interventions are separate and distinct. Incompetence is not determined by the seriousness of a patient's situation, but the justification for overruling a refusal is. Approaches that simply sort patients into two groups, the competent and the incompetent, seem to consider that no further justification is needed to overrule the refusals of incompetent patients.

2. Unlike the view that irrational decisions of competent patients can be over-ruled, this definition is consistent with the legal tradition. On definition C, all persons who persist in making seriously irrational decisions are correctly regarded as incompetent.

3. Although we define competence as the ability to make a rational decision, the incompetence of a person to make a kind of rational decision is never determined simply by the irrationality of her decision in the present case. A person is competent to make a rational decision only if both of the following are true: (a) she does not have a cognitive disability that prevents her from understanding and appreciating the relevant information or coordinating that information with her own stable values, and (b) she does not have a mental disorder that takes away her ability to make a rational decision. If none of these disabilities, including having a relevant mental disorder, is present, she is competent to make a rational decision, even if she is presently making an irrational decision. Of course, persisting in a seriously irrational decision would show that the person has a mental disorder that takes away her ability to make a rational decision and hence is incompetent to make that kind of decision. However, if, for example, a person overcomes a volitional disability that prevents her from consenting to ECT and consents, then she is competent to make that kind of decision.

The ability to make a rational decision of a certain kind is what people should have had in mind when they accorded "competence" the primacy it has in the consent process. They did not realize that the bare-boned U+A of the information presented could exist in the presence of mental disorders that took away from people the ability to make a rational decision of a certain kind. Definition C simply makes explicit what most people already hold. It is understandable that understanding and appreciation were initially selected as criteria for competency: they are fairly easily assessed, and they usually do agree with our intuitions about particular cases; the overwhelming majority of patients who lack the ability to make a kind of rational decision lack it because they don't understand and appreciate the relevant information. However, cases like #1 and #2 force us to realize that U+A does not capture the full meaning of the concept of competence as the ability to make a rational decision.

Definition C provides the correct account of the relationship between U+A, the rationality/irrationality of the patient's treatment choice, and the concept of competence as an essential feature of valid consent. Neither U+A by itself nor the rationality/irrationality of the patient's decision provides an adequate explanation of the meaning of competence. Combining the two provides a definition of competence that (1) accords with most persons' intuitions about what should be done in particular cases, (2) is linked with a coherent theory about the paternalistic justification of overruling some patients' treatment decisions, and (3) is consistent with the prevailing legal account of the role of competence in valid consent.

NOTES

1. Chell (1998) frames the definitional issue similarly: "The trick is to define [competency] so that it helps us do the job that needs to be done. The job in this context is to make decisions involving decision making. We must decide whether or not we will allow the patient to decide. Thus, what are the proper considerations we must keep in mind in making decisions? What criteria should be reflected in a proper definition?"

2. Dame Elizabeth Butler-Sloss (2002) apparently holds such a position. In a recent highly publicized case in England, this presiding judge wrote, quoting her own words in an earlier case, "a mentally competent patient has an absolute right to refuse to consent to medical treatment for any reason, rational or irrational, or for no reason at all."

3. Gert et al. (1997: 141).

4. In fact, the state in which she was hospitalized (New Hampshire) had a statutory definition of competence that explicitly defined competence in terms of understanding and appreciating, just as these criteria have been defined here. Lawyers who were familiar with the case were of the opinion that the patient should be classified as competent to refuse by New Hampshire standards.

5. Gert et al. (1997: 140).

6. See Gert (1998) or Gert et al. (1997) for a discussion of irrational fears and irrational desires.

7. Normative terms other than "irrational" could be used: "pointless," "needlessly harmful," "dangerous," and so on. We prefer the term "irrational" because its definition has been carefully elaborated (Gert 1998).

8. Other formal criteria could be suggested. "Expressing a choice" is sometimes mentioned (Grisso and Appelbaum 1998). A patient, for example, might be able to U+A the relevant information but for some neurological or psychological reason be unable to express his choice in any way and therefore understandably be deemed "incompetent to consent or refuse." Another formal criterion sometimes mentioned is the patient's ability to reason logically in justifying her consent or refusal in terms of her general goals. However, all formal criteria have the same problem: it is possible for a patient to satisfy them and yet make a seriously irrational decision that most observers would feel should be overriden. For example, a seriously depressed patient's most important general and overriding goal may be to die, and thus his refusal of treatment would be a logical extension of his goal.

9. For a full discussion of the definition of mental disorder, see Gert and Culver, "Defining Mental Disorders," chapter 29 in this volume.

10. This is a position that was put forward by Culver and Gert (1982).

11. See Culver and Gert (1982) for a full explanation of the conditions under which irrational decisions can be paternalistically overruled.

12. Although that legal tradition itself seems vague and confused; see Culver and Gert (1990: 641–42).

13. This position has been advocated by Roth et al. (1977), Drane (1985), and Buchanan and Brock (1989).

14. For a lengthier analysis of shifting-definition approaches, see Culver and Gert (1990: 632–39).

15. See Gert et al. (1997) for a full discussion of this definition.

16. Volitional disabilities are conditions like addictions and phobias that can interfere with a person's ability to make a rational decision. For example, a patient with a phobia about needles might not be able to consent to have her blood drawn even if she herself

acknowledges that it is irrational not to consent to such a low-risk diagnostic intervention. The woman in Case #1 who dreaded ECT so strongly that she was not able to consent to the one treatment that would probably save her life was suffering from a similar malady and would be judged incompetent on this definition of competence.

REFERENCES

Buchanan, Allan B., and Brock, Dan W. (1989) *Deciding for Others: The Ethics of Surrogate Decision-Making.* New York: Cambridge University Press.

Butler-Sloss, Dame Elizabeth (2002) *Re B* (Adult: Refusal of Medical Treatment) [2002] EWHC 429 (Fam), [2002] 2 A11 ER 449.

Chell, Byron (1998) "Competency: What It Is, What It Isn't, and Why It Matters." In John F. Monagle and David C. Thomasma (eds.), *Health Care Ethics: Critical Issues for the 21st Century.* Gaithersburg, MD: Aspen, pp. 117–27.

Culver, Charles M., and Bernard Gert (1982) *Philosophy in Medicine.* New York: Oxford University Press.

Culver, Charles M., and Bernard Gert (1990) "The Inadequacy of Incompetence." *Milbank Quarterly* 68: 619–43.

Drane, James (1985) "The Many Faces of Competency." *Hastings Center Report* 15: 17–21.

Gert, Bernard (1998) *Morality: Its Nature and Justification.* New York: Oxford University Press.

Gert, Bernard, Culver, Charles M., and Clouser, K. Danner (1997) *Bioethics: A Return to Fundamentals.* New York: Oxford University Press.

Grisso, Thomas, and Appelbaum, Paul S. (1998) *Assessing Competence to Consent to Treatment.* New York: Oxford University Press.

Roth, Loren H., Meisel, Alan, and Lidz, Charles W. (1977) "Tests of Competency to Consent to Treatment." *American Journal of Psychiatry* 134: 279–84.

CHAPTER 18

DANGEROUSNESS

"The General Duty to All the World"

DANIEL N. ROBINSON

THE most recent decade has featured a dramatic shift in the issues that once dominated the interface between psychiatry and law—a shift away from solicitude over those judged to be in need of care and treatment and toward those classified as dangerous to others (Applebaum 1988). Two factors are chiefly responsible for this. First, legislative reforms, designed to respect the rights of those judged to be mentally ill, resulted in the release of thousands of hospitalized mental patients, some of whom proved to be and might well have been predicted to be dangerous to others. Second, the general increase, or at least widely believed increase, in violence has led to a more active legislative interest in therapeutic theories and practice. Clear and unavoidable tensions arise within the overall context. Democratic regimes, respectful of the dignity and liberty of persons, hold themselves to the highest juridical standards where dignity and liberty are at issue. All regimes of law, with the duty to protect persons in their lives and property, must exercise coercive force and related police powers where harmful actions are reasonably expected. The rights of the mentally disordered as patients must be reconciled with the rights of vulnerable citizens. Nonetheless, mere eccentricity cannot be the basis on which to deny persons their liberties (Robinson 1973). Moreover, actions presumably caused by mental disease are worthy of treatment rather than punishment. In all, then, the subject of dangerousness presents a panoply of issues drawn from medicine and the social sciences, jurisprudence, philosophy of mind, and action theory. One essay of moderate length cannot do justice to the full range of issues or, for that matter, to any one of them down to its roots.

A further complication arises from the fact that ascriptions of "dangerousness" do not have a common base. Some are inferences drawn from reliable observations and calling for no special skills or preparation. The repeat offender, whose actions routinely imperil life and limb, is understood, without benefit of theory or special assessment, to be dangerous. Here classification is based on actual biographical facts. On other grounds, dangerousness is imputed to those whose mental conditions or disturbances are associated with violent behavior, though the latter has not occurred. Here the grounds are statistical or "actuarial" but to some extent are drawn from a sample of biographies. Thus, the prediction that persons with temporal lobe focal epilepsies are more likely to engage in antisocial behavior is based not on a developed theory regarding the functions of the temporal lobe but on the incidence of such behavior in samples made up of patients with such lesions.

The melding of the biographical and the statistical—combined with various checklists, personality inventories, depth interviews, and *relata*—results in higher predictive efficiency, but the overall record still remains less than encouraging. Clinical predictions fare especially poorly. A systematic review of the literature 20 years ago found clinical predictions of violence to be accurate less than a third of the time, even when these predictions were made about the behavior of those already institutionalized and with a record of violence (Monahan 1981). The very recent Macarthur Study of Mental Disorder and Violence, published as *Rethinking Risk Assessment* (Monahan et al. 2001) is more promising, but only slightly. The study's major conclusion is worth quoting directly:

> Of the scores of variables whose relationship with violence we studied in this project, many (indeed most) had some significant association with future violence. None of these relationships was sufficiently strong, however, for it to be fairly said that a given variable constituted *the* cause of violence, even for a subgroup of patients. . . . Nor . . . does any single concatenation of variables account for violence as a unitary phenomenon. . . . People will be violent by virtue of the presence of different sets of risk factors. There is no single path in a person's life that leads to an act of violence. (Monahan et al. 2001: 142)

The implications for adjudication are clear. Granting that among the most momentous of state actions is the suspension of a citizen's liberties, requiring the most stringent standards of procedural and substantive due process, it becomes questionable whether psychiatric and psychological appraisals and predictions actually work in the interest of justice.

This duly noted, it must be granted further that clinical experience and available diagnostic tools can render predictions more accurate and that, however slight the gain, it is only prudent for the courts to avail themselves of these. But to what extent and with what measure of confidence? When one is judged as dangerous before the fact, and on grounds at once shifting and uncertain, liberty is hostage to theory. When those who are in fact dangerous are permitted to enter the civic world unimpeded, the safety of others is hostage to yet another theory. It is not for psychology or psychiatry to determine where the fulcrum is to be set in order to balance the freedom of the individual and the safety of others. This is the task of law, which can be informed but not ruled by the shifting perspectives of the healer. It is instructive to examine the actual operation of the law to illustrate the special burdens and duties faced by psychiatrists and psychologists who are called on to assess and manage those judged to be dangerous.

I. A Case Study

On April 1, 1996, two days after obtaining a weekend pass from the VA hospital in Augusta, Georgia, Geoffrey Hodges phoned the police to report that he had just choked and stomped his mother to death, though he was unsure as to whether she was dead. He expressed the hope that she was dead, for, he insisted, she wasn't his mother but someone who had kidnapped him at birth and thus had to be killed.[1]

Who is Geoffrey Hodges? By the time of the lethal assault, he had been in and out of prisons and mental hospitals for 17 years, bearing a repeatedly confirmed diagnosis of "paranoid schizophrenia." After his discharge from the U.S. Navy in 1979 for violent behavior, he began a history of making threats against members of his family, and these were serious enough to lead to his court-ordered confinement in the Athens, Georgia, General Hospital (November–December 1979). Within two months of his release, he was again arrested for making terrorist threats and was again confined in psychiatric facilities. After this release, he was found threatening to kill a person from whom he had purchased a van, leading to yet additional months under court-ordered treatment. During this time, he made threats against his mother, promising to cut her to pieces for being in bed with an alien. In 1983, he was arrested for taking an ax to his trailer and running in the woods naked for three days; in 1984, for obscene language, burglary and assault, and other violations. This time, the finding of not guilty by reason of insanity resulted in psychiatric confinement for a period of five years.

By 1990, Hodges had been shuffled from prison to hospitals and from one hospital to another, with each reassignment based on additional episodes of violence and threats of violence. On April 12, 1992, after a violent fight, he was placed in the Georgia Regional Hospital on a physician's certificate, only to be discharged two days later but on orders to take prescribed medicine. Within three months, he was back in the Georgia Regional Hospital, the medical record showing that "he was not compliant with his medications and he was becoming violent and hostile. . . . Homicidal ideation toward President Bush . . . previous suicide attempt by drug overdose . . . required seclusion and restraints at one time." After fewer than 90 days, he was again discharged. This pattern would repeat itself another ten times between 1992 and March 1996, when he came under what the court referred to as "interdisciplinary" treatment. The records available left no doubt that Geoffrey Hodges was a violent, delusional, and dangerous person, with a specific and paranoid animus toward his mother.

On March 17, 1997, Sheila Spence and Sheryl Jones, daughters of the deceased, filed a claim of wrongful death against the Department of Veterans Affairs. Failing at that level, they then brought suit against the United States in the U.S. District Court for the Middle District of Georgia.[2] The burden of the claim was proof of negligence, which in Georgia (as in nearly all jurisdictions) requires the plaintiff to establish the following:

1. A legal duty on the part of the defendant to conform to standards of conduct raised by the law for the protection of others against unreasonable risks of harm
2. A breach of that standard
3. A legally attributable causal connection between the breach of the standard and the resulting injury
4. A loss or damage to the plaintiff's legally protected interests as a result of the alleged breach

The plaintiffs' contention was that the issuing of a weekend pass to Geoffrey Hodges was causally responsible for the death of their mother and that the decision to issue the pass constituted a failure to conform to applicable medical standards. In specifying the principle that grounds the legal duties embraced by the concept of negligence, the Georgia court relied on the earlier decision reached in *Bradley Ctr., Inc. v. Wessner.*[3] In that case, too, a wrongful death action was instituted for a murder following the issuing of a weekend pass to a patient under psychiatric supervision. One of the defenses available in such actions is found in that provision of the law of torts that imposes no burden whatever on a third party to prevent someone from causing harm to others (Restatement, *Torts*, 2d, § 315). In *Bradley Ctr.*, however, the court noted an established exception; viz.,

> One who takes charge of a third person whom he knows or should know to be likely to cause bodily harm to others, if not controlled, is under a duty to exercise reasonable care to control the third person to prevent him from doing such harm. Restatement, *Torts*, 2d, § 319. n1. See also Prosser, *Handbook of the Law of Torts*, § 56, p. 349.

Thus, "where the course of treatment of a mental patient involves an exercise of 'control' over him by a physician who knows or should know that the patient is likely to cause bodily harm to others, an independent duty arises from that relationship and falls upon the physician to exercise that control with such reasonable care as to prevent harm to others at the hands of the patient."[3] On the matter of negligence itself, the court in *Bradley* reached conclusions deeply rooted in common-law understandings and unaffected by the special nature of medical practice:

> The legal duty in this case did not arise out of this "consensual transaction" between doctor and patient, however, so there is no basis for a requirement of priv-

ity. *The legal duty in this case arises out of the general duty one owes to all the world not to subject them to an unreasonable risk of harm.* This has been expressed as follows: ". . . negligence is conduct which falls below the standard established by law for the protection of others against unreasonable risk of harm." (Restatement, *Torts*, 2d, § 282;[4] italics added)

The rationale is directly applicable to *Smith and Jones v. United States.* The physician in charge of Geoffrey Hodges had a duty arising from the very power he had over the patient. It was the physician's decision to issue or withhold the weekend pass. As the pass was the causal antecedent of the death, it remained only to establish whether or not such an outcome was reasonably foreseeable. On this question, the case law and the juridical principles that guide it are various and subtle but lead nonetheless to a generally coherent and applicable set of standards. Part of the complexity is rooted in what might be called the "standing" of various third parties, especially in relation to injurious actions committed by others. Suppose, for example, that Roberta sees Robert (a total stranger) about to steal Jennifer's car. Granting that it would be both decent and ethical for Roberta either to discourage the theft or to alert its imminent victim, Roberta would suffer no legal liability for failing to warn Jennifer. Even after the fact, Roberta might decline to participate as the police begin their investigation. In general, it is not tortious to withhold assistance from victimization at the hands of others. Suppose, however, that Roberta has an agreement with Jennifer that calls for the latter to provide her with transportation and that imposes severe financial penalties just in case Jennifer fails to honor the agreement. The theft now stands to be of considerable benefit to Roberta and thus gives her a quite different standing. In this example, Roberta actually sees the theft developing. Surely the physician treating Geoffrey Hodges had no such vantage point, but he did have a vantage point: the one established by Hodges's record of violence and by regular therapeutic contact. As reasoned by the Georgia court in *Smith*, sustaining a complaint for negligence does not require proving that the defendant should have foreseen the particular action or outcome:

> Instead, all that is required for liability to attach is that the defendant, exercising ordinary prudence, "might have foreseen that some injury would result from his act or omission, and that consequences of a generally injurious nature might result." Id. (quoting *Emory Univ.*, 104 S.E.2d at 243). In other words, "negligence is predicated on what should have been anticipated rather than on what happened."

II. Prediction and Liability

The court in *Smith* heard conflicting testimony from psychiatrists on both sides and recognized that this was yet another "battle of the experts."[4] The court's own understanding was clear:

Psychiatrists are not clairvoyant. . . . No one has shown that psychiatrists have any special powers in so far as predicting dangerousness. The American Psychiatric Association has spent a great deal of effort trying to convince courts, attorneys, and law enforcement agencies that psychiatrists do not have special powers to predict dangerousness. Clearly, the profession itself is fully aware of its limitations in this area. It is also clear that police agencies, judges, parole boards and citizens at large are also unable to make these predictions with any great accuracy.[5]

Though not clairvoyant, psychiatrists are expected to possess a far greater than ordinary capacity to assess the severity of mental disorders and to render judgments on which civil authorities have reason to act. The *Smith* court found the psychiatrist who had treated Hodges to be actionably negligent to a degree unmitigated by the imprecise nature of psychiatric assessment. Before issuing the weekend pass, the attending psychiatrist should have performed a "dangerousness assessment" in light of Hodges's history and disorder. Expert testimony delineated the specific elements in such an assessment. These would have included the degree of Hodges's paranoia, his capacity to empathize with past and potential victims, his insight into his own prior misconduct, his current degree of anger or hostility, the current status of his mental illness, his tendencies toward depression or suicide, and so on. The plaintiff's expert in *Smith* concluded that the failure to undertake such an assessment prior to granting a weekend pass constituted a quality of practice that fell below professional standards of care.

It is doubtful, however, that the application of this list of considerations would be generally effective, even if practicable. It is unlikely that even experienced clinicians would reach precise agreement on factors such as a patient's "empathy" and "insight," or even the current "degree" of paranoia. Using a list of risk factors before issuing or refusing to issue a pass almost certainly would lack the concrete validity of judgments made based on the patient's *career* of activities under various circumstances and pressures. Grove and Meehl (1996) have made droll reference to *broken leg countervailings* in these areas: an elaborate and validated assessment instrument leads to the conclusion that Mr. Jones will attend the opera tomorrow night. Early the next day, Mr. Jones breaks his leg and is wrapped in an immobilizing cast. Mr. Jones is now seen by all as one who will assuredly *not* go to the opera. For a clinician to rely on risk-assessment instruments over and against what is conveyed by what Grove and Meehl refer to as an "overwhelmingly prepotent fact" (1996: 307) would simply be silly. Countervailing influences are, of course, the order of the day and conspire to defeat predictions based on the most searching of assessment techniques.

At play in such contexts is the trade-off between type 1 and type 2 errors, or, in the idiom of signal detection theory, between correct detections and false alarms. There is only one strategy that will guarantee that a radar system will *never* fail to report "missile": *it must identify everything as a missile*. There is only one strategy that will guarantee that a radar system will never wrongly identify objects as missiles: *it must call nothing a missile*. One can improve the "hit" rate in any system designed to make fine discriminations. The greater the system's repository of relevant facts about missiles and nonmissiles, the greater the rate of correct detections, with no corresponding increase in false alarms. To know, for example, that any missile entering the earth's atmosphere will have a descent velocity in excess of 3000 mps — and that no duck has ever attained such velocities — establishes with near certainty that the approaching object (descending at 18,000 mps) is not a duck.

Apart from developing a library of relevant information (apart from increasing the system's *memory*), there are other ways of differentially altering rates of correct detection and false alarm. Principal among these is by way of the "payoff" matrix built into the system's decision processes. One can assign far greater penalties for false alarms than for missed targets, and vice versa. The decision made in the matter of Mr. Hodges was based on the judgment that he had been improving under medication. Had the medical staff operated under a payoff matrix that severely penalized missed targets — those who subsequently committed violent acts — Hodges never would have been permitted to leave the facility. Had the medical staff operated under a payoff matrix that severely penalizes false alarms — judging as "dangerous" those who, over a course of years, never endanger anyone — there is a chance Hodges never would have been hospitalized *until* he caused great harm to another.

Staying with the idiom of signal detection theory, it may be said that, in the matter of dangerousness and confinement, the payoff matrix must be established through the political process, for it is not an essentially medical or scientific matter. Rather, society, though elected legislatures, must finally decide on the level of risk beyond which the confinement of allegedly dangerous fellow citizens is first tolerable and then obligatory.

III. Prediction, Labels, and Liability

Liability cuts both ways, of course, and declaring a person to be dangerous before the fact of any violent or antisocial conduct may well be construed as defamatory. For example, consider the provisions of the Fourteenth Amendment to the U.S. Constitution in the matter of due process. Among other protections, the amendment is intended to safeguard the given citizen against enduring a state-imposed burden unique to that person. This includes defamatory characterizations claimed or proven to be false, with the additional feature of altering the status of the person as citizen. Taken together, these two elements constitute the *stigma plus* test, which seeks to determine whether a challenged characterization is stigmatizing and whether it alters the legal status of the person thus stigmatized.

The application of this test to actual cases illustrates the contexts in which psychiatrists, functioning under the color of law, may find diagnostic labels subjected to constitutional scrutiny. Perhaps the area richest in such possibilities is that associated with "Megan's Law," which requires sex offenders to register with state authorities as a condition of their release from prison.[6] Typically, the law also provides for the full disclosure of data included in the registry, thus allowing communities to identify those who have been convicted of the crimes covered by the law.

The nature of the burden is evident in the provisions of the relevant statutes in the state of Connecticut. Registrants who change their address must notify the commissioner of public safety within five days. If they travel to or reside within another state temporarily for purposes including, but not limited to employment or schooling, they must notify the Connecticut commissioner and register with the appropriate agency in the other state. Registrants must provide blood samples for DNA analysis and must appear at specified locations to be photographed whenever the commissioner requests. Failure to abide by any of these requirements constitutes a felony, punishable by up to five years in prison. A ruling in a recent challenge to the Connecticut statutes in this area found them unconstitutional. In the class-action suit, *John Doe v. Dept. of Public Safety*,[7] the Court of Appeals affirmed rulings by a lower court, which found Connecticut law in violation of the due process clause of the Fourteenth Amendment. The court thereupon granted declaratory and permanent injunctive relief to the appellants against the disclosure of any information contained in the registry, ruling that Connecticut statutes altered an offender's legal status and were "governmental in nature." On the "plus" aspect of the *stigma plus* test, the principle is precise: Could the statutory requirements ever be imposed by a private actor in a position analogous to state officials? If the answer is affirmative, it is then sufficient to show the duties imposed to be extensive and onerous.

It is instructive in this light to consider the position of state-appointed psychiatrists or those who practice within a government-controlled facility. Psychiatrists in such contexts who classify a patient as dangerous and as requiring confinement before the fact of any violent or antisocial action surely might trigger the *stigma plus* test in the United States or versions of it in other jurisdictions. The characterization "dangerous" is not only stigmatizing (Walker 1980) but clearly subject to challenge, given the statistical and clinical records of prediction within psychiatry. When such a characterization proceeds under the color of law, carrying with it constraints and burdens on the patient that could not be imposed by a private actor (doctor) in the same capacity, the entire procedure may be judged as "governmental in nature." Here again, therefore, the otherwise legitimate attempt to safeguard the public, confronted by the law's equal concern for the preservation of rights, sets up what is finally a collision course.

U.S. law at both the state and the federal levels has undergone any number of refinements that, on the whole, seem to have rendered both diagnosis and adjudication rather more impressionistic. The "sex offender" is again the most instructive example, for the statutes covering dangerousness have been especially carefully crafted to meet this problem. Moreover, compared to the incidence of other forms of violent behavior, these offenders have particularly high rates of recidivism, understood as the result of a "mental" disorder the significantly diminishes powers of self-control. It is on this basis that the law makes a fundamental distinction between sexual assaults punishable under criminal statute and those that warrant civil commitment. Indeed, the U.S. Supreme Court has held that the Constitution forbids the civil commitment of offenders where the state has failed to make the "lack-of-control" determination. The Court has noted that such determinations cannot reach the level of "mathematical precision." It is sufficient to establish a "serious difficulty" in controlling behavior. The pivotal case was *Kansas v. Hendricks*.[8] The Court would revisit its reasoning in *Hendricks* in *Kansas Petitioner v. Michael T. Crane*,[9] noting:

> In *Hendricks*, this Court did not give "lack of control" a particularly narrow or technical meaning, and in cases where it is at issue, "inability to control behavior" will not be demonstrable with mathematical precision. It is enough to say that there must be proof of serious difficulty in controlling behavior. The Constitution's liberty safeguards in the area of mental illness are not always best enforced through precise bright-line rules. States retain considerable leeway in defining the mental abnormalities and personality disorders that make an individual eligible for commitment; and psychiatry, which informs but does not control ultimate legal determinations, is an ever-advancing science, whose distinctions do not seek precisely to mirror those of the law. Consequently, the Court has sought to provide constitutional guidance in this area by proceeding deliberately and contextually.
> . . . That *Hendricks* limited its discussion to volitional disabilities is not surprising, as the case involved pedophilia—a mental abnormality involving what a lay person might describe as a lack of control. But when considering civil commitment, the Court has not ordinarily distinguished for constitutional purposes between volitional, emotional, and cognitive impairments.

It is not argumentative to acknowledge the highly subjective and shifting standards likely to obtain as psychiatrists, jurors, and judges consider whether the repetition of a violent assault carries with it the property of "self-control" on the part of the assailant. It is doubtful that any such repetitive activity is independent of powerfully motivating states, but it is also doubtful that repeat offenders within the ambit of criminal law are not similarly motivated. Is, then, the signal criterion that of "mental illness"? If so, there must be a credible means by which to establish, first, that the actor suffers from such an illness; second, that the illness is causally responsible for the action; and third, that the mental illness is of that specific nature that robs the actor of the degree of self-control envisaged by the rule of law itself. Applied to the wide and various domain of "dangerousness," these three conditions appear to fall far beyond the competence of contemporary psychiatry, at least to the extent that psychiatric findings in this area would reach the level of "evidence" as customarily understood.

IV. CAVEATS

As noted in the introduction, politics has become a more audible and active participant in the domain of mental health, drawn to it by the understandable fears and concerns of society at large. Increasing pressure is being brought to bear on psychiatrists and psychologists to identify the dangerous and on legislatures to establish the means by which those thus identified can be effectively removed from those whom they would (allegedly) endanger. With each grotesque victimization of the young, the weak, the defenseless, a predictable cry goes up for the authorities to "do something." Where the offenses are patently criminal, that cry is heard, and long-established procedures are in place to remove the offender. Where the offenses either have not yet occurred or are judged to be the result of uncontrollable impulses arising from mental illness, society again insists that some effective mode of quarantine be instituted.

The problem, of course, is that there is little by way of parallels between the established procedures in criminal law and what is called for by judgments of "dangerousness." The imprisoned criminal is one who has committed the crime, not one who was merely "likely" to do so. Imprisonment is the outcome of an adversarial trial procedure, governed by rules of evidence and by the heavy burden of proof that must be borne by the accuser. The term of imprisonment must "fit" the offense and be determinate. The defendant, after all this, retains options for appeal, retrial, parole, and other remedies.

Although great progress in mental health law has improved the civic status of those judged to be mentally ill, there are far fewer safeguards against injustice available to the psychiatric patient. Accordingly, the fulcrum that would seek to balance the potentially conflicting rights of the individual and the collective should be set at a point that is clearly advantageous to the former. As Nigel Walker has noted, "When we exercise the right to detain someone, not because he deserves it, or for longer than he deserves, but solely for the sake of other people's safety, this is in a sense human sacrifice, and puts us under an obligation to that person" (1994: 190).

It is now a veritable maxim that, considered in light of the rights enjoyed by citizens, it makes little difference whether a place of confinement is called a hospital or a prison. There is, needless to say, much to recommend in that "therapeutic state" that would approach the offender as a congeries of treatable conditions that, unattended, constitute a threat to society and an obstacle to a contributory life. Nonetheless, this very approach, granting the generous motives that may direct it, is not without its own costs. In a now classic essay, Herbert Morris affirmed the *right* to punishment: "The primary reason for preferring the system of punishment as against the system of therapy might have been expressed in terms of the one system treating one as a person and the other not" (1968/1975: 588).

Considered in this light, the wiser course, where doubt exists, may well be for psychiatric diagnosis to lean strongly toward the presumption of volitional and cognitive competence and strongly away from the presumption of mental and volitional impairment. This is the wiser course chiefly because it leads to the potential patient's retention of the status of *citizen*, and thus not only of that dignity but also of the myriad resources with which to preserve liberty.

NOTES

1. For its timeliness and its centrality to the issues at hand, I've chosen the Georgia case of *Spence and Jones v. United States* (132 F. Supp. 2d 1061; 2001 U.S. Dist.; Decided February 2, 2001).

2. Although as a sovereign state the United States must expressly agree to be subject to suit, immunity is waived for claims involving certain kinds of tortious conduct committed by federal employees in the course of their employment. 28 U.S.C.S. §§ 2671–80.

3. *Bradley Ctr., Inc. v. Wessner* (250 Ga. 199, 296 S.E. 2d 693, 695; Ga. 1982).

4. Courts have made their peace with this arrangement, perhaps more by default than by principle.

5. *Smith and Jones v. U.S.*

6. "Megan's Law" memorializes the seven-year-old child in New Jersey who was sexually assaulted and murdered by a neighbor in 1994. The assailant had two previous convictions for sexual offenses.

7. 271 F. 3d 38, 2001 U.S. App.

8. 521 U.S. 346, 369, 138 L. Ed. 2d 501, 117 S. Ct. 2072.

9. 122 S. Ct. 867; 151 L. Ed. 2d 856; 2002 U.S.

REFERENCES

Applebaum, P. (1988) "The New Preventive Detention: Psychiatry's Problematic Responsibility for the Control of Violence." *American Journal of Psychiatry* 145: 779–85.

Grove, W., and Meehl, P. (1966) "Comparative Efficacy of Informal (Subjective, Impressionistic) and Formal (Mechanical, Algorithmic) Prediction Procedures: the Clinical-Statistical Controversy." *Psychology, Public Policy and Law* 2: 293–323.

Monohan, J. (1981) *The Clinical Prediction of Violent Behavior.* Washington, DC: Government Printing Office.

Monohan, J. et al. (2001) *Rethinking Risk Assessment: The Macarthur Study of Mental Disorder and Violence.* New York: Oxford University Press.

Morris, H. (1975) "Persons and Punishment." In Joel Feinberg and Hyman Gross (eds.), *Philosophy of Law.* Encino, CA: Dickenson.

Robinson, D. N. (1973) "Therapies: A Clear and Present Danger." *American Psychologist* 28: 129–33.

Walker, N. (1980) *Punishment, Danger and Stigma.* London: Rowman and Littlefield.

Walker, N. (1994) "Dangerousness and Mental Disorder." In A. Phillips Griffiths (ed.), *Philosophy, Psychology and Psychiatry.* Cambridge: Cambridge University Press.

CHAPTER 19

TREATMENT AND RESEARCH ETHICS

RUTH CHADWICK
GORDON AINDOW

WHAT, IF ANYTHING, IS SPECIAL ABOUT TREATMENT AND RESEARCH IN PSYCHIATRY?

IN considering the ethics of treatment and research in psychiatry, a number of different kinds of question need to be addressed: To what extent are the ethics of treatment and research specific to this field, and to what extent are they the same as or analogous to ethics in other areas of medicine? What are the relevant issues in both treatment and research, and what are the appropriate ethical frameworks for addressing them? In this chapter we concern ourselves with analyzing the ethical considerations relevant to these issues. Although we do not aim to offer coverage of legislation in different countries in the field, we do attempt to look at how current scientific developments in genetics might have an effect on such psychiatric ethics.

One further preliminary clarificatory point is in order. We are not, here, addressing the ethical issues associated with diagnosis. As far as the ethics of treatment are concerned, what is at issue is the treating of those who have been diagnosed (for the purposes of this chapter, we presume correctly) as suffering from a mental disorder. In the research context, there will be issues about whether it is acceptable for those so correctly diagnosed to participate in clinical trials.

One marked difference between psychiatric care and other areas of medicine concerns the nature of the therapeutic relationship in this context and the multiple obligations to which health-care professionals (HCPs) might feel themselves subject. What must be examined is whether there is a basis for this in the nature of psychiatric illness itself. We consider two possible reasons for the view that there is a relevant difference between the context of psychiatry and other areas of medicine: (1) the stigma of mental illness and (2) a presumption of an association between mental illness and impairment of autonomy. In our view, these are not unrelated:

> *Stigma* Despite considerable advances in degrees of enlightenment, there is
> still stigma associated with psychiatric disorder, and this is only exacerbated
> by the prominence in the media of stories of violent episodes initiated by
> patients. Stigma may arise from lack of understanding. Kathy Wilkes has
> written, of schizophrenia, that it is "difficult if not impossible to see the
> world through the mind of the schizophrenic, in terms of which the way he
> behaves seems, and might be shown to be quite rational; and he for his part
> has temporarily, or perhaps permanently, lost the ability to see the world as
> we do" (1988: 90). Thus, she suggests, there is a perception of difference.
> But, as Wilkes further points out, "we must note that the mentally ill . . . are,
> since they belong to they same species, as much like us as it is possible to
> be" (98). She makes the interesting suggestion that it is in our capacity for
> mental illness that we are distinctive as a species. While these points have
> some force, they in fact presuppose a "them" and "us" divide, which may in
> itself be regarded as stigmatizing.
>
> *Capacity for autonomy* Arguably another, if not the primary, reason why it
> might be thought that the issues are different is that there is an important
> presumption in treatment and research in other contexts, at least where we
> consider the case of adults:[1] that is, the adult is presumed to be an individ-
> ual with a capacity for autonomy—in other words, capable of thinking and
> deciding whether to accept a course of treatment or to participate in a re-
> search trial. From an ethical point of view, the *principle of autonomy* sug-
> gests that this capacity should be respected. In practice, respect is imple-
> mented by acting in accordance with the decisions the individual makes. It
> is not clear that this presumption is present in psychiatry, partly because of
> the stigma of mental illness, but it is important to be careful about what
> might be the implication of saying that the presumption is not present. We
> consider various interpretations of this thesis next.

Strong Thesis

A strong version of the thesis is a presumption that the capacity for autonomy is *lacking* in a person diagnosed with psychiatric disorder. This might be supported by an argument that psychiatric disorder undermines an individual's capacity for autonomy because the condition in question may be understood as, in itself, an interference with thought processes and with rational decision making. Richard Lindley, for example, argues that the mentally disordered person who has irrational beliefs is incapable of making rational decisions about his welfare: "What is special about someone who has radically irrational beliefs of this kind is that he is likely, unwittingly, to get into all kinds of dangers. The person who believes he is indestructible might well walk into the middle of a busy road . . . he would not be moved by one's reasoning" (1978: 41).

Two caveats are appropriate here. The first is that Lindley's example is a "hard" case where the person in question appears to be making a decision that is clearly irrational and not receptive to any counterargument or evidence to the contrary— namely, that he is indestructible. However, it may be argued that for most people the issues are less dramatic and, consequently, present more of a challenge in deciding whether specific decisions are irrational. The point about specific decisions leads to the second caveat: examples concerning persons so disordered in their mental state that they are unmoved by any reasoning about threats to their safety may suggest a global, rather than a local (i.e., relative to a specific context or circumstance), incapacity to reason appropriately. It would take much more argument to support the view that the nature of psychiatric illness is such that it can support a presumption of global incompetence: that is, an inability to take any autonomous decisions at all. As the Nuffield Council on Bioethics points out:

> Even at its worst . . . mental disorder is rarely a matter of comprehensive incapacity; it is commonly a matter of impaired or intermittently impaired capacities. Most people can continue, throughout the duration of their disorder, to take all decisions for themselves with no more assistance than a person without mental disorder. Accordingly, no general case can be made for those suffering mental disorders to be exceptions to the usual requirements for informed consent, or to other aspects of respect for persons. (1998: s. 1.25)

Weaker Thesis

Considering the global/local distinction, a weaker thesis would be that, although there is little if any basis for a presumption of a global lack of capacity for autonomy in one diagnosed with psychiatric disorder, there is likewise no basis for a presumption that the individual in question has the capacity for autonomy to support any particular local decision. This means that the burden of proof shifts toward demonstrating that the individual has the capacity.

Arguably, the burden of proof should not shift in this way: there should be a presumption that the capacity is present until proved otherwise. There are, after all, arguments to suggest that in general people who are ill have diminished capacity for autonomous decision making, and yet we do not think it right that health-care professionals should act on that assumption.

The concept of competence is clearly relevant here, and it is also important to take context into account. As Beauchamp and Childress point out, while autonomy and competence differ in meaning, attributions of autonomy and competence depend on similar criteria. While competence is task-specific, "two plausible hypotheses are that an autonomous person is (necessarily) a competent person (for making decisions), and that judgments of whether a person is competent to authorize or refuse an intervention should be based on whether the person is autonomous" (1994: 135). A person may be competent to perform a task at one time and not at another. It is potentially sobering to consider how well any person might meet the criteria for complete rational autonomy, when we reflect on the power of pain, passion, sadness, and loss, which are part of the experience of everyone.

In light of these considerations, therefore, it appears unjustifiable to presume that the person who has been (correctly) diagnosed with mental illness lacks the capacity for autonomy, while at the same time taking the view that the presumption in favor of autonomy for persons not so diagnosed holds.

Against this, it might be argued that this is fair up to the point of diagnosis, which has its own attendant ethical issues. Arguably, where psychiatric illness has been diagnosed, autonomy is more vulnerable than in the case of physical illness. It is not clear that this point is sufficient, however, to shift the burden of proof.

Still Weaker Thesis

In light of these considerations, a weaker thesis again than the preceding one can be put forward: in the case of psychiatric disorder, the diminishing of a person's capacity to take autonomous decisions *may* be symptomatic. This does not undermine the need for evidence of an individual's local incompetence relating to any specific decision.

TREATMENT

Ethical issues concerning treatment in psychiatry have traditionally been concerned with (a) the possible justifications of compulsory treatment, which are to a certain extent associated with the issues discussed in the preceding section; (b) the character of some of the treatments themselves (e.g., ECT) and their insecure scientific foundation (in the years since the introduction of the care-in-the-community policy, other issues have come to the fore of the debate); (c) treatment "in the community" and what that means; the use of drug therapy and its long-term effects, and evidence-based medicine; and (d) the nature of the therapeutic relationship in this context, arising out of the multiple obligations of HCPs.

Justification of Compulsory Treatment

The default position with competent adult patients is that they have the right to refuse treatment. It is also the case that competent adults cannot be compulsorily detained and subjected to interventions on the grounds that they might pose a danger to themselves or to others. While it is beyond the scope of this chapter to discuss the grounds for detention as such, the question of compulsory treatment is clearly related to that of detention; indeed, there is a more general point to be made about the need to consider the setting in which treatment is given.

Detention and constraint of people with mental illness is typically argued on grounds of potential harm to themselves or to other people, so it is clear that the interests of the patient are *not* the sole consideration. We do not discuss here the ethical issues concerned with intervening to prevent harm to self, as in potential suicide. We do consider that, on the grounds of preventing harm to others, closer scrutiny of particular situations may arguably show that the grounds for detention or constraint appear to be based more on the potential for offense than on the risk of physical harm — and this, again, is associated with the stigma of mental illness. People may be troubled by behavior that appears unusual or bizarre and feel that this constitutes a threat requiring action, even if closer observation of particular situations might suggest limited potential for harm by the patient. Consequently, practitioners may then feel themselves charged with intervening and offering treatment. While this may be argued from the perspective of a duty of care on the part of a practitioner, it may seem more akin to a duty to protect the interests of other relevant parties (e.g., caregivers, neighbors, police, health-care workers) before the interests of the patient. The practitioner may be in a position of "jailer" as much as caregiver and at least has to have regard for the complexities of the double role of regulatory and therapeutic agent (cf., Unsworth 1987; Davis 1978).

Right to Refuse Treatment

A question that has given rise to a considerable amount of debate is whether patients compulsorily detained have the right to refuse treatment. There are different possible scenarios:

- The patient has the capacity and consents to treatment.
- The patient lacks the capacity to consent to treatment.
- The patient has the capacity but refuses treatment.

The most complex situation here is the third. In other medical settings, such a refusal should and, we assume, would be respected. Some argue that even if a patient is competent to make a specific local decision, this decision should not always be respected — for example, when a decision, although competent, is irrational (see discussion in Sherlock 1983; Lesser 1983). For example, they may refuse a treatment because they regard it as a form of torture, punishment, or poison. Harry Lesser argues:

> Only if the phobia, or the depression or indecisiveness, is evidently preventing the patient from thinking clearly at all, or if it is combined with an inability to give any reason for his or her expressed preference, is one justified in regarding the preference . . . as irrational . . . and the patient—however irritating this may be to some doctors—should be considered "rational until proved irrational." (1983: 145)

Lesser's argument here is in accord with our earlier points about where the burden of proof lies. When the patient is competent, the fact that HCPs do not agree with a decision is not a ground for overruling it.

Troubling Treatments

Some of the treatments in psychiatry have been regarded as particularly troubling from an ethical point of view; these tend to be those that involve physical intervention, such as psychosurgery (Missa 1998), rather than "talking therapies" (Clarke 1995). The depictions of such treatments in novels such as Marge Piercy's *Woman on the Edge of Time* and Ken Kesey's *One Flew over the Cuckoo's Nest* have presented them in an unfavorable light. Electroconvulsive therapy (ECT), for example, has been regarded as particularly controversial, even if, overall, more physical harm is caused by drug therapies. While there are clearly ethical issues associated with the potential effects of drug therapy (Dawson 1998), there are several objections, beyond physical harm, that might be made to ECT: for example, as an assault on the dignity of the person, it is wrong in itself (Clarke 1995). Nevertheless, supporters of ECT have defended it for consequentialist reasons, on the grounds that it "works." The problem with this argument is twofold: first, there are also negative consequences to be considered, such as memory impairment; second, in an era of evidence-based medicine, claims about the efficacy of ECT are insufficiently supported. In light of these points, it may be questioned whether it is irrational to refuse this treatment. This is important in light of a further objection to ECT that relates to the wider context of delivery of treatment: What does it mean to say it "works"? What are the criteria for success? As Clarke notes: "Decisions about ECT are fraught with social considerations in the sense that the treatment is often aimed at re-establishing norms of behaviour within settings that partly determine such considerations" (1995: 329). This suggests doubts about whether the interests of the patient, either from a welfare point of view or from the perspective of restoring impaired autonomy, are always the paramount consideration.

Treatment in the Community

The debate about refusal of treatment took a new twist with the move toward care in the community. Community care is not just a question of moving people out of institutions and into smaller units but is arguably a challenge to traditional psychiatric theory and practice (Pilgrim and Rogers 1993: 116). The underlying philosophy of community care may differ according to whether care *in* the community or care *by* the community is what is envisaged (Coombes 1998). Care in the community, while it may permit a greater involvement by patients in their own care, may also exchange a large institution for a mini-institution or a quasi-institutional setting. Care by the community implies a greater degree of professional withdrawal, using the client's own network of relationships and self-care (Coombes 1998). Among the factors that encouraged the policy were increasing realization of the disempowering effects of institutionaliation and the availability of drug treatments that make treatment in a hospital unnecessary. In the early years after the policy of community care was adopted, two themes emerged. The first concerned plans for short-term treatment rather than long-term admission; the second was a plan for a network of hostels and home accommodation, social work support, day care, and sheltered housing to provide a "real" alternative to institutionalization (Murphy 1991). Community care was explained in the following way, as autonomy-enhancing: "Community care means providing the right level of support to enable people to achieve maximum independence and control over their own lives. For this to become a reality the development of a wide range of services provided in a variety of settings is essential" (Department of Health 1989).

Community care was not intended necessarily to involve a change in the treatment given—there continued to be a need for long-term support—but the setting of treatment was a significant issue in itself. The ethical issue then turned to situations where patients who, discharged into the community after having earlier been detained for compulsory treatment, subsequently either omitted to, or refused to, continue their medication. Debate focused on the issue, well put by David Brindle: "If mentally ill people can be treated compulsorily in hospital, one side argues, why not also in the community now that more and more of them are living there? Because, retorts the other side, people deemed well enough to live in the community have the right to decide their own medication" (1990).

The first view is supported by the argument that it is in the interests of the patient to avoid compulsory readmission and that therefore compulsory treatment orders should be available. This appears to be a justification for overriding autonomy in the short term, by not accepting a refusal of treatment, in the interests of longer-term autonomy, in the sense of freedom to live in the community, and on the grounds of "best interests" in terms of health and well-being. These different considerations are not always easy to distinguish in the debate.

In the United Kingdom, for example, compulsory community treatment was recommended, in 1979, by the British Association of Social Workers and then, in 1987 and 1983, by the Royal College of Psychiatrists when the government of the time was forced to confront the issue by a range of fatalities and high-profile incidents (Heath 1998). It was thought that the use of such new powers might benefit some patients in, for example, cases of early-onset schizophrenia where effective, promptly delivered community treatment could forestall the need for hospital admission and might indeed improve the patient's prognosis. Some reporters on models of compulsory community treatment orders in the United States, including Bean (2001), also state that these orders may be seen as acting as a relief from the perhaps more repressive conditions of some hospitals: community treatment orders (CTOs) assist the promotion of dignity for the patient and can reduce the need for frequent readmission to a hospital. Furthermore, CTOs may be seen as relieving pressure on relatives and other caregivers by intervening before a patient relapses and possible crisis ensues. This last point shows that the interests of third parties are becoming a consideration, as they traditionally have been in the case of compulsory treatment in hospitals.

Therapeutic Relationship

A further issue in treatment concerns not only what treatment is given but also who gives it (i.e., which health-care professionals) and how. This gives rise to the need to discuss the therapeutic relationship and the possibility of trust within it. In the past ten years, a body of work has suggested the need for inclusion, partnership, and collaboration between services and users (see, for example, Repper et al. 1994). Yet this liberal emphasis, while it may be attempting to escape the shadow of old-style institutionalization, may be overshadowed by a different shift toward increased legislation and control.

The Sainsbury Centre for Mental Health (SCMH 2001) observes that an increased emphasis on legislation such as CTOs in care delivery could distract managers and clinicians from the fundamental role of improving services and care. There remains the potential for users to distrust services, with the possibility that they will see clinicians as controlling, their central role having become the supervision of compliance with medication and other forms of treatment (a return in another guise of the "jailer" role alluded to earlier). It is curious to note a perverse incentive for HCPs to utilize CTOs: designating a service user as a "risk" within the parameters of these powers may actually procure greater services and benefits (e.g., housing, financial support).

Advocacy

Advocacy is deemed an important role for HCPs; however, with the tensions associated with serving the interests of so many powerful stakeholders, it appears highly problematic for the HCP to act as an advocate for a patient. The wishes and interests of the patient may be in stark contrast to those of other interested parties. It may become practically difficult to promote the interests of the patient ahead of the wishes of other influential voices. Indeed, the contractual obligations of HCPs require them to countenance the goals of their organization. These mixed obligations may present obvious tensions when placed in conflict with the goals of the individual patient. To whom is the HCP in service? To whom is his or her loyalty due? These issues present a dilemma for trust and rapport.

During conflicts of interest, the HCP may actually act on behalf of parties other than the patient. These other parties may include the HCP's employer, which will wish to avoid risks and possible litigation. Parents and caregivers may also have very different wishes for the patient than those the patient him- or herself expresses. All these other interests may act as a bar to the patient's being appropriately advocated for. Indeed, under such duress, the HCP's only route to avoid further conflict may, paradoxically, be to advocate that the patient receive the support of an independent advocate in order to minimize conflict.

RESEARCH

Where research is concerned, analogous conflicts of both interests and ethical principles arise. First, however, it is important to note that the distinction between treatment and research is not always clear-cut: some research has the potential to have therapeutic effects, and it may be difficult to draw the line between innovative treatment and research. Research has been defined in the following way: "Where an activity involving a patient is undertaken with the prime purpose of testing a hypothesis and permitting conclusions to be drawn in the hope of contributing to general knowledge" (Royal College of Physicians 1990).

Once again we have to consider the extent to which the issues in psychiatry are different from those that obtain for other medical research. In research ethics generally, the interests of the research subject are protected by both autonomy and welfare considerations, and these are reflected in the doctrines of informed consent and minimal risk, respectively. In the case of research in psychiatry, we encounter the same general problem concerning the possibility of impaired decision-making capacity on the part of research subjects. The issue here may be construed in terms of the question whether this fact should give rise to *special* protections for research subjects. It has been argued, for example, by the U.S. National Bioethics Advisory Commission (NBAC), established during the administration of President Bill Clinton, that there is a cogent case for special protections in this field, as with other vulnerable groups (NBAC 1998). NBAC acknowledged that research provides significant opportunities to develop new therapies and that failure to do research on particular groups can produce "therapeutic orphans" (Hattab 1998).

In addition to autonomy and welfare considerations, NBAC added others, such as the soundness of research design: "Unless the researcher is a competent investigator and the research design is sound, it is inappropriate to engage persons as research subjects, regardless of the level of risk" (NBAC 1998: 9). This is a requirement of morally acceptable research in general. Consideration is also given to the principle of justice in the context of urging that this population of potential research subjects not be *exploited* — for example, by shouldering the risks and burdens of research from which the benefits would largely accrue elsewhere. This consideration, while not exclusive to research in psychiatry, is especially relevant to vulnerable populations.

In line with the argument put forward earlier, it seems clear that, where the subject has the necessary capacity, his or her informed consent to participate should, if sought, be respected. The difficult questions concern the extent to which it is permissible to enroll research subjects in a trial (a) in the absence of seeking informed consent or (b) when the subject does not have the capacity to consent:

a. Is informed consent always necessary? There are some types of research, generally speaking, for which informed consent need not be sought — for example, certain epidemiologic research that poses minimal risk to participants. It is difficult to see an argument for the view that research dealing with psychiatric disorders should be different in regard to informed consent, provided that there are appropriate confidentiality protections in place.

b. Is it permissible to enroll research subjects who do not have the capacity to consent? Table 19.1 shows a number of possible scenarios according to the degree of risk to the subjects on the one hand and the identity of the potential beneficiaries on the other. To take this view that the issues could be resolved through a risk-benefit analysis would be too simplistic. (We should also note, if only to set it on one side for the purposes of this chapter, that the terms "minimal" and "more than minimal" risk are not transparent.) It is necessary also to pay attention to how the benefits are distributed, which is where the issues of justice are relevant. Further, autonomy considerations are by no means totally absent. To say that the subject lacks the capacity to consent is insufficiently informative. There might be what we shall call autonomy-related *evidence*. He or she might have expressed a view at a period of intermittent capacity; although lacking the capacity to consent, he or she might register a strong objection; authority might be vested in a surrogate decision maker.

One possibility is that research protocols should be assessed on a case-by-case basis and that the issue reduces to one of what the *process* should be and who should make the decisions. There are questions, however, as to whether, in relation to certain cells in the diagram, some considerations should be regarded as trumps over others, whatever the merits of the individual case. For example, in light of the possible need for special protection to research subjects in this area and the danger of exploitation, justice considerations suggest that where the potential benefits will accrue to others but not to the research subjects (whether these potential benefits are humanitarian goods or simply advances in knowledge), research should not proceed. Where the research imposes more than minimal risk, welfare considerations point in the same direction. But what about the case where the risk is minimal? There may be a dif-

Table 19.1. Research: Distribution of Risks and Benefits

	Minimal Risk	More than Minimal Risk
Potential benefits to subjects	Acceptable unless autonomy-related evidence to the contrary	Above all "do no harm"? Or trade-off?
Potential benefits but not to subjects	Room for trade-off?	Justice considerations prevail

ference of opinion as to whether justice considerations act as trumps here or whether there is room for a trade-off. It is conceivable that some research protocols may have very great potential benefits for research—for example, there may be the possibility of producing therapeutic benefits for another group that suffers from a disorder as serious as, though different from, that which affects the potential subjects. Here, in light of the "special protection" and exploitation considerations, however, the burden of proof will lie with those who would justify it, and there would need to be a very high standard of justification. Here it might be relevant to consider whether there is any autonomy-related evidence regarding the subjects' wishes. To guard against the possibility of overstating the potential benefits of the research in an era in which science is held to promise much, it is arguable that all such decisions should be informed by representatives of mental health service users.

Let us consider the top row of the table, where the potential benefits accrue to the research subjects themselves. Here the justice problem encountered earlier is absent. If testing a new form of therapy has the potential to benefit the research subjects, where there is minimal risk, then welfare considerations suggest that the research is acceptable, unless there is other autonomy-related evidence to tip the balance, such as a strong objection. Where there is more than minimal risk, the issues are more complicated. One possibility is that we should allow the avoidance of potential (more than minimal) harm to trump the possibility of benefit. If the possibility of trade-off is considered at all, however, again it will be important to pay attention to the views of service users in the decision-making process, the likelihood of the potential harms as well as the degree, the potential for benefit, and any autonomy-related evidence.

GENETICIZATION

Cutting across the different categories outlined earlier is the contemporary issue of geneticization, or introducing genetics as a form of explanation of phenomena. The

Human Genome Project and the advent of geneticization have far-reaching implications because of the potential for predictive testing and gene therapy. Surely, this might seem to avoid some of the traditional problems in psychiatry. Suppose, for example, a predictive test were found for a severe mental disorder x, considered to undermine an individual's capacity for autonomous decision making, and there was an effective preventive therapy available. The individual could then make an autonomous decision to have the therapy before symptoms appear, thus avoiding any worries about informed consent. Even setting aside queries about the predictive power of a given test, however, this possibility only gives rise to new ethical issues. All this assumes relatively high sensitivity and specificity of the test and does not take into account the psychological costs of testing. Both true and false negatives *and* positives have costs and benefits (Shickle and Chadwick 1994). The costs of a result, whether a positive or a negative, might be raised anxiety, increased distress, damaged self-image, and damaged image in the eyes of others.

Geneticization also gives rise to special issues with regard to research. Despite the arguments for the importance of research on psychiatric disorders, some arguments might count against the desirability of genetic research in this area. For example, research on the genetic basis of psychiatric disorders might be held to reinforce not only a medical model but also a deterministic one (cf. Nuffield Council on Bioethics 1998). Genetic research in general has a number of potential problems associated with it because of the potential uses and misuses, by third parties, of genetic information about individuals. The potential dangers of this in the psychiatric context are clearly exacerbated by the possibility of stigmatization, although stigmatization is also an issue in the case of genetic disorders that are not psychiatric in character.

ETHICAL FRAMEWORKS: COMMUNITARIANISM

In health-care ethics generally, at least during the last 20 to 30 years of the twentieth century, autonomy has been considered the supreme principle. But in the case of mental health, there has been more willingness to intervene for the patient's own protection. What is also striking is the attention traditionally given in this context to the protection of others, and this, as we have seen, has posed problems for HCPs.

It is worth noting that the emphasis on autonomy in health-care ethics may not have helped the interests of patients with a psychiatric disorder, in light of the facts we have noted about presumptions, or the absence of presumptions, of a capacity for global or local autonomy. The predominance of the "four-principle" approach to health-care ethics has recently come under criticism because it is an approach to ethics that very much concentrates on the individual patient, and there are others to consider, including formal and informal caregivers and the wider community in which community care takes place. A communitarian ethic urges us to regard the individual as necessarily situated within a network of relationships. The individual's autonomy has to be negotiated within a context. Families, for example, can play an important part in identifying needs and supporting patients. Such an approach might make sense of the need to think about the interests of others, as well as those of the patients themselves (and thus may provide a way of mediating between different interests in, for example, the difficult issue of confidentiality, such as in the famous Tarasoff case in the United States). In discussions of mental health care, as shown in the example of detention, consideration has always been given to the protection of others, but the ethical basis of this has not always been clear. The central questions are what and whose interests are at stake and how they can best be protected. If the principle of autonomy will not do the work of protecting the interests of patients, research subjects, and others, then what will? Would a communitarian approach be the way forward?

We are not arguing for a replacement of autonomy and welfare considerations by a communitarian approach. But it is important to respect the insights from alternative frameworks, such as communitarian and feminist bioethics, which emphasize relatedness and mutual dependency in addition to autonomy. The ideal of the autonomous individual may need to be at least rounded out to take into account the network of relationships in which an individual exists, including the wider social context.

NOTE

1. In this chapter we do not consider special cases such as child psychiatry and psychogeriatry.

REFERENCES

Bean, P. (2001) *Mental Disorder and Community Safety*. Houndmills, Basingstoke: Palgrave.

Beauchamp, T. L., and Childress, J. F. (1994) *Principles of Biomedical Ethics*, 4th ed. New York: Oxford University Press.

Brindle, D. (1990) "Keep Taking the Tablets." *Guardian* (3 January).

Clarke, L. (1995) "Psychiatric Nursing and Electroconvulsive Therapy." *Nursing Ethics* 2(4): 321–31.

Coombes, L. (1998) "Mental Health." In R. Chadwick (ed.), *Encyclopedia of Applied Ethics*. San Diego: Academic Press, pp. 197–212.

Davis, A. J. (1978) "The Ethics of Behavior Control: The Nurse as Double Agent." *Issues in Mental Health Nursing* 1: 2–16.

Dawson, A. (1998) "Psychopharmacology." In R. Chadwick (ed.), *Encyclopedia of Applied Ethics*. San Diego: Academic Press, pp. 727–34.

Department of Health (1989) *Caring for People: Community Care in the Next Decade and Beyond*. London: Her Majesty's Stationery Office.

Hattab, J. (1998) "Psychiatric Ethics." In R. Chadwick (ed.), *Encyclopedia of Applied Ethics*. San Diego: Academic Press, pp. 703–26.

Heath, T. (1998) "Compelling Arguments," *Mental Health Care* 2(1): 10–11.

Lesser, H. (1983) "Consent, Competency, and ECT: A Philosopher's Comment." *Journal of Medical Ethics* 9: 144–45.

Lindley, R. (1978) "Social Philosophy." In R. Lindley, R. Fellows, and G. Macdonald (eds.), *What Philosophy Does*. London: Open Books, pp. 1–52.

Missa, J-N. (1998) "Psychosurgery and Physical Brain Manipulation." in R. Chadwick (ed.), *Encyclopedia of Applied Ethics*. San Diego: Academic Press, pp. 735–44.

Murphy, E. (1991) "Community Mental Health Services: A Vision for the Future." *British Medical Journal* 302: 1064–65.

National Bioethics Advisory Commission (NBAC) (1998) *Research Involving Persons with Mental Disorders That May Affect Their Decisionmaking Capacity*. Rockville, MD: Author.

Nuffield Council on Bioethics (1998) *Mental Disorders and Genetics: The Ethical Context*. London: Author.

Pilgrim, D., and Rogers, A. (1993) *A Sociology of Mental Health and Illness*. Buckingham: Open University Press.

Repper, J., Ford, R., and Cooke, A. (1994) "How Can Nurses Build Trusting Relationships with People Who Have Severe and Long-Term Mental Health Problems? Experiences of Case Managers and Their Clients." *Journal of Advanced Nursing* 19: 1096–1104.

Royal College of Physicians (1990) *Research Involving Patients*. London: Royal College of Physicians.

Sainsbury Centre for Mental Health (1997) *Pulling Together: The Future Roles and Training of Mental Health Staff*. London: Sainsbury Centre for Mental Health.

Sainsbury Centre for Mental Health (2001) *Executive Briefing 14: Reforming the Mental Health Act*. Available at www.sainsburycentre.org.uk

Sherlock, R. (1983) "Consent, Competency and ECT: Some Critical Suggestions." *Journal of Medical Ethics* 9: 141–43.

Shickle, D., and Chadwick, R. (1994) "The Ethics of Screening: Is Screeningitis an Incurable Disease?" *Journal of Medical Ethics* 20(1): 12–18.

Unsworth, C. (1987) *The Politics of Mental Health Legislation*. Oxford: Clarendon Press.

Wilkes, K. (1988) *Real People: Personal Identity without Thought Experiments*. Oxford: Clarendon Press.

CHAPTER 20

CRIMINAL
RESPONSIBILITY

SIMON WILSON
GWEN ADSHEAD

THIS chapter examines the relationship between criminal responsibility and mental disorders. Other legal excuses, such as mistake, self-defense, and duress, are not explored here. The broader notion of moral responsibility, of which criminal responsibility is perhaps a subclass, is also not discussed. We have a powerful intuition that the insane, among others, are sometimes not responsible for their behavior. Psychiatrists have been involved in assisting the courts in making determinations of who is and who is not "criminally responsible" for their actions since the trial of Hadfield in 1800 (Green et al. 1991). What "criminal responsibility" might mean and how it might be measured has caused a good deal of discussion among psychiatrists, philosophers, and lawyers. There is general agreement that the term is problematic. There is not general agreement on the source of the problem. We begin by reviewing the legal evolution of the concepts of criminal responsibility and mental excuses.

LEGAL EVOLUTION OF CRIMINAL RESPONSIBILITY

Aristotle, in the Nicomachean Ethics (Elliott 1996), recognized two classes of involuntary actions: those that stemmed from ignorance (not knowing what one was doing) and those that stemmed from compulsion (knowing what one was doing but being unable to help it). This was the root of the complicated legal concept of criminal responsibility, and the medical defenses of insanity and diminished responsibility.

Mens rea

Henri de Bracton, a thirteenth-century legal scribe to Henry II, made the first reference to the requirement for a "guilty mind" in committing a criminal offense (Green et al. 1991). The law requires both a "guilty act" (actus reus) and a "guilty mind" (mens rea) for most criminal offenses, and so mental problems may affect the "guiltiness" of one's mind and hence the criminality of one's conduct. Some jurisdictions explicitly codify different sorts of mens rea, forming a hierarchy of degrees of culpability. The American Model Penal Code of 1962 describes four such degrees of mens rea (Section 2.02(2)): purposely—the actor intends a harmful outcome; knowingly—the actor knows harm is very likely but proceeds anyway; recklessly—the actor consciously disregards a substantial and unjustifiable risk; and negligently—the actor is unaware, but ought to be, of a substantial and unjustifiable risk.

English common law makes similar distinctions, although they are not so explicitly codified (Smith 1999). We might view these degrees of mens rea as translating into a hierarchy of criminal responsibility—a person being more responsible for an act done purposely than for one done negligently. Certainly the degree of blame and severity of punishment are closely linked, whereas the legal mechanisms for excusing the mentally disordered are not found in this hierarchy. The law treats the mentally disordered as being irrational.

Actus reus

In rare cases, where one behaves unconsciously (for example, following a head injury), the law considers that no actus reus has occurred, and the accused is acquitted on the grounds of automatism.[1] The law assumes that one cannot perform actions unconsciously, and this stance is reminiscent of the philosophers' distinctions between actions and mere bodily movements (White 1968).

Insanity

This is not the place to review the history of the insanity defense in detail (see Hamilton 1986). Legal insanity has largely been seen as a cognitive matter, concerning reason, or rather lack of reason, and this should be seen in the context of the traditional legal view that reason controls behavior (Bowden 1983). The insanity defense was codified by the M'Naghten Rules of 1843, which require, for insanity, that "at the time of committing the act, the party accused was laboring under such a *defect of reason*, from *disease of the mind*, as *not to know the nature and quality* of the act he was doing, or if he did know it that *he did not know that what he was doing was wrong*." This remains the test of insanity in English law, and it forms the basis of insanity defenses in many or most other Anglo-American jurisdictions. Psychiatrists have been unhappy with the strict and narrowly cognitive definition of criminal irresponsibility of the M'Naghten Rules, which are rarely met by even the most psychotic of defendants (Mackay 1995). Philosophers have tended to be more satisfied with this definition, though (Kenny 1986; Gendin 1973).

At other times in its history, insanity was seen as a status (like being a child), rather than an excuse (Mackay 1995). And, at other times and places, causation has been seen as key to insanity. Lord Denman, in *R v. Oxford* (1840), stated that "a person may commit a criminal act and not be responsible. If some contributory disease was in truth the acting power within him, which he could not resist, he would not be responsible" (cited in Green et al. 1991). The American Durham Rule excused conduct caused by mental disease: "an accused is not criminally responsible if his unlawful act was the product of mental disease or mental defect" (*Durham v. United States D.C. Cir.* 1954). Causation has been dismissed as the "fundamental psycholegal error" (Morse 1999). Such definitions of insanity seem perilously deterministic, as though, simply because behavior is caused, it should be excused. Irrationality is what matters, Morse (1999) argues. However, *pace* Morse, causation is not totally beside the point, as illustrated by an example from Kenny (1986) of an academic who is suffering from paranoid delusions that his colleagues are persecuting him and who decides to poison his mother-in-law to inherit her fortune. It is hard to see why one set of crazy beliefs that make him irrational should excuse an apparently calculated motive.

Diminished Responsibility

Diminished responsibility was introduced into English law by the Homicide Act of 1957. It was already well established in Scotland and had been since the case of Dingwell in 1867 (Green et al. 1991). Section 2 of the 1957 act states: "Where a person kills . . . he shall not be convicted of murder if he was suffering from such an *abnormality of mind* (whether arising from a condition of arrested or retarded development of mind or any inherent cause or induced by disease or injury) as *substantially impaired his mental responsibility* for his acts." This is a partial defense to a charge of murder, reducing the crime to manslaughter if successful. The wording of this act has caused considerable difficulties for psychiatrists. Strictly speaking, the psychiatric expert is supposed to confine his testimony to the issue of "abnormality of mind," the question of "substantial impairment of mental responsibility" being the ultimate issue and therefore a matter for the jury, not the expert.[2] It has not worked like this in practice, however, with psychiatrists frequently being pressed to address the ultimate issue (e.g., Masters 1985). Walker (1968) has suggested that diminished responsibility brought together a number of diverse mental states that had previously been excused under the pretext that they "do have something in common—an impairment of some mental faculty which is called 'responsibility' " (152). Griew gives this idea short shrift:

> One distinguished psychiatrist recently remarked to me: "I don't think we know very much about mental responsibility." He had, I believe, been seduced into thinking that this was a meaningful remark by long experience of being invited, as an expert, to opine about the state of a defendant's "mental responsibility"—as though it were indeed a specific faculty. My answer should have been: tell me what would count as "knowledge about" mental responsibility, so that it might enable you to give more authoritative evidence to the effect that it was substantially impaired; what exactly is it about which you seek knowledge? (1986: 19)

Griew believes that impaired "mental responsibility" (and, by extension, criminal responsibility) really contains two ideas: that of diminished liability (a legal conclusion) due to reduced culpability (a moral conclusion). Psychiatry has nothing to say about these matters.

CRIMINAL RESPONSIBILITY

What then of criminal responsibility? Morse provides a definition by exclusion of criminal responsibility that assigns criminal responsibility to a defendant "if the state can prove beyond a reasonable doubt that the defendant's behavior satisfied the definitional 'elements' (criteria) of the crime charged and no affirmative defense of justification or excuse can be established" (1999: 148). So one is criminally responsible if one has behaved in a way defined by the state as criminal, and without any state-sanctioned excuse for doing so. But why should the state sanction certain excuses? And why is madness so universally seen as exculpating?

We are back to our initial, powerful intuition that some people are more responsible for their behavior than others. But we have also seen something of the criticisms of the notion of "mental responsibility" in the 1957 English Homicide Act and the suggestion that the concept is confused with ideas about blame and punishment rather than being a separate, objectively identifiable condition that might have consequences in terms of blame and punishment.

Thought Experiments

Let us start with our intuitions and a thought experiment. Consider Jane, who often calls the red-haired John, whom she barely knows, "You red-headed bastard wanker." We are shocked. When we learn that Jane suffers from Tourette's syndrome,[3] that seems to make all the difference. We believe that Jane is less responsible for, and has less choice about, her actions than if she were simply someone who is habitually rude. Furthermore, let us stipulate that Jane and John are living in a society where using profane language is a criminal offense. We would, I believe, consider Tourette's syndrome an excuse from a conviction for using profane words, an insanity defense, perhaps. Rudeness seems less likely to afford such a defense. So there is a difference between Tourette's Jane (T-Jane) and rude Jane (R-Jane).

The contrast between T-Jane and R-Jane provides useful insights into our intuitions about criminal responsibility. Although it has the advantage of being simple, it is a poor and atypical example of a mentally disordered defendant. This is a weakness-of-thought experiment, and it would be more helpful to have a back-up real-life example for more detailed analysis.[4] Let us also bear in mind, therefore, the case of Mr. M. Mr. M is a man in his 30s with an unremarkable upbringing and no previous violent behavior. Over the past few months, his behavior has altered; he is disheveled, talks to himself, and is late for work. He kills a coworker by cutting her throat. When asked about this, he gives a rambling and difficult-to-follow account of believing that his victim was controlling his mind. He had come to know that she had been using drugs to increase her "brain power" and was able to cause his heart to skip a beat, and she could make light bulbs stop working. He suspected she might be a Romanian spy and was convinced she was evil. He went to work early one morning in order to kill her. He does not regret his actions and instead has been rather surprised not to be offered some kind of reward. Mr. M is found guilty of manslaughter on the grounds of diminished responsibility.

There are two extreme positions in considering these cases and criminal responsibility: what we shall call a "realist" approach and an "antirealist" approach. Finally we explore the "psychiatric/pragmatic approach."

Realist Approach

There is something called "criminal responsibility," and it is this that distinguishes T-Jane from R-Jane and Mr. M from a sane killer. The difference between T-Jane and R-Jane is something to do with their responsibility for their verbal behavior — T-Jane has much greater difficulty controlling her verbal behavior than R-Jane. T-Jane's profane utterances may not even be actions of hers, being more like tics than purposeful actions, although the fact that the content of the utterances does contain some accurate information about her surroundings might seem curious in this case. In other words, R-Jane is more responsible for her verbal behavior than T-Jane. R-Jane has free will and can choose how to behave. T-Jane's behavior is determined and beyond her control.

This is beginning to touch on the confusing issues of free will and determinism (Williams 1980; Hospers 1990). Both free will and determinism struggle with the question "How can any of us be responsible for our actions?" For determinists, an actor is merely one part of a long causal chain stretching back to the beginning of the universe. For the free-will supporter, there must be uncaused events originating within the actor that cause actions: How can the actor be responsible for uncaused events? We have a powerful sense of our own ability to freely choose our behavior, and this is the common-sense view of the law. Nineteenth-century psychiatrists, such as Esquirol, believed that some psychiatric disorders disabled one's volition and hence one's responsibility (Smith 1979). Foucault (1978) has demonstrated the ridiculous circularity of some of these conditions, such as homicidal monomania, which were evident only in terms of a criminal act. Confused thinking about the nature of determinism and free will reached its acme in a form of hard determinism whereby all criminal behavior was viewed as fair game for psychiatry (e.g., Hubert and East 1939). Hard determinism leads to the view that no one is responsible for his behavior, and so we have lost our initial intuition that some people (such as the mentally ill) are less responsible than others. The determinism of psychiatry contrasted with the free-will position of the law has led Stone to assert that there is a "contradiction between the law's enduring free-will theory or morality of action and psychiatry's deterministic theory of causes" (1978: 656). This is probably confused thinking. Although we intuitively believe there is something different between T-Jane and R-Jane, we cannot simply be determinists when thinking about T-Jane and free-will supporters when thinking about R-Jane. Either all our behavior is determined or none of it is. We need to be able to distinguish between T-Jane and R-Jane from within the same model. We also need a model that allows people to behave badly without automatically and circularly labeling them as mad.

The metaphysical approach seems to suggest that there is a difference between T-Jane's brain and R-Jane's brain, and that that something is "mental responsibility." This view has to answer Griew's (1986) criticism that the notion of "mental responsibility" has become a piece of mental machinery. There are different approaches to this. Some would argue that T-Jane has a disorder of will; she is unable to control her behavior because of a damaged will. For example, Robinson (2001) has argued that the law requires two assumptions: nomological indeterminacy (things could have been otherwise) and agentic power (people have control over things). T-Jane has a lack of agentic power and hence a legal excuse. This does not really deal with Griew's objections; "mental responsibility" is simply replaced by a fancier-sounding term, "agentic power," which is really Aristotle's excuse of compulsion rehashed: "I knew what I was doing, but I couldn't help it." This might be a good representation of T-Jane's situation—an irresistible impulse to utter profanities. The law, though, has been reluctant to admit such a defense on the grounds that the difference between "I couldn't resist" and "I didn't resist," while making all the difference to the law, may be impossible to determine empirically (as with Lord Parker in the case of Byrne (R v. Byrne (1960) 2 QB 396, 44; Cr App R 246).

There is a weakness in the thought experiment because T-Jane is an unusual mentally disordered defendant, compared to Mr. M. Did Mr. M have a disorder of will? This seems much less likely: he was able to choose to follow a particular course of action—namely, killing his victim—and to carry it out. There was nothing robotic or coerced about his actions. He intended to kill his victim and then did it. Morse has argued that the problem lies not with the will but with practical reasoning. He states, "mental disorder may compromise rationality because its signs and symptoms can give people crazy reasons for action that are not susceptible to correction by reason" (1999: 148). This seems to fit Mr. M's case better: he is partially excused because his actions are motivated by crazy reasons that are untouched by evidence to the contrary. We are still left with the original problem, though. Why should crazy reasons excuse when rational ones do not? Morse argues that irrationality may be used as an excuse insofar as it impairs a person's ability to properly follow the law.

Yet another way of viewing the difference between T-Jane and R-Jane is in terms of explanations. T-Jane's behavior is better accounted for by a mechanistic explanation, in terms of disordered brain circuitry, whereas R-Jane's behavior is better explained by her intentions and reasons. Dennett (1967) has called these two types of explanations the "physical stance" and the "intentional stance," respectively. T-Jane is diseased and broken, and so a physical explanation may work better. R-Jane is functioning normally but behaving badly. This manner of describing the ill and the diseased differently may date back to the medical psychologists of the nineteenth century (Smith 1979). T-Jane is mad; R-Jane is bad. This is a peculiarly enduring dichotomy, and one that is not especially helpful in the real world. Is Mr. M mad or bad? He is certainly mad, but then other mad people with similar beliefs may not have chosen to kill. Why did he not move far away from the victim? Why did he not tell the police what she was doing to him? A "physical stance" explanation does not seem to work well with Mr. M; it is easier to explain his behavior by referring to his (mad) beliefs and desires.

Antirealist Approach

There is no "criminal responsibility," or if there is we don't need to rely on it—this is the antirealist line. The difference between T-Jane and R-Jane, and between Mr. M and a sane killer, is that we believe both T-Jane and Mr. M should be exempt from punishment and blame. Criminal responsibility is simply an ex post facto argument to bolster our initial intuitions about who should be punished and who should be treated. There is nothing fundamentally different inside T-Jane and R-Jane; what distinguishes them is our beliefs about what should happen to them. Hart (1968) has stated that "for criminal responsibility there must be 'moral culpability,' " so Mr. M is less morally culpable than a killer without crazy reasons, and T-Jane is less morally culpable than R-Jane. Culpability (i.e., blaming and punishing) is what matters, not "responsibility." This view is given weight by, for example, Swedish law, according to which insanity is not an excuse (does not affect "criminal responsibility") but merely alters disposal (treatment rather than punishment; Felthous 1999). This view is also given weight by Green et al.'s (1991) assertion that criminal responsibility has lost its importance to a large extent in English law since the advent of the Mental Health Act of 1959, which enabled offenders convicted of offenses (other than murder) to receive a hospital disposal, regardless of their degree of "responsibility" for the offense. Such legislation does not exist in America, and hence the American preoccupation with "criminal responsibility," they argue.

Bayles (1982) has argued for three general philosophical approaches to blaming and excusing. The first is Bentham's utilitarian approach, where one excuses those for whom punishment would be inefficacious. Critics have objected to this on the grounds that the advantages of the general deterrence of others by punishing an individual might eliminate excuses. The second is Kant's influential view that one must excuse those who could not have avoided performing a criminal act and punish only those who had the capacity and a fair opportunity, to conform their behavior to the law.[5] The third is Hume's view, which holds that blame and punishment are not for acts but for character traits, so that those who act out of character are excused (this is reminiscent of Foucault's [1978] comments about changes to the law in the nineteenth century). Gillett (1991) has also argued along similar lines, suggesting that we are interested in people's intentions for their behavior because intentions have to do with character and, hence, blameworthiness. This approach seems to fit with Mr. M, who is clearly mentally ill and has behaved out of character. He needs treatment and not punishment. What about T-Jane, though? She, just as much as R-Jane, is forever going around uttering profanities, and so on a Humean view we should punish her just as rigorously as R-Jane. The Kantian approach would rescue her because T-Jane could not have avoided uttering profanities unlike R-Jane.

An alternative antirealist solution to the problem of criminal responsibility is a radical behaviorism–type approach, where one does away with "criminal responsibility" by confining one's talk to observable behaviors. Miller (1979) argues that much of the problem with talk of "criminal responsibility" is a category mistake. Mental illnesses are discussed as though they are the sorts of things that can cause criminal behaviors. Miller argues that mental illness is simply shorthand for a constellation of behaviors: "It is not that some occult entity, mental illness, affects a person's actions, it is that a person's actions is [sic] his mental illness." Miller calls this an "anthropomorphic error," meaning that mental illnesses are reified and are thus transformed from shorthand (i.e., "schizophrenia" is the name given to odd verbal and physical behaviors of a particular sort) into things. Things can then be causally efficacious.

There is clearly something to this argument, although it is also reminiscent of the radical behaviorism of the 1950s, which attempted to do away with mental states altogether for the good of the science of psychology. Miller's point that mental illnesses are descriptions, not things, and therefore are not capable of causing anything is well taken. However, it is also beside the point, according to Morse (1999). Causation is irrelevant to excusing. All behavior is caused, so to argue that one is excused because one's behavior was caused rather than chosen freely is "the fundamental psycholegal error," in Morse's language. This is returning to the free will and determinism arguments explored earlier.

Yet another antirealist approach is to view responsibility, blaming, and punishment as all socially constructed. Backlar (1998) asks where blame should properly lie when a psychiatric patient acts criminally: with society, with the patient for not taking his medication (see also Mitchell 1999), with the family, or with the community? Miller (1979), too, states that "it is conceivable for the law to decide that the accused is not criminally responsible because he is poor and sick and comes from a broken home." In other words, it may not be too much of a leap to imagine a society where these sorts of things are seen as just as exculpatory as mental diseases.

Psychiatric/Pragmatic Approach

Psychiatrists identify and describe abnormal mental states in the same way that physicians identify and describe abnormal physical states. This is the standard "medical model" of psychiatry, most trenchantly criticized by Szasz (1974). A particular criticism for Szasz arises in relation to criminal responsibility. Since medieval times, it has been assumed that abnormal mental states affect criminal responsibility by reducing it. If this is correct, then abnormal mental states can do this (a) by restricting the capacity to make intentions that others hold blameworthy, (b) by restricting the capacity to be autonomous more generally, and (c) by restricting the capacity to reason morally.

In English courts, psychiatrists are therefore invited to give an opinion on whether a "mental abnormality" or "disease of the mind" is present; then they may be invited to give an opinion on how that affected the defendant's criminal intent. As we have seen, for an insanity defense to be successful, the psychiatrists must connect a mental disease with failure to know or appreciate certain information about the intention. For diminished responsibility (in British law), there must be an "abnormality of mind" that "substantially impaired" the defendant's responsibility.

How do psychiatrists relate their diagnostic identification of mental abnormality to responsibility? There are many conceptual difficulties. First, there is no agreed definition of what it is to be criminally responsible: that is, what mental capacities might be necessary. Further, even if a checklist of capacity criteria could be drawn up, the courts, in their role as social commentator, might still wish to retain the ultimate privilege of determining who is responsible for a defendant's actions, rather than deputing this to medical doctors.

How do psychiatrists decide what is "abnormal" in relation to criminal behavior? In the case of Byrne, abnormality of mind was defined as "a state of mind so abnormal that the reasonable man would term it so"—which rather suggests that this apparently diagnostic question could also be left to the jury. What is also not clear is whether the abnormality is related to the individual in question (i.e., is it out of character for him?) or whether it is a social abnormality (i.e., does it break group norms?). A focus on an individual's abnormality raises a conventional medical question; a focus on group norms makes the question more moral: What sort of behavior, although statistically abnormal, is not acceptable to the group? This question itself is not so simple; social groups set different thresholds for responsibility for different types of criminal action (as can be seen in the different legal approaches to intention/mens rea).

Even if psychiatrists can agree on what constitutes "abnormality," it is not clear how these abnormalities affect moral reasoning. A dichotomous approach (normal/ abnormal) may not do justice to the psychological complexity of forming intentions. In this sense, the adversarial process of Anglo-American criminal law is inimical to the diagnostic process of psychiatry (Eastman 1992).

It is also not clear that psychiatric explanations for criminal behavior are sufficiently robust. There have been many and varied criticisms of the M'Naghten test of insanity (e.g., Reznek 1997), not least because it fails to address the most common pathological effects that the mentally ill experience. Some have argued that it is too cognitively based: that moral reasoning is not just a matter of "knowing" things but also involves feeling things. The pathology of action found in mental illnesses rarely involves a state in which one is not conscious of what is being done; rather, it is the interpretation and genesis of the action that gives it its symptomatic quality (Fulford 1989). Returning to Mr. M, one might argue that his practical reasoning is at fault, the way that he weighs up different kinds of evidence and makes a choice (Fulford 1996). Mr. M might prefer to argue that his delusions excuse him because he feels compelled by them, or that his delusions mislead him into error and ignorance of the true situation—both classic Aristotelian excuses.

It is not clear to what extent various psychiatric symptoms do, in fact, result in a sense of compulsion or the experience of ignorance. Individuals with impulse control disorders (DSM-IV-TR) are said to "fail to resist"; but, indeed, the most successful treatment for some compulsions involves "response prevention"—simply telling the person not to do it. The most successful treatment for addiction involves simply getting support for not taking the desired substance. Individuals with command hallucinations obey their "voices" in only 50 percent of cases. Finally, individuals who have committed actions of which they later feel ashamed seek to distance themselves from ownership of their actions: "It wasn't me, it was my illness." Psychological therapy with offenders often involves helping patients come to terms with the fact that they did make such a choice (Cox 1991).

If we now think about error and ignorance, then delusions do provide the sufferer with a false picture of the world on which to base important decisions. However, there are still a number of difficulties with the argument that the presence of delusions could provide the basis for reduced responsibility. First, there is a question of the strength of the belief. Although a delusion is classically defined as a fixed belief that is not amenable to rational argument or evidence to the contrary, recent research into therapy for delusions suggests that cognitive therapy, which uses rational argument, can help individuals reduce their certainty about their delusions (e.g., Garety and Freeman 1999), which seems contradictory. Second, patients do not always hold their beliefs with complete absolute tenacity but, like many ordinary people, seem sometimes to waver in their beliefs. Third, the presence of delusions does not necessarily reduce capacity to make treatment decisions or decisions to participate in research. Does the decision to commit a crime require a higher degree of capacity, and on what grounds?

Buchanan (2000) suggests that psychiatric evidence excuses insofar as it provides a medical explanation for a "bad" choice (choice theory) or explains a defendant's choice in terms of his character (character theory). He goes on to explore the strengths and weaknesses of each position and concludes that psychiatry probably has more evidence to adduce about choice making than about character. However, Buchanan notes four problems: (1) mental faculties are affected relatively, not absolutely, by mental disorders; (2) mental faculties affect one another and are interconnected—beliefs affect feelings, which affect beliefs; (3) some mental state changes are under conscious control, or at least some degree of control, which may fluctuate over short periods of time; and (4) relatively minor impairments may have large effects, psychologically.

Character theory is of interest, insofar as it is relevant to the defense of provocation. In British law, the character of the accused is relevant to whether it was reasonable for him to be provoked by the actions of the victim. Recent legal arguments have examined the extent to which psychiatric disorders could be part of the character of the accused (e.g., R v. Smith (Morgan)).

Character theory might also be relevant to the vexed question of the extent to which having an abnormal personality might excuse responsibility. For example, it is well known that people with personality disorders often offend against others because they lack empathy. This lack of empathy is (probably) the result of an interaction of acquired brain damage at birth and abusive parental care. We also know that normal people can, as it were, "switch" empathy "on and off." Here again are the familiar questions: Is a lack of empathy the kind of thing that should excuse responsibility, and if so, does it matter how one came to lack it?

Some psychiatrists have sought to limit their evidence to "brain" rather than "mind" disorder, suggesting that only psychiatric conditions that have an organic basis can excuse responsibility and, by extension, that where there is brain disease, there will also be mind disorder. Fulford (1996) discusses the metaphysical limits of this argument, suggesting that the subjective experience of illness is an important aspect of experience. Because this subjectivity distinguishes pathology from health, it may therefore also be relevant to the diagnostic process. Arguments based on the brain/

mind distinction also do not deal with the question of whether the presence of a brain tumor that gives rise to odd decisions should excuse those decisions, if they are morally and legally wrong, any more than any other mental condition that gives rise to similar decisions.

Forensic psychiatrists, in the pursuit of objectivity, may look at previous records of illness or behavior (especially crime) in attributing exculpating mental illness. But, again, in the context of a criminal charge, it may prove difficult to avoid hindsight bias. The psychiatrist may also be influenced by previous knowledge of the accused, or by the charges, or by the legal bodies that instruct him. Even though he strives for "objectivity," which is the province of the "expert," there may be so many competing accounts of the accused that no single "objective" truth may exist. The adversarial legal system assumes that there are different accounts of the truth, and the court will decide for the account that is best argued on the day. This approach to establishing "truth" is very different from the traditional empirical method with which psychiatric experts are familiar in research or the diagnostic processes that they use clinically.

It is also not clear that current approaches to diagnosis are sufficiently subtle in terms of relating mental illness to intention. This is particularly clear in relation to the distinctions often made between mental illness and personality disorder. Persons with mental illnesses are seen as "having" a disease, which in a sense possesses their brain/mind and controls their behavior in a global way. Persons with personality disorder are seen as "being" personality disordered; their behavior is a function of their identity and character and is therefore to some extent chosen and identified with by them. Toombs (1995) discusses the impact of chronic illness and disability on personal identity and argues that doctors do not always appreciate how patients with disabilities experience themselves not as having disorders but as being disabled.

The distinction between mental illness and personality disorder commonly made by mental health professionals may also be understood in terms of "illness behavior" (Mechanic 1978). Mental disorders like schizophrenia fit the model better: nobody would want to be schizophrenic, and patients with the illness want to get better. Even a lack of insight ("there's nothing wrong with me") may be understood as a symptom. Personality disorder, however, fits the model much less well. Persons with a personality disorder appear not to think they have a problem except with other people. They may not see themselves as "ill," in the conventional psychiatric sense, but still present themselves as needing "help." They may also ask for help in difficult ways and not comply with advice that the professionals think will make them feel better.

It has to be said that mental health professionals do not necessarily apply their thinking about mental illness and responsibility in consistent ways. Those professionals who work with patients with histories of violence are often engaged in day-to-day judgments about moral responsibility and the capacity of the patient to "choose" to behave well or badly. A patient with schizophrenia who has been excused his offenses on the grounds of his mental illness may still be held responsible for "bad" behavior on the ward on the grounds that "he knew exactly what he was doing"—which is one limb of the insanity defense.

One of the obvious difficulties in psychiatric testimony about responsibility is that it is just one narrative in a complex set of narratives, each with its own moral implications. Furthermore, often the psychiatrist has to rely heavily on what is said to him by the accused, whose narratives are likely to vary over time and by context (Adshead 1998). The medical model of psychiatry requires psychiatrists to get information from (apparently) independent informants, who may be more reliable than a person with a mental disorder. However, in the case of criminal charges, there are rarely such people as independent informants. In the theater of the criminal court, all speaking parts are important.

CONCLUSIONS

We have a strong intuition that some people are less responsible for some of their actions than others, which underpins the legal tradition of excusing the mentally ill their criminal behavior in certain circumstances. Exactly what is meant by the term "criminal responsibility," though, is far from clear. Some have argued that it is a real mental quality, which can be more or less present during a piece of criminal behavior, presumably in the mind of the perpetrator. Others have argued that it is an artificial social construction that allows society to withhold punishment from those whom it deems not to deserve punishment and instead to require treatment. This essay has considered some of these arguments in more detail.

Recent research into the abnormal experience of agency, such as "alien limb syndrome," has suggested that a number of brain areas contribute to the performance of consciously chosen or willed actions (Spence and Frith 1999), especially the dorsolateral-prefrontal cortex. Such research findings can be used to argue that our intentions can be explained in terms of (or even determined by?) brain function. What is not clear is how such research will be able to distinguish between morally different intentions: choosing to move one's hand to wave goodbye is not the same as choosing to wave one's hand with a knife in it. Such a reductionist approach seems only to move the threshold for assessing the culpability of intentions to a different level, rather than providing an exculpatory account.

Similarly, published research on moral reasoning in offenders, which shows that they have "lower" levels of reasoning than nonoffenders, does not address the real question of responsibility: namely, what is the "right" level of moral reasoning for blameworthiness? Any notion of "levels" of reasoning presupposes a threshold that will be socially constructed and thus is arbitrary, not simply a function of the individual.

A different account of excuse that uses psychological explanation based on childhood experience has developed—what Dershowitz (1997) calls "the abuse excuse." In these cases, it is argued that the defendant could not have acted other than he did, because of the impact on him of early adverse childhood experience. In stark contrast to Aristotle's premise, it is argued that a man is not responsible for his "bad" character if it is the result of traumatic experience. Of course, such an argument does not address the converse: Can a man not be praised for his "good" deeds if they are the result of good experience? Similarly, there are clearly many people who have experienced childhood trauma who do not have "bad" characters—although this is yet another version of psychological determinism, in this case citing external rather than internal events. It seems that victims of childhood adversity can use this experience as both a justification and a psychiatric explanation for later violence.

Psychiatrists involved in the assessment of responsibility seem to move between physical and intentional explanations for "bad" intentions. The physical fits more easily with the medical role but, as we have seen, may not do justice to the claims of social processes. The intentional stance may fit better with a psychological approach to choices but may make it impossible for psychiatrists to avoid making moral judgments in the courtroom.

NOTES

1. The law is more complex than this, distinguishing between insane and noninsane automatisms on the basis of whether the cause of the automatism was internal or external to the accused. In the case of insane automatism, the accused is pronounced not guilty by reason of insanity; in the case of noninsane automatism, one is acquitted.

2. L. J. Lawton in *R v. Robinson* said, "We cannot stress too strongly that these cases of homicide are to be tried by judges and juries and not by psychiatrists" (cited in Griew 1986).

3. Tourette's syndrome is a neuropsychiatric condition with an onset in childhood; it is characterized by multiple motor and vocal tics, often including swearing (coprolalia).

4. Some of the philosophical papers in the literature founder for just this reason. For example, Wolf (1989) gives the example of JoJo, the son of a military dictator, who develops views of the world under his father's influence, ending up a vicious and tyrannical leader himself. Wolf expects us to believe that JoJo would not be held responsible for his murder and torture in a court of law. This thought experiment is far removed from the reality of insanity acquittees, and almost no one would actually consider JoJo to have an insanity defense, a point eloquently made by Wilson (1996).

5. This Kantian view seems close to Morse's (1999) arguments that irrationality is exculpating because it impairs one's ability to follow the law.

REFERENCES

Adshead, G. (1998) "The Heart and Its Reasons: Constructing Explanations for Offending Behaviour." *Journal of Forensic Psychiatry* 9: 231–36.

Backlar, P. (1998) "Criminal Behavior and Mental Disorder: Impediments to Assigning Mental Responsibility." *Community Mental Health Journal* 34: 3–12.

Bayles, M. D. (1982) "Character, Purpose, and Criminal Responsibility." *Law and Philosophy* 1: 5–20.

Bowden, P. (1983) "Madness or Badness?" *British Journal of Hospital Medicine* 83(Dec.): 388–94.

Buchanan, A. (2000) *Psychiatric Aspects of Justification, Excuse and Mitigation: The Jurisprudence of Mental Abnormality in Anglo-American Criminal Law.* London: Jessica Kingsley.

Cox, M. (1991) "Psychopathology and Treatment of Psychotic Aggression." In P. Bowden and R. Bluglass (eds.), *Principles and Practice of Forensic Psychiatry.* London: Churchill Livingston.

Dennett, D. C. (1967) *Brainstorms.* Montgomery, VT: Bradford Books.

Dershowitz, A. (1997) *The Abuse Excuse.* Boston: Little, Brown.

Eastman, N. (1992) "Psychiatric, Psychological, and Legal Models of Man." *International Journal of Law and Psychiatry* 15: 157–69.

Elliott, C. (1996) "Key Concepts: Criminal Responsibility." *Philosophy, Psychiatry, and Psychology* 3: 305–7.

Felthous, A. R. (1999) "Introduction to Mental Illness and Criminal Responsibility." *Behavioral Sciences and the Law* 17: 143–46.

Foucault, M. (1978) "About the Concept of the 'Dangerous Individual' in 19th-Century Legal Psychiatry." *International Journal of Law and Psychiatry* 1: 1–18.

Fulford, K. W. M. (1989) *Moral Theory and Medical Practice.* Cambridge: Cambridge University Press.

Fulford, K. W. M. (1996) "Responsibility, Mental Illness and Psychiatric Experts." In H. Tam (ed.), *Punishment, Excuses and Moral Development.* Avebury: Aldershot.

Garety, P. A., and Freeman, D. (1999) "Cognitive Approaches to Delusions: A Critical Review of Theories and Evidence." *British Journal of Clinical Psychology* 38: 113–54.

Gendin, S. (1973) "Insanity and Criminal Responsibility." *American Philosophical Quarterly* 10: 99–110.

Gillett, G. R. (1991) "Intent in Law and Medicine." *New Zealand Law Journal* 91(April): 115–21.

Green, C. M., Naismith, L. J., and Menzies, R. D. (1991) "Criminal Responsibility and Mental Disorder in Britain and North America: A Comparative Study." *Medicine, Science and the Law* 31: 45–54.

Griew, E. (1986) "Reducing Murder to Manslaughter: Whose Job?" *Journal of Medical Ethics* 12: 18–23.

Hamilton, J. R. (1986) "Insanity Legislation." *Journal of Medical Ethics* 12: 13–17.

Hart, H. L. A. (1968) *Punishment and Responsibility: Essays in the Philosophy of Law.* Oxford: Clarendon.

Hospers, J. (1990) *An Introduction to Philosophical Analysis,* 3rd ed. London: Routledge and Kegan Paul.

Hubert, W., and East, N. (1939) *Report on the Psychological Treatment of Crime.* London: Her Majesty's Stationery Office.

Kenny, A. (1986) "Anomalies of Section 2 of the Homicide Act 1957." *Journal of Medical Ethics* 12: 24–27.

Mackay, R. D. (1995) *Mental Condition Defences and the Criminal Law.* Oxford: Clarendon.

Masters, B. (1985) *Killing for Company: The Case of Dennis Nilsen.* London: Arrow.

Mechanic, D. (1978) *Medical Sociology.* Glencoe, IL: Free Press.

Miller, G. H. (1979) "Criminal Responsibility: An Action Language Approach." *Psychiatry* 42: 121–30.

Mitchell, E. W. (1999) "Madness and Meta-Responsibility: The Culpable Causation of Mental Disorder and the Insanity Defence." *Journal of Forensic Psychiatry* 10: 597–622.

Morse, S. J. (1999) "Craziness and Criminal Responsibility." *Behavioral Sciences and the Law* 17: 147–64.

Reznek, L (1997) *Evil or Ill? Justifying the Insanity Defence.* London: Routledge.

Robinson, D. N. (2001) "Madness, Badness, and Fitness: Law and Psychiatry (Again)." *Philosophy, Psychiatry, and Psychology* 7: 209–22.

Smith, J. (1999) *Smith and Hogan: Criminal Law,* 9th ed. London: Butterworths.

Smith, R. (1979) "Mental Disorder, Criminal Responsibility, and the Social History of Theories of Volition." *Psychological Medicine* 9: 13–19.

Spence, S. A., and Frith, C. D. (1999) "Towards a Functional Anatomy of Volition." *Journal of Consciousness Studies* 6: 11–29.

Stone, A. A. (1978) "Psychiatry and the Law." In A. M. Nichols Jr. (ed.), *Harvard Guide to Modern Psychiatry* Cambridge, MA: Harvard University Press.

Szasz, T. (1974) *Law, Liberty and Psychiatry.* London: Routledge and Kegan Paul.

Toombs, K. (1995) *Chronic Illness.* Indianapolis: Indiana University Press.

Walker, N. (1968) *Crime and Insanity in England.* Vol. 1: *The Historical Perspective.* Edinburgh: Edinburgh University Press.

White, A. R. (ed.) (1968) *The Philosophy of Action.* Oxford: Oxford University Press.

Williams, C. (1980) *Free Will and Determinism: A Dialogue.* Indianapolis, IN: Hackett Publishing.

Wilson, P. E. (1996) "Sanity and Responsibility." *Philosophy, Psychiatry, and Psychology* 3: 293–302.

Wolf, S. (1989) "Sanity and the Metaphysics of Responsibility." In J. Christman (ed.), *The Inner Citadel.* New York: Oxford University Press.

CHAPTER 21

RELIGION

BROOKE HOPKINS
MARGARET P. BATTIN

IN *Of Two Minds: The Growing Disorder in American Psychiatry*, T. M. Luhrman describes the ongoing career of John Hood, a peer counselor in the locked unit at a California psychiatric hospital. Thirty years ago, Hood was diagnosed as paranoid schizophrenic. Although he is a strong advocate of alternative approaches to mental illness besides the pharmacological one, he has been on antipsychotic medication since the period of his original diagnosis. He has never heard voices, but he does hear the walls "creak loudly and repeatedly."[1] According to Hood, the creaks are supernatural in origin: "They are God telling me what I am doing wrong."[2] As a consequence of the mental suffering he has undergone over the years, including various kinds of paranoid delusion, Hood thinks of himself as a shaman. Yet Hood's success as a healer and as an advocate for consumers in the California mental health system led to his being named Mental Health Person of the Year in 1998 by the State of California.

Hood's story raises many questions about the relationship between psychiatry and religion.[3] For example, on what grounds could one argue that Hood's claim that the creaks he hears are "supernatural in origin" is false? Is there some way in which Hood's belief that he possesses shamanistic powers actually *aids* him in his ability to relieve the condition of those he counsels in the locked unit of the hospital where he spends some of his time? Are there, as Hood believes, limits to the "medical model" of psychiatric illness that leave room for other, more religiously based approaches to mental suffering? Is this a matter of two deeply different discourses, which Hood, unlike most people, is able to employ more or less simultaneously in understanding his "illness"? These introduce the kinds of questions we want to address in this chapter.

Whatever its character, the relationship between psychiatry and religion is immensely complex. Psychiatry itself, as a branch of modern medical science, is by no means homogenous, and it is not the only contemporary discipline that deals with mental phenomena: psychoanalysis, psychology, neurology, counseling, social work, brain science, and cognitive science also seek to describe, explain, and sometimes alter such phenomena. Religion is a still more broadly encompassing concept, covering an immense spectrum of experience, belief, tradition, and institutional structure not only in the monotheistic cultures of Judaism, Christianity, and Islam but also in the diverse religious cultures of Hinduism, Buddhism, and Confucianism, and in preliterate cultures in many parts of the world.[4] In all of these, questions arise about the authenticity of religious experience, about how to identify what counts as true religion, how to distinguish religious from cultural practice, how to recognize religious practitioners and institutions, how to tell religious figures from secular pretenders, and how to know whether one's own experience is genuinely religious. But because psychiatry began as a branch of Western medicine and has developed relatively recently within the religious and cultural environment of Europe and America, its connections to Western religion, both in content and in institutional structure, are stronger than its links to other traditions. Indeed, much of the academic discussion in philosophy of psychiatry has Western traditions in mind when it addresses issues concerning religion.

It is the overlap of essentially clinical, curative elements in both psychiatry and religion that allows a comparatively unified point of departure into a wildly diverse terrain. As Don Browning and Ian Evison put it, "From the moment modern psychiatry emerged as a distinct profession, psychiatry and religion have overlapped and at times overtly competed. The reason for this is clear: both seek to heal forms of brokenness that stand on the ambiguous borderline between body and what is variously referred to as 'psyche' or 'spirit.' "[5] This is not to say that psychiatry and religion perform the same function—that is part of the issue for discussion here. But it is to say that the overlap between psychiatry's goal of making it possible for patients to live with less suffering in their lives and religion's aim of relieving fear, suffering, and meaninglessness in human life provide an initial starting point for discussion. To quote the philosopher K. W. M. Fulford: "Religion and psychiatry occupy the same country, a landscape of meaning, significance, guilt, belief, values, visions, suffering and healing."[6] This is the region, or at least part of it, that is now opening to new, philosophically informed exploration. In this chapter we consider what we think are the five principal questions that arise in this terrain.

1. How Can We Tell the Difference between Religious Experience and Psychiatric Symptoms?

Socrates spoke of hearing a voice that would tell him when he was about to do wrong.[7] St. Paul wrote in the third person that he had been uniquely "caught up into the third heaven . . . into paradise, and heard unspeakable words, which it is not lawful for a man to utter."[8] The medieval mystics Teresa of Avila and Julian of Norwich recounted their visions in detail, including intense personal experiences of seeing and being with their religion's savior.[9] In Bedlam, one of the earliest asylums for the mentally ill, inmates heard voices and saw visions, sometimes of religious figures, sometimes of devils, and sometimes of fantastical objects with no apparent rooting in reality.[10] The founder of the Quaker religion, George Fox, hearing "the Word of the Lord" outside Lichfield, took off his shoes and wandered into the city, where he saw what seemed to him to be "a channel of blood running down the streets, and the market place like a pool of blood."[11] The English poet Christopher Smart had the habit (for which he was confined to what we would now call a mental institution) of dropping to his knees in public places like St. James Park to pray aloud.[12]

Many people claim to hear voices, see visions, feel themselves to be outside their bodies or to have other paranormal experiences. Some of these experiences are understood as religious, and others are labeled psychotic and pathological; but it is not clear how to tell the difference between them. Further complicating the issue, different religious traditions assign quite different roles to these sorts of experiences. Zen Buddhism, for example, has no place for visions or voices, while charismatic evangelical Christianity, in contrast, makes the state of experiencing Jesus directly, or being "born again," fundamental to true religious conversion.

Inaugurating many of the contemporary discussions of this issue in his Gifford Lectures, delivered at Edinburgh just 100 years ago, William James (1842–1910) sought to offer a philosophical answer to the problems that arise when religion, or, to be more precise, religious experience, is challenged by what he calls "medical materialism," or what would now be called modern neuroscience.[13] Yes, James acknowledges, "every religious phenomenon has its history and its derivation from natural antecedents,"[14] is "brain-based,"[15] to use more modern terminology, but what counts in the human realm is the difference such a phenomenon makes for the person who experiences it. If it is a difference that proves consoling, strengthening, or enabling, then the experience can be said to be religious in the positive sense; if it produces anguish, pain, or an intolerable restriction of one's horizons, it is pathological.[16] In what has become a *locus classicus* in recent discussions of the relation between psychiatry and religion, James writes,

Religious mysticism is only one half of mysticism. . . . In delusional insanity, paranoia, as they sometimes call it, we may have a *diabolical* mysticism, a sort of religious mysticism turned upside down. The same sense of the ineffable importance
in the smallest events, the same texts and words coming with new meanings, the
same voices and visions and leadings and missions, the same controlling by extra-
neous powers; only this time the emotion is pessimistic: instead of consolations we
have desolations; the meanings are dreadful; and the powers are enemies to life. It
is evident from the point of view of their psychological mechanism, the classic
mysticism and these lower mysticisms spring from the same mental level, from that
great subliminal or transmarginal region of which science is beginning to admit
the existence. . . . To come from thence is no ineffable credential. What comes
must be sifted and tested, and run the gauntlet of confrontation with the total context of experience, just like what comes from the outer world of sense. Its value
must be ascertained by empirical methods, so long as we are not mystics ourselves.[17]

Many of the most useful recent discussions of the relationship between psychiatry
and religion have tried to carry out the program of sifting and testing proposed by
James, who judged the validity of so-called religious experience on the basis of its
benefits and not on the basis of its origins in the workings of the brain, which for
him was an indisputable given. Did the experience originate in a chemical "imbalance" or in an "abnormal" pattern of electrical activity in the brain? — for James, this
was not the right sort of question to ask. The right question to ask is: Is its outcome
for the individual, and possibly even for a larger social group, a positive or a negative
one?[18]

To be sure, contemporary critics like Wayne Proudfoot have claimed that the
whole notion of "religious experience" is so vague and overly general as to make the
possibility of ever finding an adequate definition of it futile.[19] Nevertheless, a number
of contemporary theorists have followed James's lead in exploring the relations between psychotic and religious experiences, among them Michael Jackson, K. W. M.
Fulford, and Roland Littlewood. For example, Jackson, using case studies collected
by the Alister Hardy Research Centre, in Oxford, argues for a "problem-solving"
approach to the question of the differences between "benign spiritual experience"
and "acute psychotic experience," claiming that both involve "a sequence in which
a cognitive or emotional impasse triggers an altered state of consciousness which
releases a potentially resolving insight or solution to the impasse, often in symbolic
form."[20] The difference is that "in benign cases, the insight successfully resolves the
triggering crisis and the process is self-terminating," whereas in pathological cases
"the insight increases the sense of crisis, triggering a further cycle of experiences and
a spiral away from reality into full-blown psychosis."[21] Among the factors that determine these two contrasting results, Jackson argues, are "the individual's level of
schizotypy, their appraisals of the social feedback their insight produces, and the
quality of the insight experience involved."[22] In another paper by Jackson, co-authored
with Fulford, some of the same cases are used to argue, within the context of a much
more extensive discussion of the limits of a purely medical model of psychiatry and

its systems of classification, that a more refined approach needs to be taken to the issue of the relationship between psychopathology and spiritual experience, one that recognizes the embeddedness of such phenomena "in the structure of values and beliefs of the person concerned."[23]

Adding to the discussion of difficulties in differentiating between religious and pathological experience, Littlewood's *Pathology and Identity: The Work of Mother Earth in Trinidad* (1993) offers a book-length study of the impact of the teachings of a religious charismatic on the community she had gathered around her. Trained in both anthropology and psychiatry, Littlewood is as interested as Jackson and Fulford in the need to recognize the culturally mediated nature of the psychiatric classifications used in understanding the relations between psychopathology and religious experience. However, Littlewood emphasizes the way in which the innovative teachings of a religious or spiritual leader (who may be considered "crazy" by the medical establishment) are received by those around her. He formulates the basic question this way: "Can the extreme personal experiences of what medicine terms psychosis, when taken in part as some random, 'natural' event, give shape to society? May such arbitrary intrusions actually have a place in social innovation, sometimes serving as a charter for new departures?"[24] Such concerns about "religious" experience are implicit in the work of Jackson and Fulford (as they are in James); they are at the ethical center of Littlewood's study.

At work in many of the discussions of putative differences between religious experience and psychiatric symptoms are at least three central assumptions, present to a greater or lesser degree in the work of various authors. Often playing a central role is (1) the unexamined assumption that religion and psychiatry are mutually exclusive, that the question about supranormal experience is an either/or question to which the answer may be that the experience is religious, or that it is psychotic, but that it cannot be both. This assumption is challenged by only a few authors, notably Littlewood and to some extent Jackson and Fulford. Also frequently playing a significant role is (2) the tacit assumption that the answer to the question of veridicality actually matters: that it is important whether the entity seen in a vision or heard in a voice is "really real." Probably because they assume that the things seen in visions are not real—like the streets of Lichfield running with channels of blood—many authors appear to sidestep or ignore this issue of evidence, and even William James in his rejection of the question seems to fail to entertain it. And finally, central in the work of many authors, though openly challenged by Jackson, Fulford, and Littlewood, is (3) the assumption that there is such a condition as "normal" and that departures from normalcy are disvalued and should, if possible, be restored to the normal condition. Cultural contexts and expectations play a role, it is generally recognized in all these discussions, but what is not always examined is the extreme degree to which differing cultural contexts can account for the difference between the "religious" and the "insane." While these assumptions have varying but important roles in the literature concerning each of the five basic questions raised in this chapter, the studies discussed here have moved a long way in identifying, challenging, and supporting or discarding them.

2. Is Religion a Symptom of Mental Illness (or Vice Versa)?

As a branch of psychiatry, psychoanalysis has always stood in an ambivalent relationship to religion. Perhaps more than any other single figure, its founder, Sigmund Freud (1856–1939), is associated with the question of whether religion and mental illness go hand in hand, and his answer, while not a direct yes, comes very close. Together with Emil Kraepelin (1855–1956) and Eugen Bleuler (1857–1939), Freud stands at the beginning of the differentiation of research psychiatry and the clinical practice of psychoanalysis into discrete fields that occurred at the beginning of the twentieth century, and thus Freud may be in part responsible for the assumption of mutual exclusivity discussed earlier, as well as various other problematic assumptions.[25]

Freud attacked religion as a symptom of man's inability or unwillingness to face the harsh realities of life and death, "a regression to primary narcissism." In Freud's view, religion constitutes a kind of "group neurosis," an institutionalized form of mental illness in the face of civilization's "discontents."[26] For Freud, the impact of religious systems is largely detrimental; religion shields the individual from recognizing his own situation by pretending to offer divine compassion, forgiveness, and hope of a better life when in fact no such thing is the case. Similarly, the contemporary psychiatrist Samuel Klagsbrun, though otherwise sensitive to the positive role religious practice can play in the lives of those who hold strong beliefs, adds to Freud's skepticism the observation that religion often breeds repression. In religious families, communities, and organizations, Klagsbrun says, "unacceptable thoughts are considered a sin and are pushed away, put in a mental repository where they go unexamined. . . . [In such communities] there is a tendency to hide mental illness as much as they can until they can't hide it anymore."[27] Freud did admit the possibility of so-called oceanic feelings,[28] but he particularly dismissed institutional religion as a counterproductive throwback.

Freud's negative view of religion stands in particular contrast to William James's open-minded, constructive view, and perhaps for this reason James's view has played a much larger part in recent discussions of the issues in psychiatry and religion. Freud's view is now largely treated as a side event, while James's is still viewed as mainstream. Freud also shared the assumption—another of the many assumptions that are inadequately examined in this literature—of a specific model of history: namely, that history is in progress in the transition from religion to science. This view reinforces the bifurcating either/or view of psychiatry and religion: religion is understood as primitive, uninformed, a type of neurotic compensation, while the advance into the scientific understanding of mental phenomena offered by psychiatry is just that—an advance.

Freud's negative view of religion makes a variety of additional assumptions, also inadequately examined. It assumes that it is possible to identify neurosis and group neurosis. It assumes a causal theory of experience that identifies the institutions and cultural patterns that human beings establish as responsible for their experience. And it conflates the notion of cause with that of association, in the process also confusing the notion of primary causes with that of contributory factors. Even if religious belief, practice, and institutional activity do form a sort of "group neurosis," this does not entail that religion has *caused* the neurotic condition.

Psychoanalysis, however, has been anything but monolithic on the topic of religion, and other thinkers, rejecting Freud's negative view, have sought to stress religion's positive impact on mental health. Karl Jung (1875–1966) was the leading spokesman for such a view, "that our evolutionary history has freed up sexual libido so that it has become available for such cultural interests as architecture, religion, etc."[29] For Jung and his followers, religion has provided indispensable benefits. It offers a sense of embeddedness within a tradition. Its myths, rituals, and collective community provide the strength that faith in something greater than the individual affords. In addition to Jung, the British object-relations theorist D. W. Winnicott, while acknowledging the tendency of certain religions (those "that have made much of 'original sin' ") to "deplete the individual of an important aspect of creativeness,"[30] stresses the crucial importance for human health of what he calls the "capacity to believe."[31] This includes belief in the "illusions" of art and religion, which create a "potential space" within which individuals and groups experience their most "creative living."[32] And Klagsbrun, while seeing religion's potential to generate repression, also sees its importance in contributing to an individual's sense of identity.

Some thinkers who reject Freud's largely negative view hold that their religion can provide meaning in life, a sense of purpose, an understanding of community, a higher goal. Religion is not a symptom or product of mental illness. On the contrary, it can also reinforce important social values: responsibility for one's own actions, concern for one's neighbor and charity toward others in general, the condemnation of those who intentionally cause suffering, and the acceptance of society in general as a good. It is religion, on this more favorable view, that teaches that human life is important and that the fruits of divine creation are to be respected; religion is the source and basis of ethical concern among human beings for one another.

In addition, evolutionary accounts of the early history of religion typically claim that religion has developed in societies because of its selective advantages: it provides a mechanism of social control, a way of managing fears, a set of explanations about the world (and, for early traditions, explanations of natural phenomena like lightning, thunder, and floods), and furthers group cohesiveness, though they may hold either that such mechanisms of social control are adaptive now or that they have been adaptive in the past but are no longer so in modern information-based, technological societies.[33] An aesthetics-based account might hold that religion is the source and basis of human creativity, as believers seek to express their devotion in art, music, literature, and other forms of worship: what might have been "madness" is transformed into inspiration; despair becomes hope, and hope fuels work for a better world; each single individual comes to see himself or herself as a focus of divine love. Such accounts hold that without religion, the lot of humankind might have been chronic neurosis and pervasive mental illness; religion offers a group cure, by making possible the transformation of isolation and despair into community and hope.[34]

Of course, these positive views also rest on a variety of assumptions that are inadequately examined. As in Freud's negative view, they also make assumptions about causation; they tend to conflate the notions of causation and association; they sidestep the issue of what counts as neurosis or mental illness in the first place; and they assume that it is meaningful to speak of the condition of humankind in the absence of religion, as if this counterfactual could be empirically assessed. Nevertheless, these accounts do offer a counterpart to the influence of Freud and open the way to continuing inquiry into the overall "effects" of religion — whether these effects are in general negative or positive either for society or for the individuals of whom societies are composed.

3. WHAT ARE THE INSTITUTIONAL RELATIONSHIPS BETWEEN PSYCHIATRY AND RELIGION?

"Psychiatry was Religion before it was Psychiatry," writes Michael Stone.[35] Many theorists of religion, partly but not exclusively in the tradition of Freud, have seen the institution of religion in the past as playing the role now occupied by psychiatry: both, as we saw Browning and Evison saying earlier, "seek to heal forms of brokenness."[36] However, it is the similarity of institutional structures between religion and psychiatry that attracts the notice of some, Thomas Szasz being the most vocal and persistent.[37] At least in the West, religious traditions have developed organizational patterns of authority, hierarchy, and subordination that are mirrored in the institutional structures of psychiatry. The priest, surrounded by acolytes and ministering to the dependent, subordinate laity, becomes the psychiatrist, supported in his authority by the institutions of medicine, treating patients who need him. The religious institution understands the laity as sinful and offers ways to overcome this fall from grace — prayer, penitence, faith — while the psychiatric institution understands its patients as ill and offers treatment to relieve this condition: psychoactive pharmaceuticals, talk therapy, or, if all else fails, electroconvulsion. In both institutional religion and institutionalized psychiatry, rules of practice (written and unwritten) govern the behavior of practitioners; in both cases, money flows from the recipients of services to the practitioners. And, in both cases, it is the practitioners who define the condition of the subordinate populace as in need of their services and who determine what is to be done to relieve their condition.[38] Similarities between psychiatric and religious structures are also heightened in some groups that reject conventional, "physicalist" notions of health and illness, like Christian Science, or that tend to rely on internal rather than professional counseling for many forms of mild mental illness, for example, Mormonism. Although religion and psychiatry may be in competition in specific cases—someone hears a voice, and religion and psychiatry offer quite different accounts of what this means and what is to be done about it—nevertheless, the institutional structures of religion and psychiatry and their underlying power relationships are very much the same.

Critics also assert that related areas of professional practice exhibit even greater similarities to religious structures. Psychoanalysis, for example, is described as remarkably like a religion itself: it has sects, orthodoxies, heretics; its practice revolves around a form of extended confession; it insists on sectarian loyalties to specific schools of practice and demands long-term commitment (not to mention ongoing financial contribution) from its communicants. Of course, such critics rarely observe that the official objective in psychoanalysis (while it may not be adhered to in all cases of treatment) is to render the patient capable of existence independent of further treatment, an objective not shared by religious groups, but the critique is telling just the same.

4. ETHICAL ISSUES OF PSYCHIATRIC PRACTICE WITH RELIGIOUS PATIENTS OR RELIGIOUS PSYCHIATRISTS

As an institutional practice, psychiatry also raises issues of professional ethics, frequently discussed in public and professional spheres, that may be exacerbated when matters of religion are involved.[39] Paramount are issues about confidentiality: whether the psychiatrist may ever divulge a client's apparent intentions of harm or self-harm, an issue decided in the affirmative by the well-known Tarasoff case.[40] While this issue has been discussed at length in secular contexts, it may be intensified when the client's religious background includes expectations of confessional confidentiality (as, for example, in Catholicism) or when the client understands the psychiatrist's role in ways roughly analogous to that of the priest, a (mis)understanding the psychiatrist may be tempted to exploit.

Additional ethical issues in psychiatric practice—including such matters as abuse or sexual abuse of patients, setting of fees, and discontinuing therapy or dismissing patients—may be intensified in religiously heightened contexts. And there are some situations in which religious prohibitions may affect treatment: for example, when discontinuing a psychologically stressful pregnancy cannot be contemplated for religious reasons (e.g., a prohibition of abortion) or when gender roles stipulated by a religious tradition do not conform to a patient's personal values or social setting (for instance, the subordination or seclusion of women in Islam). Psychiatry as a profession has not always been sufficiently alert to the differences that religious commitments on the part of either the practitioner or the patient may make in these issues.

Nor has psychiatry always been sufficiently alert to the role the therapist's own religious commitments or absence thereof may play in shaping his or her understanding of the patient's problem. Since the days of Freud, Kraepelin, and Bleuler, psychiatry has been largely secular and scientific, largely devoid of religious terminology or categories in its theoretical framework. However, many practitioners find that their own conceptions of guilt, sin, transcendence, forgiveness, love, and the like still play a role in their response to patients, despite training in secular psychiatric or psychoanalytic methods. And many practitioners have embraced specific religious commitments of their own, such as Buddhism or other persuasions that involve, for example, the practice of meditation, which may influence their treatment of patients. Whether they have religious commitments of their own, however, many psychiatrists are unwittingly influenced by their own conceptions in the treatment they provide. This engenders what Jennifer Radden (personal communication) describes as a kind of built-in framing that they would do well to acknowledge and examine, a framing parallel to the (other) hidden value assumptions that guide them.

Classificatory systems such as DSM categories, billing codes, and forensic assessments also raise ethical issues, since they may be only imperfectly appropriate for a given patient. These inadequacies may be exacerbated when the patient's "condition" or "mental illness" includes ostensibly religious states. As hinted in the first section of this volume, still deeper dilemmas arise in some cases of psychiatric treatment for symptoms ambiguously describable as "religious" or "psychotic." Should you medicate somebody who has visions? What about the patient who values or may seek such experience?[41] Ought the therapeutic effort be to eliminate the occurrence of "psychotic"/"religious" experience, to cope with it, to intensify it, or what?

5. ARE PSYCHIATRY AND RELIGION COMPATIBLE?

The largest of the questions that the issue of religion and psychiatry raises is the question of whether they are compatible or whether, instead, they constitute two different and competing human systems. This question not only returns to the dichotomizing either/or assumption discussed earlier but raises again—at a deeper level—perhaps the most difficult of the issues in philosophy of psychiatry. This is not just the issue of whether religion or psychiatry can better address matters like visions and voices, or whether the effects of religion (and for that matter psychiatry) are in general destructive or constructive, or whether the institutional structures of religion and psychiatry are alike in basic ways. Rather, this is the issue of whether psychiatry, insofar as it is or seeks to be a science, is compatible with religion, when religion so often insists that it stands apart from science—that it opens an area of human experience where "mere" science is inadequate to speak. William James's pragmatic approach to the question of the validity of religious experience in an age of scientific rationalism and biologically oriented psychiatry is no longer adequate here, nor is Freud's summary dismissal of the problem.

This issue is rooted in the deeper problem of how we are to understand human consciousness itself. After all, it is human consciousness that experiences visions and voices, guilt, awe, a sense of doom or a feeling of faith, as well as shame, anxiety, depression, feelings of paranoia, grandiosity, and omnipotence, and in general all experience both "religious" and "secular," both "pathological" and "normal"—indeed, *all* human experience. This is what Fulford describes as "the central mystery of the mental, how patterns of blind molecular movement in my brain and yours are, at the same time, the conscious experience of me writing and you reading these words."[42] But we do not fully understand the nature of human consciousness, or the nature of human intentionality, or for that matter other alleged paranormal experiences such as prescience, synchronicity, telepathy, and the like, if indeed they occur. Nor is it clear whether "scientific" progress in neuroanatomy, brain chemistry, evolutionary biology, and similar fields can be expected to yield the answer, or whether scientific accounts of this sort must inevitably fall short of seeing what is involved in certain kinds of *religious* experience.

One way around this impasse, associated with postmodernism, is to see it as the result of a difference of discourses: on the one hand the discourse of religion and religious experience and on the other the discourse of medical science and the underlying discourses of biochemistry and psychobiology. (This would have its roots in the conflict between the discourses of science and of religion that characterizes much of the modern period.) On this view the discourses are distinct; most people employ one or the other (or still others besides religion and medical science) as a way of explaining phenomena they experience or observe, and comparatively few individuals are able to function within both language games or explanatory systems. But this postmodern approach still begs the question: it is the nature of human consciousness itself that still remains the mystery, the mystery that must be resolved if the question of the relationship of psychiatry and religion is ever to be settled.

6. CONCLUSION: THE CIRCULARITY OF THE ISSUE

Psychiatry's relationship with religion raises more complex and less well resolved issues than its relationships with perhaps any other area of human reflection or experience—more than, for example, psychiatry's relationship with art, with science, with politics, or with play. Two deep central questions lie beneath all the issues discussed earlier, raising the basic issue of circularity.

First, psychiatry attempts to achieve or restore "healthy" or "normal" functioning for individuals who suffer from mental illness, but it cannot conclusively answer the question of whether religious belief and religious experience are healthy and normal or the product of idiosyncratic or institutionally shaped pathology. Hence the problem of circularity: Is religion itself, or at least some religious belief and experience, normal or pathological, and hence is it inside or outside psychiatry's reference class for the goal—health and normalcy—it seeks to achieve?

Second, and related, is the question of the relevance of social consequences. As we've seen, writers on religion have made a huge variety of claims about these consequences, from the Freudian claim that religion functions as a group neurosis; to the claim that it can promote deeper and more autonomous self-reflection and ethical self-regulation on the part of a population, thus making a more humane and responsible society possible; or again to the claim that it creates artificially constricted categories of moral prohibition, thus grossly limiting human freedom. Such claims about the social consequences of religion raise the fundamental question of the relevance of religion's social consequences to psychiatry, a question made more difficult by the assumption that psychiatry is in no position to establish the truth or falsity of religious claims. What is the relevance for psychiatry of religion's social effects? If religion's consequences are on the whole beneficial to society, does that mean that psychiatry should regard religion as "normal" and "healthy" and therefore promote religious involvement and experience for its patients—whether or not it can establish the truth of religious claims? If the contrary, ought psychiatry work to discourage religious experience and belief—that is, try to "cure" people of their religiosity? Thus these issues, too, are associated with the circularity that the issue of psychiatry and religion ultimately involves, the central theoretical challenge this question presents. We began by saying that, in practice, both psychiatry and religion seem to involve both clinical and curative elements, but it remains unclear, either for individuals or for societies in general, whether this is evidence of a deep commonality of vision or whether, instead, it papers over an unbridgeable gap.

NOTES

1. Luhrman, *Of Two Minds*, 268.
2. Ibid.
3. It is important for the sake of clarity to acknowledge at the outset the difference between the term "religion," which refers to a set of beliefs, practices, and institutional arrangements, and the much broader term "spirituality," which has recently been defined by the Special Interest Group on Spirituality and Psychiatry sponsored by the Royal College of Psychiatrists as "the essentially human, personal and interpersonal dimension, which inte-

grates and transcends the cultural, religious, psychological, social and emotional aspects of the person" (www.rcpsych.ac.uk/college/sig/spirit/2). The terms overlap, of course, but had this chapter been titled "Spirituality" rather than "Religion," it would have taken quite a different shape.

4. For discussions of the relationship between psychiatry and other, "non-Western" religions, see Part II of Bughra, *Psychiatry and Religion*.

5. Don Browning and Ian Evison, "Introduction," to Browning et al., *Religious and Ethical Factors in Psychiatric Practic*, 3–4.

6. Fulford, "Religion and Psychiatry," 5. This essay is the most philosophically sophisticated treatment of this topic.

7. Plato, *The Apology*, 437.

8. II Corinthians 12:2, 4.

9. See Wapnick, "Mysticism and Schizophrenia."

10. MacDonald, *Mystical Bedlam*.

11. James, *Varieties of Religious Experience*, 8.

12. Cf. Screech's claim that "madness and Christianity go hand in hand," in "Good Madness in Christendom," 25.

13. James, *Varieties of Religious Experience*, 13. For an excellent account of James's text against the background of the history of the relationship between popular religious culture and early attempts to explain certain religious phenomena like trances and visionary experience, see Taves, *Fits, Trances, and Visions*.

14. James, *Varieties of Religious Experience*, 4.

15. Jackson and Fulford, "Spiritual Experience and Psychopathology," 50.

16. This point was made more recently by Watson in "Aspects of Personal Meaning in Schizophrenia," 175–89.

17. James, *Varieties of Religious Experience*, 426–27.

18. See Henry Maudsley, whom James cites: "What right have we to believe Nature under any obligation to do her work by means of complete minds only?" *Varieties of Religious Experience*, 19.

19. Proudfoot, *Religious Experience*.

20. Jackson, "Benign Schizotypy," 247.

21. Ibid.

22. Ibid.

23. Jackson and Fulford, "Spiritual Experience and Psychopathology," 54.

24. Littlewood, *Pathology and Identity*, xii. For another case of the relationship between "madness" and "religious innovation," see Littlewood, "Psychopathology, Embodiment and Religious Innovation," 178–97. For further clarification of Littlewood's ideas on this topic, see his "Commentary on 'Spiritual Experience and Psychopathology,'" 67–73.

25. See Part 1 of Browning et al., *Religious and Ethical Factors in Psychiatric Practice*, for discussions of this topic from different religious perspectives.

26. Freud, "Obsessive Actions and Religious Practices," 126–27; Freud, *Civilization and Its Discontents*.

27. Fuchs, "Finding Faith's Place in Psychiatric Treatment,". A16, an interview with Samuel Klagsbrun on the topic of the positive role religion can sometimes play in the lives of the mentally ill.

28. Freud, *Civilization and Its Discontents*, 11.

29. John Turner, personal communication.

30. Winnicott, "Morals and Education," 94.

31. Winnicott, "Children Learning," 143. For a full discussion, see Hopkins, "Winnicott and the Capacity to Believe," 485–97.

32. Winnicott, "Location of Cultural Experience," 103.

33. See chapter 22 by Dominic Murphy, this volume.

34. As noted in note 11, there is now a considerable literature on the positive impact of religious beliefs and practices on mental health. See especially Koenig, *Handbook of Religion and Mental Health.*

35. Stone, *Healing the Mind,* xi.

36. Browning et al., *Religious and Ethical Factors in Psychiatric Illness,* 4.

37. See especially Szasz, *Myth of Mental Illness.* For a strong version of Szasz's argument in a nutshell, see "Deviance and Control: Religion and Psychiatry," 308–15.

38. For an extended analysis of ethical dilemmas that arise within the structures of institutional religion, see Battin, *Ethics in the Sanctuary.*

39. For a more personal exploration of some of these ethical issues see, Drury, "Madness and Religion," 115–37.

40. *Tarasoff v. Regents of the University of California,* 1976.

41. See, e.g., Salzman, *Lying Awake.*

42. Fulford, "Religion and Psychiatry," 14; see also Fenwick, "Neurophysiology and Religious Experience," 167–77.

REFERENCES

Battin, Margaret P. (1990) *Ethics in the Sanctuary: Examining the Practices of Organized Religion.* New Haven: Yale University Press.

Bhugra, Dinesh (ed.) (1996) *Psychiatry and Religion: Context, Consensus, and Controversies.* New York: Routledge.

Browning, Don, Jobe, Thomas, and Evison, Ian (eds.) (1990) *Religious and Ethical Factors in Psychiatric Practice.* Chicago: Nelson-Hall.

Drury, Maurice O'Connor (1996) "Madness and Religion." In *The Danger of Words and Writings on Wittgenstein.* Bristol: Thoemmes Press.

Fenwick, Peter (1996) "Neurophysiology and Religious Experience." In Dinesh Bhugra (ed.), *Psychiatry and Religion: Context, Consensus, and Controversies.* New York: Routledge, pp. 167–77.

Freud, Sigmund ([1930] 1961) *Civilization and Its Discontents.* Translated by James Strachey. New York: Norton.

Freud, S. "Obsessive Actions and Religious Practices." In *The Standard Edition of the Complete Works of Sigmund Freud,* vol. 9. London: Hogarth Press, pp. 126–27.

Fuchs, Marek (2002) "Finding Faith's Place in Psychiatric Treatment." *New York Times,* April 27, A 16.

Fulford, K. W. M. (1996) "Religion and Psychiatry: Extending the Limits of Tolerance." In Dinesh Bhugra (ed.), *Psychiatry and Religion: Context, Consensus, and Controversies.* New York: Routledge, pp. 5–22.

Hopkins, Brooke (1997) "Winnicott and the Capacity to Believe." *International Journal of Psycho-Analysis* 78(3): 485–97.

Jackson, Mike, and Fulford, K. W. M. (1997) "Spiritual Experience and Psychopathology." *Philosophy, Psychiatry, and Psychology* 4(1): 41–65.

Jackson, Michael (1997) "Benign Schizotypy: The Case of Spiritual Experience." In Claridge Gordon (ed.), *Schizotypy: Implications for Illness and Health.* New York: Oxford University Press, pp. 227–50.

James, William ([1902] 1941) *The Varieties of Religious Experience*. New York: Longmans.

Koenig, Harold (ed.) (1998) *Handbook of Religion and Mental Health*. San Diego: Academic Press.

Littlewood, Roland (1993) *Pathology and Identity: The Work of Mother Earth in Trinidad*. Cambridge: Cambridge University Press.

Littlewood, Roland (1996) "Psychopathology, Embodiment and Religious Innovation: An Historical Instance." In Dinesh Bhugra (ed.), *Psychiatry and Religion: Context, Consensus, and Controversies*. New York: Routledge, pp. 178–97.

Littlewood, Roland (1997) "Commentary on 'Spiritual Experience and Psychopathology.' " *Philosophy, Psychiatry, and Psychology* 4(1): 67–73.

Luhrman, T. M. (2000) *Of Two Minds: The Growing Disorder in American Psychiatry*. New York: Knopf.

MacDonald, Michael (1981) *Mystical Bedlam: Madness, Anxiety, and Healing in 17th Century England*. Cambridge: Cambridge University Press.

Plato (1999) *The Apology*. In *Great Dialogues of Plato*. Translated by W. H. D. Rouse. New York: Signet.

Proudfoot, Wayne (1985) *Religious Experience*. Berkeley: University of California Press.

Salzman, Mark (2000) *Lying Awake*. New York: Vintage.

Screech, M. A. (1985) "Good Madness in Christendom." In W. F. Bynum, Roy Porter, and Michael Shepherd (eds.), *The Anatomy of Madness: Essays in the History of Psychiatry*, Vol. 1. London: Tavistock Press, pp. 25–37.

Stone, Michael (1997). *Healing the Mind: A History of Psychiatry from Antiquity to the Present*. New York: W. W. Norton.

Szasz, Thomas (1961) *The Myth of Mental Illness: Foundations of a Theory of Personal Conduct*. New York: Hoeber-Harper; rev. ed. (1974). New York: Harper and Row.

Szasz, Thomas (1987) "Deviance and Control: Religion and Psychiatry." In *Insanity: The Idea and Its Consequences*. New York: Wiley.

Taves, Ann (1999) *Fits, Trances, and Visions: Experiencing Religion and Explaining Experience from Wesley to James*. Princeton: Princeton University Press.

Thompson, C. (ed.) (1987) *The Origins of Modern Psychiatry*. New York: Wiley.

Watson, J. P. (1982) "Aspects of Personal Meaning in Schizophrenia." In Eric Shepherd and J. P. Watson, *Personal Meanings*. Chichester: Wiley.

Wapnick, Kenneth (1990) "Mysticism and Schizophrenia." In Richard Woods (ed.), *Understanding Mysticism*. Garden City, NY: Doubleday.

Winnicott, D. W. (1971) "The Location of Cultural Experience." In *Playing and Reality*. New York: Basic Books.

Winnicott, D. W. (1986) "Children Learning." In *Home Is Where We Start From*. New York: W. W. Norton.

Winnicott, D. W. (1994) "Morals and Education." In *The Maturational Processes and the Facilitating Environment*. Madison, CT: International Universities Press.

PART IV

THEORETICAL MODELS

CHAPTER 22

DARWINIAN MODELS OF PSYCHOPATHOLOGY

DOMINIC MURPHY

ONLY crackpots doubt that human beings evolved, but the significance of evolution for the sciences of the mind is bitterly contested. We can distinguish three different evolutionary explanations of psychopathology. The three explanations are not mutually exclusive, in the sense that one theory could make use of all of them (e.g., Murphy and Stich 2000). But they involve more or less strong commitments to evolution as important to psychiatry.

First, the overall picture of the normal mind should be that of a mind that has been shaped by natural selection. This is a very minimal concession to evolution, and it is one that pretty much all parties accept. But spelling out the details in terms of particular research programs introduces substantial complications. It is a matter of great controversy whether the mind's evolutionary past is of much theoretical importance in contemporary psychology, and among theorists who accept the importance of evolution there is no consensus on the right version of evolutionary psychology. The most obvious way in which this minimal commitment to evolution enters the picture in psychiatry is that it might lead us to conceive the function of neurological and psychological structures in explicitly teleological terms. Hence, a mental disorder, on this view, is the failure of some part of our psychology to perform its evolutionary function (Papineau 1994; Wakefield 1996).

Second, an evolutionary perspective may lead us to reconceive the nature of a disorder as resting on a mechanism that was once adaptive but is no longer adaptive because of changes in the environment. This view does not identify a system within the person as malfunctioning but locates the pathology in a mismatch between the environment the system was originally adapted for and our current environment.

Third, there exists at least the theoretical possibility that some disorders represent patterns of behavior that are adaptive even in the current environment. It could be that psychological adaptations evolved to respond to properties of the environment that have not changed so as to render those mechanisms currently dysfunctional, and this raises the possibility that forms of what we currently take to be pathology are in fact straightforwardly adaptive in the current environment, just as they were in the ancestral environment in which our minds evolved.

The second and third of the explanations I have distinguished are often taken to be definitive of an evolutionary psychiatry. However, an evolutionary psychiatry that employed only these sorts of explanations would be in the unfortunate position of arguing that none of our psychopathology should be explained in terms of something going wrong with our minds. But our minds can malfunction, just as our bodies can, and an evolutionary perspective on psychiatry needs to take that into account: it is questionable how much of our psychopathology can be explained in terms of mismatches or adaptations, rather than simple breakdowns. I discuss these three types of evolutionary perspective in turn.

To begin with, then, let's look at the idea that our psychology is an evolved product prone to breakdown. The most familiar form of this hypothesis is the view that the mind consists of a large number of domain-specific modules, each with a proprietary database and a function that evolved in an ancestral environment to solve a specific problem (Tooby and Cosmides 1992; Pinker 1997). This picture offers a simple way to understand mental disorders: as failures of modules to perform their evolutionary function. Depending on one's theoretical commitments, the evolutionary-modular picture can be transformed in a variety of ways. The evolution of the mind is compatible with many cognitive architectures besides the heavily modular one stressed by evolutionary psychologists. The evolutionary psychologists' picture also presents evolution as working very directly on the cognitive architecture, but one may also assume that evolution works not by selecting modules but in other ways, such as via the regulation of events in brain development. Both the specifics of how the mind is organized and the way evolution has worked on that organization represent degrees of freedom in the development of an evolutionary psychology, and the picture of psychological breakdown assumed by an evolutionary psychopathology varies, depending on how the normal mind is understood.

This approach to psychopathology sees evolution as significant because it underwrites the picture of the normal mind that psychiatry depends on, and evolution may suggest the existence of mechanisms that we would not otherwise have expected. However, this account can also incorporate many proposals for explaining psychopathologies that are not developed with an evolutionary perspective in view; all that is required is an account of the function of some part of our mind and a theory of how that function fails to be performed.

Heavily modular accounts of the mind, such as those offered by evolutionary psychology, have the further appeal that a clear partition of the mind into discrete systems offers the chance to avoid issues about the role of our values in diagnosis by turning diagnostic questions into fully objective questions about malfunction. The prospects for a fully objective psychiatry thus depend on how far the cognitive neurosciences can carry out their program for the understanding of cognition, and evolutionary considerations may have an important part to play in completing that program.

Although some theorists within psychiatry do think of psychological and neural structures as adaptations, many do not. But the assumption that the function of some part of the mind/brain is adaptive often does not change the theory significantly, and much work is easy to integrate within an evolutionary approach, since according to this first perspective evolutionary considerations do not play a prominent role in the explanation of psychopathology. It is the dysfunctions that explain psychopathology, not the fact that normal functions are adaptations. I now discuss putative explanations for psychiatric disorders that appeal directly to evolutionary considerations. The research programs I look at first do not locate the malfunction from which psychiatric patients suffer in their modules; rather, they blame a mismatch between the present environment and the environment that the modules evolved to deal with. There are two forms of this strategy: the first takes a trait and argues that this particular trait was designed to serve a particular function in a past environment but that, in the present environment, it is no longer adaptive. The second strategy is to argue that a mental disorder was never adaptive itself but is a by-product of genes that normally influence the development of a trait that does have an adaptive history, even though it no longer serves a useful function.

Examples of the first strategy for explaining the existence of environment/adaptation mismatches include work on the anxiety disorders (Marks 1987; Marks and Nesse 1994) and several recent discussions of depression (Hagen 1999; Nesse and Williams 1995; Price et al. 1994). The second strategy is represented here by the theory of schizophrenia presented by Stevens and Price (1996). These theories deny or do not assume that the psychological conditions they discuss are adaptive in the contemporary world, although in some cases that possibility is consistent with the evolutionary scenario they employ. If that possibility were taken seriously, then we would be better off including these conditions in the third category.

Marks and Nesse (1994) begin their argument that some anxiety disorders are hangovers from once adaptive behaviors by noting that situations that typically cause phobias are the ones we would expect if we were adapted to be afraid of situations that were dangerous in ancestral environments. They urge that in the ancestral environment a fear of public places and a fear of being far from home might well have been adaptive responses "that guard against the many dangers encountered outside the home range of any territorial species" (251). A fear of heights accompanied by "freezing instead of wild flight" (251) would have had obvious adaptive value, too. In a modern urban environment, however, people who become extremely anxious when they are away from home, in public, or in high places find it difficult or impossible to live normally. Thus, because the modern environment is so different from the ancestral environment, people who are toward the sensitive end of the distribution of phenotypic variation may be incapable of coping with many ordinary situations, despite the fact that all of their mental mechanisms are functioning in just the way that natural selection designed them to function.

This is not quite the argument Marks and Nesse give. I now develop their argument in what I take to be its strongest form, in which the idea of an environment/selection mismatch plays an important role. Then I look at the evidence.

Marks and Nesse certainly do argue that the nervous system "has been shaped so that anxiety arises in response to potential threats" (254). In effect, we are biologically predisposed to find certain stimuli scary on very little basis, so that fear "develops quickly to minimal cues that reflect ancient dangers" (254). This is an important point, because it aligns the hypothesis with a well-attested body of research in a variety of species that documents the speed with which certain associations can be learned. All sorts of phobic associations can be acquired, but some are acquired much more quickly and commonly than others, and these are the phobias that Marks and Nesse try to explain. Their basic idea is that we possess psychological mechanisms that are designed to react to certain stimuli in ways that prepare us for the appropriate response (freezing in some cases, flight in others, for example). The problem that Marks and Nesse attribute to sufferers from phobia is an overactive set of anxiety-producing mechanisms that produce dysfunctional amounts of anxiety in some individuals. As they note, this implies that there ought to be individuals out there who suffer from too little fear, but they do not show up in treatment. (They might show up when medals are being given out, though.)

Sometimes Marks and Nesse appear to argue that phobics suffer from broken modules, with the result that they become unduly anxious. But what seems to be their preferred meaning is that, like most traits, forms of anxiety could be expected to show considerable phenotypic variation. Individuals toward the sensitive end of these distributions—those who become anxious more readily when far from home or when they find themselves in high places—might well have functioned quite normally in ancestral environments. However, these same sensitive individuals might find themselves at a disadvantage in contemporary environments that have changed, relative to the ancestral environment, in ways that make these anxiety-producing mechanisms less valuable than they once were. This does not mean that they have no value: it does pay to be careful when picking one's way along a cliffside, after all. In the majority of cases, though, situations in which we nowadays confront once-dangerous stimuli are not perilous any more. Most of our modern perceptions of ourselves as at a considerable height above the ground are due to looking out of windows, not peering over the edge of a cliff.

So the second reading of the claim that phobics suffer from an excess of normal anxiety is, first, that phobics are toward the sensitive end of the normal distribution of functioning in this regard, and, second, that the environment has changed so that most of our encounters with stimuli that were formerly a threat are no longer dangerous.

The idea that phobias are expressions of prepared evolved responses toward stimuli that it was once adaptive to avoid does rest on a solid comparative basis, although the matter cannot be regarded as settled: many different lineages, including our own, display a readiness to respond to some stimuli rather than others, and the stimuli are ones that it is or would have been adaptive to avoid. Humans seem to share this general capacity; for example, it is not at all uncommon for us to avoid certain substances after they have made us ill just once, as anyone who drank too much Southern Comfort as a teenager can testify. The pattern of the most common phobias is consistent with the evolutionary hypothesis, as is the general tendency of humans and other animals to selectively learn to avoid certain stimuli on the basis of very brief exposure. The stimuli that count are ones that would have been dangerous once but that, because the environment has changed sufficiently, are now largely harmless, so that a hair-trigger response is now no longer of use.

The second way to argue that a disorder is related to a once adaptive trait is represented by Stevens and Price, who argue that the predisposition to schizophrenia must be adaptive: "natural selection has fixed it as an enduring component of the human genome" (1996: 142). They do not think that schizophrenia itself, the full-blown psychosis, is ever adaptive, but they do argue that there must be an adaptive trait to be found somewhere on the schizophreniform continuum, which includes schizotypal and paranoid personality types.

Stevens and Price make two assumptions. First, they argue that a mild form of schizoid behavior must have been adaptive. Second, they argue that schizophrenia sufferers are victims in the same way that sickle-cell anemics are victims; they have a greater number of genes for the relevant trait, and this combination is what leads to the expression of the disorder. If there were fewer copies of the relevant allele present, schizophrenics would have the adaptive trait. However, the analogy with sickle cell is doubly flawed: sickle-cell trait protects against malaria in some contemporary environments, and Stevens and Price do not assume that schizotypal behavior is currently adaptive; more important, it is not the case that people with only one copy of the allele are a little bit anemic, whereas people with two copies are a lot more anemic. That's the story that Stevens and Price want to tell for schizoid behavior, and the analogy does not hold.

The main interest in the hypothesis, which seems very implausible on its face, is the idea that certain disorders may be inevitable by-products of adaptive traits, rather than the adaptive traits themselves. This does seem to be a theoretical possibility, although the justification that Stevens and Price offer is completely speculative and, on the face of it, highly implausible. Stevens and Price offer what they call a group-splitting account of schizophrenia. They argue that our ancestors lived in groups that would have grown to a point at which they outran available resources, whereupon the group would have to split up. The adaptive value of mild schizoid symptoms, they assert, comes at that point; they contend that mildly schizoid individuals would have been regarded as charismatic and hence able to draw followers away with them to start a new group; this would have been good for the group. They claim that "the schizoid genotype is an adaptation whose function is to facilitate group splitting" (1996: 152).

Now, this counts as a selection/environment mismatch hypothesis, in the sense that human groups no longer need to split for this reason, and so the adaptation is no longer needed. As well as traits that are selection/environments mismatches, though, we might also ask about adaptations to features of the ancestral environment that are still adaptive today.

The hypotheses we have just looked at assume that environmental changes may render well-designed systems pathological. However, we don't have to suppose that the environment has changed in every respect during human evolution. The last hypothesis we examine argues that some putative pathologies are adaptive in the current environment, just as they were in the ancestral environment in which our minds evolved. This has recently been proposed as a possible explanation for some personality disorders.

Personality disorders are patterns of experience and behavior that are culturally very deviant, persistent, and inflexible; arise in adolescence or early adulthood; and lead to distress or impairment. McGuire and Troisi (1998) suggest that two personality disorders in particular may represent adaptive deviant behavioral strategies: antisocial personality disorder and histrionic personality disorder. Antisocial personality disorder is characterized by a disregard for the wishes, rights, or feelings of others. Subjects with this disorder are impulsive and aggressive and neglect their responsibilities: "They are frequently deceitful and manipulative in order to gain personal profit or pleasure (e.g. to obtain money, sex or power)" (DSM-IV-TR: 702). They may show complete indifference to the harmful consequences of their actions and "believe that everyone is out to 'help number one' " (703).

Subjects diagnosed with histrionic personality disorder are attention-seeking prima donnas. Their behavior is often sexually provocative or seductive in a wide variety of inappropriate situations or relationships (DSM-IV-TR: 711). They demand immediate satisfaction and are intolerant of or frustrated by delayed gratification. They may resort to threats of suicide to get attention and coerce better caregiving (712). Both antisocial and histrionic personality disorders are characterized by manipulativeness, although antisocial subjects manipulate others in the pursuit of material gratification and histrionics manipulate to gain nurture.

Now you might think that being able to manipulate other people so that they nurture you or further your material ends would be quite a useful trait to have, moral qualms aside. And individuals with personality disorders don't have moral qualms. That makes it easier for them to manipulate people, but it can also cause their downfall. To be diagnosed with a personality disorder, people must manifest a pattern of behavior that involves these undesirable social acts, though to satisfy the diagnostic criteria set out in DSM-IV their behavior must also "lead to clinically significant distress or impairment in social, occupational, or other important areas of functioning" (DSM-IV-TR: 689). The question is whether there exist people who are just as unsavory and manipulative but who do not suffer adverse consequences. Successful individuals with personality disorders may cheat, deceive, and manipulate but be good enough at reading social cues and understanding the structure of reciprocal exchange that they can exploit the social system and do as well, evolutionarily, as most people.

McGuire and Troisi argue that such individuals are designed to exploit others via their sensitivity to, but disregard for, the system of social exchange and that the social environment in which we currently live is similar enough to the ancestral environment that these strategies remain adaptive. Their basic idea is that a personality disorder represents an evolutionarily stable strategy. The idea of an evolutionarily stable strategy comes from the application of game theory to evolutionary biology: different behavioral strategies can evolve within a population and at some point reach an equilibrium. Such a strategy is an evolutionarily stable strategy. It is not necessary that everyone in the population play the same strategy or that everyone who plays a given strategy play it all the time. All that is needed is that a strategy be played often enough to survive in the population, even if it has seemingly few benefits to offer. Skyrms has shown how this is mathematically possible for apparently bizarre strategies such as "Mad Dog," which rejects a fair division of resources but accepts a grossly unfair one (1996: 29–31); that is, Mad Dogs punish those who play fair. McGuire and Troisi argue that personality disorders, despite the cognitive deficits that may be associated with them, may offer other benefits that maintain them in the population.

Mealey (1995) attempts to flesh out this structure with a variety of developmental and genetic evidence. She argues that the evolved strategic use of cheating in social exchange situations distinguishes primary from secondary sociopaths, the latter being amorally instrumentally rational in response to stressful environments but without the lack of emotion that characterizes primary sociopathy in her model.

This third evolutionary approach to psychopathology is the most dramatic of all: it argues that some people are designed to be antisocial in our current environments. To be attractive, this view would need to show, first, that the evolutionary environment was relevantly similar to our own and, second, that the strategy represented by the disorder of interest is robust enough to evolve across a wide variety of game-theoretic situations, since our confidence that it evolved may be shaken if the strategy requires very finely tuned initial conditions (indeed, we still have not been given any precise characterization of the strategy that the individuals we are trying to explain are supposed to be playing). But the main problem with the approach as it stands is its neglect of cognitive mechanisms. DSM-IV-TR offers a purely behavioral definition of antisocial personality disorder that raises in an acute way the question whether we are dealing with people who are pathological or merely vicious, and indeed most of the prison population would fit the diagnosis. Other researchers insist that the behavioral definition is too inclusive and obscures a genuine psychopathology, that is, psychopathy.

Hare distinguishes three behaviorally very similar groups on the basis of "personality structure, life history, response to treatment and prognosis": psychopaths, aggressive neurotics, and delinquents raised in an -antisocial subculture (1970: 9). Some researchers believe genuine psychopathy is a matter of underlying information-processing deficits. Psychopaths lack the moral emotions, and although they are at least as intelligent as nonpsychopaths, they are impulsive, irresponsible, and very poor at long-term planning. Psychological testing on psychopaths suggests they "have the capacity for genuine judgment and sound affect but that a cognitive deficiency interferes with their ability to integrate the products of these faculties with ongoing behavior" (Newman 1998: 83). Similar deficits are found in patients with frontal lobe injuries, and although lesions in the frontal lobe have not been found in psychopaths (Hare 1999), it has been argued that some sort of information-processing problems in frontal lobe systems may account for some of the cognitive shortcomings of psychopaths.

If these claims about psychopathy are correct, the McGuire-Troisi-Mealey strategy is in trouble because it will be forced to assume that the cognitive mechanisms that underlie an adaptive strategy are ones that in fact appear to be far from adaptive. McGuire and Troisi require that there be a population with the manipulativeness and ruthlessness of psychopaths but without their cognitive deficits, and perhaps with a better than normal capacity to disguise their manipulative tendencies (especially if we assume that humans evolved in small groups where repeated interactions were common); the existence of such a population remains speculative. Of course, manipulative and other antisocial behavior is widespread, and the existence of the strategy of manipulation, distributed throughout the whole population, is consistent with the game-theoretic models of population genetics. However, explaining the evolution of manipulation or antisocial behavior as a strategy is not the same as explaining the existence, in evolutionary terms, of a distinct population of manipulators.

The moral, I think, is quite general: if this approach is to work, there ought to be a theory of the specific cognitive mechanisms that underlie the behavior of interest. Otherwise, the ESS approach is open to the counterargument that the behavior is simply a normal reaction to certain circumstances or the product of abnormal psychology for which the usual explanations may be envisaged.

So an evolutionary psychiatry can make use of explanations in terms of psychological breakdowns just as readily as any other orientation on abnormal psychology. But the idea that some psychopathologies are or were adaptations is certainly a position in logical space, and in this chapter I have argued that there are two ways to fill it. A disorder may be a trait that was once adaptive but is now unadaptive, or it may be adaptive even in the current environment.

REFERENCES

American Psychiatric Association (2000) *Diagnostic and Statistical Manual of Mental Disorders*, 4th ed., Textual Revision [DSM-IV-TR]. Washington, DC: American Psychiatric Association.

Hagen, E. H. (1999) "The Functions of Postpartum Depression." *Evolution and Human Behavior* 20: 325–59.

Hare, R. D. (1970) *Psychopathy: Theory and Research*. New York: Wiley.

Hare, R. D. (1999) *Without Conscience*. New York: Guilford.

Marks, I. M. (1987) *Fears, Phobias and Rituals*. Oxford: Oxford University Press.

Marks, I. M., and Nesse, R. (1994) "Fear and Fitness: An Evolutionary Analysis of Anxiety Disorders." *Ethology and Sociobiology* 15: 247–61.

McGuire, M., and Troisi, A. (1998) *Darwinian Psychiatry*. New York: Oxford University Press.

Mealey, L. (1995) "The Sociobiology of Sociopathy: An Integrated Evolutionary Model." *Behavioral and Brain Sciences* 18: 523–99.

Murphy, D., and Stich, S. (2000) "Darwin in the Madhouse: Evolutionary Psychology and the Classification of Mental Disorders." In P. Carruthers and A. Chamberlain (eds.), *Evolution and the Human Mind*. Cambridge: Cambridge University Press, pp. 62–92.

Newman, J. (1998) "Psychopathic Behavior: An Information Processing Perspective." In D. J. Cooke, A. E. Forth, and R. D. Hare (eds.), *Psychopathy: Theory, Research and Implications for Society*. Dordrecht: Kluwer, pp. 81–104.

Nesse, R. M., and Williams, G. C (1995) *Why We Get Sick*. New York: Times Books.

Papineau, D. (1994) "Mental Disorder, Illness and Biological Dysfunction." In A. Phillips Griffiths (ed.), *Philosophy, Psychology and Psychiatry: Royal Institute of Philosophy Supplement* 37: 73–82.

Pinker, S. (1997) *How the Mind Works*. New York: W. W. Norton.

Price, J., Sloman, L., Gardner, R., Gilbert, P., and Rohde, P. (1994) "The Social Competition Hypothesis of Depression." *British Journal of Psychiatry* 164: 309–15.

Skyrms, B. (1996) *Evolution of the Social Contract*. Cambridge: Cambridge University Press.

Stevens, A., and Price, J. (1996) *Evolutionary Psychiatry: A New Beginning*. London: Routledge.

Tooby, J., and Cosmides, L. (1992) "The Psychological Foundations of Culture." In J. Barkow, L. Cosmides, and J. Tooby (eds.), *The Adapted Mind*. New York: Oxford University Press, pp. 19–137.

Wakefield, J. (1996) "Dysfunction as a Value Free Concept." *Philosophy, Psychology, and Psychiatry* 2: 233–46.

CHAPTER 23

PSYCHOANALYTIC MODELS

Freud's Debt to Philosophy and His Copernican Revolution

BETTINA BERGO

FREUD began his intellectual life with a passion for philosophy. At the university of Vienna, that passion was fed powerfully by the Aristotelian Franz Brentano. For 20 years, from the 1880s into the late 1890s (in his letters to Silberstein and to Fliess), it echoes through Freud's correspondence. Freud's path of studies meandered famously from philosophy and zoology, to medicine, to neurology, to psychopathology. However, in 1885, by the time he returned from his spring semester with Jean-Martin Charcot at the Hôpital de la Salpêtrière, in Paris, Freud had made a decision. He returned to Vienna, delivered a simple report to the Society of Physicians at the university, and unwittingly caused an unprecedented uproar. The condition of hysteria, which he had observed at length in Paris, afflicted women and men, he argued. This uniquely feminine pathology—whether its cause was anatomical or physiological—somehow overtook men, as well.

There is a remarkable connection between Freud's passion for philosophy—indeed, his debt to a few philosophers, notably Kant—and his psychological interpretation of hysteria. The connection concerns the extensions of transcendental philosophy in twentieth-century psychology. It also concerns the fate of philosophical psychology after Kant's logical destruction of the arguments for a possible thinking substance, or soul, in his "Antinomies of Pure Reason." As we will see, Freud owed a significant debt to Kant's transcendental logic, which formed the core of Kant's "Copernican Revolution." Moreover, Freud sought to prolong Kant's revolution to include, in his own dynamic psychology, normal *and* abnormal mental life *in their interrelations through the unconscious.* For that he required, in addition to the clinical "laboratory" of the analyst's couch, his own transcendental analytic and deduction, as we will see.

Kant's first *Critique* had destroyed the logical grounds for a dual substance theory (i.e., extended versus thinking substances), and, with this, the arguments for an entity called a "soul." Rational psychology after Kant had little else to do than observe the phenomena of psychic life. Now, although he was wont to profess indifference to philosophy, Freud not only was influenced by it but also adapted one of its most powerful tools in the nineteenth century: transcendental analysis and deduction. In working with his conception of a *psychical* primary process and, later, of the preconscious and the unconscious, Freud altered the nature and scope of questions for philosophy of mind.[1] At the same time, he utterly shook up rational philosophy's conception of affects and passions. He did this both by criticizing psychophysical parallelism tied to dual substance theories and by demonstrating that the so-called feminine passions could be found in men by virtue of their psyches, rather than their bodies.

The story of Freud's debt to, and impact on, philosophy was long unexplored. Yet, recent interest in Freud as a philosopher is clear. Before I sketch the unfolding of Freud's debt, recent inquiries into his relationship to philosophy should be noted.

I. Recent Work on Freud and Philosophy

In the past ten years, English-speaking philosophers, both analytic and continental, have reengaged Freud as a philosophical thinker. Commentators such as Samuel Weber, Sebastian Gardner, and Richard Boothby, among others, have reread Freud's theories of anxiety and the unconscious and his topology of id, ego, and superego. They have examined these in light of the meaning of subjective agency, the will, the nature of intentionality, the synthesis of consciousness, and so on. Indeed, Michael P. Levine's collection *The Analytic Freud* turns on the provocative wager that "the integration of psychoanalytic theory with [commonsense] philosophy [may be] necessary to both" disciplines today.[2]

Interest has also come from feminist critiques of, and dialogues with, Freud, including those of Julia Kristeva, Luce Irigaray, Marcia Cavell, Amélie Oksenberg

Rorty, Jennifer Radden, and Teresa Brennan, to mention a few.[3] Moreover, Jacques Lacan's reading of Freud's unconscious according to a structuralist logic and his insistence that Freud be understood in light of Hegel's dialectics and Nietzsche's drives have prompted both cultural studies and continental philosophy to inquire into the philosophical implications of Freudianism.[4]

II. Philosophical Influences on Freud's Psychoanalysis

This essay deliberately follows three thematic tracks. First, I explore Freud's debt to philosophy by distinguishing between the many influences on the young Freud and the formal debt he owed to transcendental philosophy. After that, I examine two important ways in which Freud challenged Kant's epistemology: the first in terms of the explanatory and diagnostic resources of Freud's model of the mind; the second in light of Freud's contribution to the structure of mental temporality. Finally, I turn to his case of male hysteria to argue that, while owing philosophy a complicated and unacknowledged debt, Freud delivered a blow to the Aristotelian-Kantian conception of affectivity and passions. By psychologizing hysteria, Freud made it impossible to hold to simple divisions of the passions into educable versus ineducable, masculine versus feminine ones—or even to argue that affectivity should be reduced to physiological events and changes in the body.

To begin, we should distinguish between influences and debts in Freud's life. At the end of the nineteenth century, philosophical influences on psychological and psychiatric thought were numerous. They were perversely clear whenever psychology pursued the scientific refutation of philosophical arguments. To that end, psychology found itself embracing either mechanisms inspired by materialist philosophies or organicist teleologies, to which Hegel had given the greatest impetus. In his early years at the University of Vienna (1873–75), Freud discovered philosophy through Franz Brentano, the proto-father of phenomenology, whom he readily qualified as a "genius."[5] Brentano's genius lay in holding Darwinism and Aristotelian teleology together, while rejecting speculative psychology and embracing a Lockean notion of simple ideas and interpreting the ego as pure act.[6] Freud's early letters to his friend Eduard Silberstein (1871–81)[7] attest to Freud's love for, and tension with, Brentano. At that time, Freud thought of himself as a materialist, while Brentano was a believer. Freud was attracted by rational psychology, while Brentano insisted that he avoid the rationalist inheritors of Descartes and read Hume and Kant instead. We learn from Freud's letter of March 7, 1875, that Brentano believed that the philosophy of his time was "in absolute chaos" and that philosophy and psychology should limit their inquiries to empirical observation. To that end, Brentano suggested that Freud avoid

Geulinx, Malebranche, and Spinoza and devote himself to Hume's skepticism and to Kantian criticism.

So considerable was Brentano's influence on him that Freud would declare, in a letter from March 15 of that year, "For the time being, I have ceased to be a materialist and am not yet a theist" (*SFES* 1990: 104–5).

To be sure, Freud's relationship to philosophy in later years showed more ambivalence than we find in his letters to Silberstein. His debts are arguably to Leibniz and Kant. They are debts because these philosophies formed the conditions of possibility for Freud's models of mental life: Leibniz, for the notion of unconscious thoughts; Kant, for the transcendental strategies. I turn to Kant in part III.

Freud's revolution turned on his discovery and mappings of what he called *das Unbewusste*, or the "Unconscious." He never claimed to have discovered the unconscious *eo ipso*, only to have grounded it on a dynamic principle of forces, or energies, potentially in conflict,[8] and to have brought a clinical method to its investigation. From his season in Paris with Charcot (1885) and his work with Josef Breuer (1893–95), Freud sought a scientific and therapeutic approach to the unconscious in light of the hysterics, male and female, observed at the Salpêtrière and under the treatment of his colleague Breuer—notably, in the latter's erstwhile patient "Anna O" in their joint work, *Studies in Hysteria*.[9]

We get a keen sense of the ultimate ambition behind Freud's mental topography from the remarks he makes in his 1926 "Self-Presentation." It meant nothing less than accounting for all psychic phenomena, normal and abnormal, conscious and unconscious. He wrote there: "Later, I ventured the attempt at a 'Metapsychology.' I gave that name to the type of observation, in which every psychic process [*jeder seelische Vorgang*] was appreciated according to the coordinates of the Dynamic, the Topical, and the Economic [in framing the unconscious], and I saw in it the most far-reaching goal that psychology could reach."[10] Now this goal included *all* psychologies, philosophical and physiological, though by the 1920s the natural scientific model was the framework behind which Freud obscured his philosophical aspiration.

To return to his influences, the development of psychoanalysis as a budding *Naturwissenschaft* [natural science] (P: 64) erected on the "science of the unconscious" took three decades. In those years, Freud's relationship to philosophy took the forms of selective borrowings[11]—including borrowed concepts such as A. Schopenhauer's conception of will, G. W. Fechner's mechanism, T. Lipps's theory of association, and modifications of Nietzsche's drives. While making his selections, Freud criticized philosophy for its two fundamental ambitions: its totalizing system building and its equation of mind with consciousness (P: 72ff; GW 8: 406). Like Brentano, Freud opposed pure speculation and insisted that no epistemology could explain nature *and* culture together. That was the luxury of what he called, derisively, a *Weltanschauung*, or worldview. His psychoanalysis remained faithful to natural science because, he argued with circular reasoning, psychoanalysis "is inapt at forming a proper *Weltanschauung*," for "it has no need for one [since] it is a part of science" (GW 15: 170; P: 69).

Freud's opposition to philosophical "worldviews" is understandable, given his philosophical influences. At the end of the nineteenth century, philosophy was certainly "in chaos." Significant contemporary figures, influenced by Darwin, had embraced forms of social Darwinism, cultural Lamarckianism, and interpretations of biogenesis, pansexualism, and psychogenesis that hierarchized cultures and races (*FBM*: 252–57, 274ff). Already in 1903, echoing the values of many intellectuals of his time, Otto Weininger, the classicist turned philosopher, decried the decadence and sensualism of Viennese arts and letters and announced the era of "*Kultur* in the place of *Zivilisation*, of the *Volk* and the race in the place of the masses, of the *Weltanschauung* in the place of skepticism, and of synthesis in the place of analysis."[12] A little more than a decade later, Oswald Spengler echoed Weininger's concerns as he began writing his *Untergang des Abendlandes* (1911).

Many intellectuals read Weininger, and Freud became painfully aware of his work. His controversial book *Geschlecht und Charakter* explored humans' ontogenetic bisexuality while it decried the recent effeminization and "Judaization" of European man. The book sold well and became the occasion for bitter arguments between Freud and his then closest friend, Wilhelm Fliess. Fliess was probably the only man to whom Freud had dared to declare in 1896, "I secretly nurse the hope of arriving by the same route [medicine] at my own *original, objective philosophy*. For that was my original ambition."[13]

Long after Weininger's suicide in 1903, Freud would declare synthesis and *Weltanschauungen* anathema to scientific endeavor. Yet, in so doing, Freud was neither consistent nor wholly dogmatic,[14] because he sought both the legitimacy of science and a legacy comparable to that of transcendental philosophy.[15]

Nevertheless, during the pre–World War I period, Freud's relationship to philosophy soured further into professions of know-nothingness. Yet, his "unconscious" philosophical sophistication astonished Ludwig Binswanger, the psychologist from Switzerland who was deeply sympathetic to psychoanalysis. Binswanger wrote, when he visited Freud in February 1910:

> I took note. . . . "None of us has acquired the habit of thinking simultaneously of the ego and conscious processes on the one hand, and the processes of the unconscious and of the sexual instinct on the other." The demand for such simultaneous thinking showed me . . . that Freud had a genuinely philosophical vein, *even though he was not aware of it.* . . .On one occasion, [Freud stated] during a Wednesday meeting that "the unconscious *is metaphysic, we simply posit it as real.*"[16]

Freud's gesture to a barebones transcendentalism was followed by a question concerning Kant's "thing in itself." Binswanger records Freud's subsequent discussion with Paul Häberlin: "Freud asked [Häberlin] whether Kant's thing in itself was not identical with the unconscious. [Häberlin] denied this, laughing, and suggested that the two notions were on entirely different levels" (*RF*: 9). In his dialogue with Häberlin, Freud was giving voice to what would prove to be his great philosophical debt. I suspect he was also casting about for legitimating antecedents to his "metaphysic" of the unconscious. Over time, Freud would work to bring Häberlin's "entirely different levels" together. The neoscience he expressed in regard to philosophy was related to his will to weave philosophical insights through his science, while criticizing philosophical constructions.

I alluded earlier to some of the "philosophies" that prompted Franz Brentano to declare the discipline in chaos in the 1880s. Needless to say, Freud kept his distance from social Darwinism, though he embraced Lamarckianism and the dusty Recapitulation theory that ontogenesis reproduces phylogenesis. But, like that of many of his peers, Freud's clinical work was shot through with philosophical influences. His speculations, like those in "Beyond the Pleasure Principle" (1920), resembled what was popularly called *Hirrenmythologie*, or informal exercises in philosophy of mind. Despite the decadence of Idealist dialectics from Fichte to Schelling, and the mysterious theories of *life force* (first popularized by the celebrated neurologist Johannes von Müller and expanded by Freud's teacher Theodor Meynert, who argued that "force" should replace Kant's *Ding an sich*), Freud employed these ideas to his own ends.[17] Despite the slippage of Darwinism into radical forms (E. Häckel)[18] and social-cosmological, evolutionist fantasies like those of Spencer, Galton, and de Gobineau — who combined notions like the "subconscious" mind with those of evolving and retarded races — Freud adapted Darwinism to his theories of sexual and cultural development. Gustave Le Bon's psychology of crowds revisited natural law in racist terms;[19] Freud cited him at length in his "Mass Psychology and Ego Analysis" (1920). But Freud's goals were unchanging: to subject these theories to correction or supplementation by depth psychology.[20] Even the philosophical imperative of the time — the improvement of the races, which grew out of biological and cultural misreadings of Darwin and which guided much empirical research — became grist for the Freudian mill that reinterpreted the social Darwinists and the sociobiological in terms of his depth psychology.[21]

If science meant for Freud insistence on observation and therapeutic efficacy (*FdL* 17: 217ff),[22] then this proved an insufficiently protected position. Freud sought legitimacy elsewhere. His use of a formally transcendental logic, along with his own case history form,[23] grounded his peculiar science. Freud's Kantian strategies themselves consisted in what we might call a transcendental analytic and deduction: that is, the *analysis* of symptoms and oneiric and linguistic signs (dream symbols, *lapsus linguae*, forgetting of names), aiming to show their conditions of possibility, and the *deduction* of the rules that order those unconscious ideas evident in dreams and psychoses, formally not so unlike Kant's a priori categories of the understanding.

III. FREUD'S DEBT TO KANT

Freud was a dualist. But he was neither a psychophysical parallelist nor a Cartesian interactionist. He rejected physical reductionism (even that of William James) and localization theories like that of the neurologist Hughlings Jackson, who had influenced him. This made Freud's particular dualism unconventional. Kant's transcendental psychology provided him a strategy against the psychophysical parallelisms popular in his time. In his 1915 lecture "The Unconscious," he addressed the primary objection to his theory of a psychic rather than a physical unconscious: the neurological or physiological nature of drives. His foils were Fechner and Meynert, but his target was ultimately Cartesian parallelism. "When all our latent memories are taken into consideration," he argued, "it becomes totally incomprehensible how the existence of the unconscious can be gainsaid. We then encounter the objection that these latent recollections can no longer be described as mental processes, but that they correspond to residues of somatic processes,"[24] rather like Descartes's pineal gland, which was mysteriously moved by both physical and psychical forces.

"Somatic residues" were a popular concept in dualist and materialist circles as Freud developed his psychoanalysis.[25] But Freud recognized that psychophysical parallelism either entailed a third-man logic that posited some intermediary instance between body and mind and then had to determine whether it was principally corporeal or mental parallelism or left to speculation how a memory became simply physical and how it could ever be subsequently brought back to consciousness. The solution required the abandonment of Cartesianism, "which breaks up all mental continuity, plunges us into the insoluble difficulties of psychophysical parallelism . . . and finally, forces us prematurely *to retire from the territory of psychological research without ever being able to offer us any compensation elsewhere*" (CP: 100). By 1926, Freud was more emphatic: "The neurotic [and the unconscious] is certainly an *undesired complication . . . for medicine. . . .* But it exists and concerns medicine closely. And for . . . its treatment, *medical training can give us nothing, but absolutely nothing.*"[26] It could offer nothing because either medicine was locked in psychophysical parallelism or it was materially reductionist.[27]

In his 1915 talk "The Unconscious," Freud expressed approval of and ambivalence about Kant's strategies. "The psychoanalytic assumption of unconscious mental activity appears to us, on the one hand, a further development of that *primitive animism* which caused our own consciousness to be reflected in all around us, and, on the other hand . . . *an extension of the corrections begun by Kant in regard to our views on external perception*" (CP: 104). Still, it was the transcendental logic — as Kant had argued it — that provided Freud with a real gain in meaning, which was, he insisted, "a perfectly justifiable ground for going beyond the limits of direct experience."[28] Better, it offered a way out of the Cartesian-Fechnerian circle of reason, in which mind investigated mind for mental contents and discovered only physical residues.

Freud sought to go further than Kant had ventured. Conceptually, Freud's "Copernican Revolution" provided a passage between mental events in normal consciousness and those characteristic of abnormal conditions. Therapeutically, Freud's "science of the unconscious" extended psychological practice to cases to which psychiatry and psychology had been unreceptive. Psychoanalysis could thus eventually provide the ground for psychology itself, rather than the reverse.[29] And Freud's psychic dynamism (conflicts), psychic economy (variations in quantities of drive cathexes), and psychic topology (metaphoric "sites" from and to which drives "move") struck a transcendental blow against Kant's temporally structured, internal intuition. If conscious life is temporally and spatially structured with a universal specificity in Kant, then conscious life, when enlarged by Freud's notions of the unconscious and the preconscious, shows us a more complex temporality than Kant's—a temporality that accounted for the persistence and somatization of traumatic memories, as well as the regressions exhibited by patients in therapy.

Hoping to bring about a contemporary Copernican Revolution,[30] Freud remained in competition with Kant and Kantianism. Binswanger's report of Freud calling the unconscious "a metaphysic," not to mention Freud's search for a *Ding an sich* that was utterly different from Kant's formal noumenon[31] lead us to wonder whether Freud was really as wrong about the difference of levels as Häberlin thought. Heuristically, the unconscious was like the thing in itself to the extent that the unconscious alone should make possible—in and despite its (noumenal) opacity—the true grasp of consciousness's unity. Formally, the unconscious was arguably more than Kant's noumenon, because it did not set a speculative limit to the possibilities of experience but instead opened certain types of experience to a systematic investigation of levels of meaning that were inaccessible to other psychologies. Yet, Freud's noumenal instance (the unconscious) cast a darker shadow across both mental life and cultural evolution. Given the unconscious drives, Freud's psychic "system" put an end, if temporarily, to aspirations at mental totalization, whether philosophical or psychological. Freud could explain the hiatuses of consciousness, but in so doing he foreclosed psychic transparency and complete integration.[32]

IV. Freud's Critique of Philosophy of the Passions: Male and Female Hysterics

I now come to the third theme of Freud's relationship to philosophy: his unwitting blow to the theory of passions. It was thus in abnormal psychology that Freud's work may have been the most radical. When Freud delivered his report to the Viennese Society of Physicians, following his stay at the Salpêtrière, and reported on Charcot's observation, classification, and treatment of hysterics—male and female—he was met with passionate opposition. German-speaking physicians, like many of their English and French counterparts, were still in thrall to one of the three persisting theories of hysteria's etiology: first, the old anatomical theory, according to which hysteria arose when the womb moved within the body, thereby influencing other organs; second, the physiological theory, according to which hysteria was a disease of drifting humors in a body conceived of as a container; third, the reflex theory of hysteria, according to which the disease was caused by the complex neurological connections between the womb and every other significant organ in a woman's body. In this last theory, when womb or ovaries became irritated, they "relayed reflex irritation to other parts of the body, causing attacks, convulsions, insensibilities, and paralyses,"or hysterical symptoms. The overlapping etiologies of hysteria and their dominant, generative metaphors justified the popular and philosophical conviction that bodily differences between men and women meant that each sex had its proper passions and virtues. As the privileged organ of pregnancy and the metonym for women's mysterious immanence, the womb accounted for "feminine virtues" like "compassion, kindness, constancy," as well as for feminine passions or vices like "religious enthusiasm, erotomania, monomania, jealousy . . . cunning."[33] Women and men were given to passions that differed in their varieties and intensities. For Freud's scandalized Viennese colleagues, hysteria was a woman's passion. It was the feminine corporeal disorder.

Freud destabilized this classification and, with it, the guiding but unreflected logic of the passions. After being shouted out of the amphitheater on October 15, 1886, and subsequently barred from many laboratories, Freud produced a male hysteric, "Herr August P.," in less than two months' time, on November 26. Evincing the characteristic anaesthesias, fainting spells, and areas of sensitivity, Herr August proved Freud's claim that there was *at least one* man in Vienna who exhibited the symptoms of hysteria. In describing his childhood and detailing the traumatic events that had preceded the outbreak of Herr August's symptoms, Freud psychologized a disease whose etiology had altered somewhat over time but had remained inflexibly biological and sex specific. The scandal was double. Not only could the male body present the symptoms of a disease that could no longer be said to originate from the uterus, but also the male psyche itself could fall prey to pathologies attributed to feminine nature. The only remaining question concerned the ultimate source of this possibility. Was masculine hysteria the result of the decadence of European culture generally—as many were arguing then, in response to the "social" turn Darwin's thought was taking?[34] Or, was this a phenomenon of specific races and groups, like the criminals studied by Cesare Lombroso, less fit for survival than others? Freud would argue that it was neither.

Despite the fact that women made up the majority of Freud's hysterics, the fact remained that Freud had upset the gendered logic of the passions, which was so entrenched that philosophers from Kant to Kierkegaard, not to mention psychiatrists of all stripes, hardly gave it a second thought. Freud weakened a structure of philosophico-therapeutic thinking that, from the Greeks to modernity, had paired passions, weak and strong, with their respective sexes and had drawn its conclusions about the possibility of educating these passions into virtues. Thus, Freud's psychology worked surreptitiously against a philosophical inheritance that had been altered first by Kant's logical demolition of the "immaterial substance" or "soul" but that had held firm to gender essentialisms concerning the relationship between reason and passions (cf. Kant's *Anthropology*). Freud's Copernican Revolution was thus more than the extension of a theory of mind into pathological mental functioning; it left man in the condition held previously by woman: prey to pathologies caused by trauma and a conflict between drives, or between drives and desires. In the matter of hysteria, no one could claim to be the enduring master in his own house of immanence. In short, Freud's debt to Kant's transcendental strategies helped him to create his psychoanalysis even as he dislodged philosophical values that distinguished mind from body, the experiential from the speculative, the masculine from the feminine.

NOTES

1. See Manson, "A Tumbling-Ground for Whimsies?" pp. 148–68.

2. Weber, *Legend of Freud*; Gardner, "The Unconscious," pp. 136–60 (this essay explores the unconscious in light of the philosophy of mind and commonsense psychology); Boothby, *Freud as Philosopher*; Levine, *Analytic Freud*.

3. Kristeva, *New Maladies of the Soul*; Kristeva, *The Sense and Non-sense of Revolt*; Kristeva, *Intimate Revolt*; Irigaray, "Poverty of Psychoanalysis"; and Cavell, *Psychoanalytic Mind*. See Rorty's discussion of the tensions between Aristotelian organicism and Hobbesian mechanism in Freud's theory of sexual development and her arguments for unconscious affects in "Affects, Mourning and the Erotic Mind," pp. 195–209. See also Radden, "Love and Loss in Freud's *Mourning and Melancholia*, pp. 211–30, and Brennan, *Interpretation of the Flesh*.

4. This is also thanks to Lacan's influence on figures such as Jacques Derrida; see Derrida, *Résistances de la psychanalyse*. See Butler, *Psychic Life of Power*, and Felman and Laub, *Testimony*.

5. Freud wrote Silberstein, on March 7, 1885: "When you and I meet, I shall tell you more about this remarkable man . . . (a believer, a teleologist (!) and a Darwinian and a damned clever fellow, a genius in fact), who is, in many respects, an ideal human being. For now, just the news that under Brentano's fruitful influence, I have arrived at the decision to take my Ph.D. in philosophy and zoology." See Boehlich and Pomerans, *Letters of Sigmund Freud to Eduard Silberstein*, p. 95; hereafter cited as *SFES*.

6. See Brentano, *Descriptive Psychology*, pp. 89 ff. The work regroups lectures delivered from 1887 to 1891.

7. Silberstein took degrees in philosophy and law and later struggled successfully against legal forms of anti-Semitism, such as denial of the right to vote and the "Jews' Oath," in his native Romania. See *SFES*, pp. 95, 103–5.

8. See Assoun's discussion of Freud's dynamic viewpoint of psychic processes as it intersects with the economic organization of the unconscious, in the metapsychology. Section 3, "Structure et principes de la métapsychologie," in his *Psychanalyse*, pp. 383–86. Hereafter cited as *P*.

9. Breuer and Freud, *Studies on Hysteria*.

10. Freud, *Gesammelte Werke*, vol. 14, p. 85. My translation. Hereafter cited in the text as *GW*.

11. A brief list of Freud's use of philosophical influences illustrates this: Goethe, Romanticism, materialist reductionism in the service of psychology, Herbart's mechanism, and Fechner's speculative physics—for the "principle of constancy" applied to the nervous system. We find here themes freely gleaned, and an undeniable competition for concepts and legitimacy.

12. See Hamann and Hermand, *Stilkunst um 1900*, cited by Le Rider, *Le cas Otto Weininger*, p. 139.

13. Cited by Zanuso, *Young Freud*, p. 81. Fliess was the Berlin otolaryngologist and amateur psychologist who claimed to have conceived the idea of bisexuality and to have shared it with Freud in their correspondence.

14. As Freud wrote to Einstein in 1932, "every natural science — including psychoanalysis — opens onto some sort of mythology. . . . We have our mythology, it is the theory of drives" (GW 16: 22; P: 70).

15. An Italian biographer described the youthful Freud as a respectful maverick and as "a philosopher and scientist intolerant of philosophy and science where these [are] closed systems dogmatically anchored in their own certitudes." Zanuso, *Young Freud*, p. 85.

16. Binswanger objected, "The labeling of the unconscious as *metaphysic* seemed to me misleading . . . because the unconscious was supposed to be the psychic *par excellence*. Freud agreed with me . . . the proper term was not 'metaphysic' . . . but 'metaconscious.' " See Binswanger, *Sigmund Freud: Reminiscences of a Friendship*, pp. 7–8. Hereafter cited as RF.

17. Fichte was J. F. Herbart's teacher. But Herbart rejected idealism in favor of a neo-Kantian mechanist psychology, whose principles were both mathematical and laid claim to observation. Many of Herbart's notions, from the static and mechanical threshold to the principle of constancy of energy, influenced both Fechner and Freud. See Wyss, *Psychoanalytic Schools from the Beginning to the Present*, pp. 97–102. Schelling's late philosophy included a neo-Platonic or emanationist *Naturphilosophie*, for which the unity of nature and spirit proceeded from the Absolute, or the "World Soul." See Ellenberger, *Discovery of the Unconscious*, pp. 202–3. For Freud's use of these ideas, see Jones, *Life and Work of Sigmund Freud*, vol. 1, p. 367. It was Herbert Spencer who used the concept of nerve force for theories of reflexes. See Ritvo, *Darwin's Influence on Freud*, p. 185.

18. See Ritvo, *Darwin's Influence on Freud*, pp. 15–19.

19. See Sternhell's remarkable discussion of Le Bon, Barrès, Sorel, and others, in *La Droite révolutionnaire*, pp. 148–50. Le Bon posited a general unconscious, governed by unknown forces. For him, "the natural condition of all beings is to be enslaved." Here, we see the relationship between reductionist mechanism and political totalitarianism.

20. See Freud, "Massenpsychologie und Ich-analyse," in GW 13: 77. Freud immediately points out that Le Bon failed to explain *why* it is that when individuals form crowds, something like a new organism, a mass-creature, is formed: "By himself, LeBon does not answer this question, he assumes the transformation of the individual in the mass and describes it in expressions that stand in good accord with the fundamental provisions of our depth psychology" (my translation).

21. This included Freud's borrowing Darwin's notion of the primal horde for his 1913 *Totem and Taboo*, to his struggle against Oswald Spengler and the German intellectuals of *Kultur*, for whom civilization evolved organically out of a given culture as the "destiny" of that culture. See Assoun, "Structure et principes de la métapsychologie," p. 575, citing Spengler, *Decline of the West*, "Introduction," Section 12.

22. See MacIntyre's classic, *The Unconscious*, p. 25.

23. See Sadoff, *Sciences of the Flesh*, pp. 24–25.

24. See Freud, "The Unconscious" (1915), in *Sigmund Freud: Collected Papers*, vol. 4, p. 100. Hereafter cited as CP.

25. In the 1870s, English psychologists like William Carpenter and G. H. Lewes spoke of "unconscious cerebrations" and "unconscious sensual and volitional processes," respectively. See Carpenter, *Principles in Mental Physiology*, and Lewes, *Study of Psychology*. Cited by Manson, "Tumbling Ground for Whimsies?" pp. 152–54 and 166.

26. See Freud, "The Question of Lay Analysis," in GW 14: 264; emphasis added.

27. See Freud, "Some Elementary Lessons in Psychoanalysis," for his last attack on parallelism, in GW 17: 143–44 and 146.

28. Freud, *General Introduction to Psycho-analysis*, p. 223. See also Wyss, *Psychoanalytic Schools*.

29. Cited by Manson, "Tumbling Ground for Whimsies?" p. 160.

30. Freud, "Difficulty on the Path of Psychoanalysis (1917)," in GW 12: 8; cited by Ritvo, *Darwin's Influence on Freud*, p. 22.

31. Binswanger, *Sigmund Freud*, pp. 7 and 9.

32. As Assoun puts it, quoting Freud's "On Psychoanalysis" (1910): "The dynamic explanation of the conscious-unconscious cleavage, effected 'through the conflict of psychic forces' as a 'result of an active struggle between two psychic groupings the one against the other' allows us to dispense with a conceptions like that of 'an innate capacity of the psychic apparatus for synthesis.'" See Assoun, "Structure et principes de la métapsychologie,"pp. 385–86.

33. Sadoff, *Sciences of the Flesh*, pp. 66., 68. Sadoff cites the British neurologist Thomas Laycock. The list is longer than I cite here.

34. This was in response to the first waves of feminism in Austria and to the rise in the Jewish population in Berlin and in Vienna, which was met with swells of anti-Semitism and variations of racial essentialisms. See Gilman, *Jew's Body*, chapter 3, "Jewish Psyche: Freud, Dora, and the Idea of the Hysteric," and Albert Lindemann, *Anti-Semitism before the Holocaust*, pp. 53–57. Also see Sternhell, *La Droite révolutionnaire*, pp. 146ff.

REFERENCES

Assoun, Paul-Laurent (1997) *La Psychanalyse*. Paris: Presses Universitaires de France.

Binswanger, Ludwig (1957) *Sigmund Freud: Reminiscences of a Friendship*. Translated by N. Guterman. New York: Grune and Stratton.

Boehlich, Walter (ed.) (1990) *The Letters of Sigmund Freud to Eduard Silberstein, 1871–1881*. Translated by A. J. Pomerans. Cambridge, MA: Harvard University Press.

Boothby, Richard (2001) *Freud as Philosopher, Metapsychology after Lacan*. New York: Routledge.

Brennan, Teresa (1992) *The Interpretation of the Flesh: Freud and Femininity*. New York: Routledge.

Brentano, Franz (1995) *Descriptive Psychology*. Translated by Benito Müller. New York: Routledge.

Breuer, Josef, and Freud, Sigmund (1966) *Studies on Hysteria*. Edited by James Strachey and Anna Freud. New York: Basic Books.

Butler, Judith (1997) *The Psychic Life of Power: Theories in Subjection*. Stanford, CA: Stanford University Press.

Cavell, Marcia (1993) *The Psychoanalytic Mind: From Freud to Philosophy*. Cambridge, MA: Harvard University Press.

Crane, Tim, and Patterson, Sarah (eds.) (2000) *History of the Mind-Body Problem*. New York: Routledge.

Derrida, Jacques (1996) *Résistances de la psychanalyse*. Paris: Editions Galilée.

Ellenberger, Henri F. (1970) *The Discovery of the Unconscious: The History and Evolution of Dynamic Psychiatry*. New York: Basic Books.

Felman, Shoshana, and Laub, Dori (1991) *Testimony: Crises of Witnessing in Literature, Psychoanalysis, and History*. New York: Routledge.

Freud, Sigmund (1959) "The Unconscious." In *Sigmund Freud: Collected Papers*, vol. 4. Translated by Joan Riviere. New York: Basic Books.

Freud, Sigmund (1972) *Gesammelte Werke*. Frankfurt am Main: Fischer Verlag.

Gardner, Sebastian (1991) "The Unconscious." In Jerome Neu (ed.), *The Cambridge Companion to Freud*. Cambridge: Cambridge University Press.

Gilman, Sander (1991) *The Jew's Body*. New York: Routledge, Chapman and Hall.

Hamann, Richard, and Hermand, Jost (1973) *Stilkunst um 1900*. Munich: Nymphenburger Verlagshandlung.

Irigaray, Luce (2002) *To Speak Is Never Neutral*. Translated by Gail Schwab. New York: Continuum.

Jones, Ernest (1963) *The Life and Work of Sigmund Freud*. Edited by Lionel Trilling and Steven Marcus. Garden City, NY: Doubleday.

Kristeva, Julia (1995) *New Maladies of the Soul*. Translated by Ross Mitchell Guberman. New York: Columbia University Press.

Kristeva, Julia (2000) *The Sense and Non-sense of Revolt*. Translated by Janine Herman. New York: Columbia University Press.

Kristeva, Julia (2002) *Intimate Revolt*. Translated by J. Herman. New York: Columbia University Press.

Le Rider, Jacques (1982) *Le Cas Otto Weininger: Racines de l'antiféminisme et de l'antisémitisme*. Paris: Presses Universitaires de France.

Levine, Michael P. (ed.) (2000) *The Analytic Freud: Philosophy and Psychoanalysis*. New York: Routledge.

Lindemann, Albert (2000) *Anti-Semitism before the Holocaust*. Essex: Longman Press.

MacIntyre, Alasdair (1997) *The Unconscious: A Conceptual Analysis*. Bristol, UK: Thoemmes Press.

Manson, Neil Campbell. (2000) "A Tumbling Ground for Whimsies? The History and Contemporary Role of the Conscious/Unconscious Constrast." In Tim Crane and Sarah Patterson (eds.), *History of the Mind-Body Problem*. New York: Routledge, pp. 148–68.

Radden, Jennifer (2000) "Love and Loss in Freud's *Mourning and Melancholia*: A Re-reading." In M. Levine (ed.), *The Analytic Freud*. New York: Routledge, pp. 211–30.

Ritvo, Lucille (1990) *Darwin's Influence on Freud: A Tale of Two Sciences*. New Haven, CT: Yale University Press.

Rorty, Amélie Oksenberg (2000) "Affects, Mourning and the Erotic Mind." In M. Levine (ed.), *The Analytic Freud*. New York: Routledge, pp. 195–209.

Sadoff, Dianne (1998) *Sciences of the Flesh: Representing Body and Subject in Psychoanalysis*. Stanford, CA: Stanford University Press.

Sternhell, Ze'ev (1978) *La Droite révolutionnaire: 1885–1914. Les Origines françaises du Fascisme*. Paris: Editions du Seuil.

Weber, Samuel (2000) *The Legend of Freud*. Stanford, CA: Stanford University Press.

Wyss, Dieter (1973) *Psychoanalytic Schools from the Beginning to the Present*. Translated by Gerald Onn. New York: J. Aronson.

Zanuso, Billa (1986) *The Young Freud: The Origins of Psychoanalysis in Late 19th Century Viennese Culture*. Oxford, U.K.: Blackwell Publishers.

CHAPTER 24

PHENOMENOLOGICAL AND HERMENEUTIC MODELS

Understanding and Interpretation in Psychiatry

MICHAEL ALAN SCHWARTZ
OSBORNE P. WIGGINS

PSYCHOPATHOLOGY AND PSYCHOTHERAPY IN PRESENT-DAY PSYCHIATRY

PSYCHIATRY is moving through a period in which its basic subject matter—namely, the experiential world of its patients—seems inaccessible and unknowable. Contemporary psychiatry does claim that there are certain aspects of mental disorders that we can know. Indeed, psychiatry is experiencing a time of steady growth of knowledge in particular areas. Neurobiology and psychopharmacology seem to be based on firm scientific foundations, and these important fields constitute a considerable part of the picture of psychiatric understanding and treatment. Moreover, psychiatry has developed manuals of diagnostic categories, the *Diagnostic and Statistical Manual of Mental Disorders* and *The Tenth Revision of the International classificatin of Diseases* (ICD-10), which are highly regarded for the rigorous procedures by which they have been constructed and revised.

It is inevitable, then, that traditional psychiatric concerns like psychopathology and psychotherapy would fall within the shadow cast by these steadily advancing fields. What is not inevitable, we think, is that, in comparison with these other fields, psychopathology and psychotherapy would fall into the disrepute into which they have in fact fallen. This disrepute is not the result of the intrinsic merits of psychopathology and psychotherapy. We believe that, for a large part, it is due to political and economic forces that today powerfully shape the reality of psychiatry. Economic forces impose limitations on the time psychiatrists can spend with patients, and political pressures enforce these limitations by dictating treatments that take no longer than the little time allowed (Schwartz et al. 2002).

Aiding the economic and political forces, however, is a particular view of psychiatric "science." It is assumed in many quarters—even in those quarters unhappy with the assumption—that the methodology used in drug trials on large populations of subjects and the methodology employed in neurobiology are the sole scientific methodologies. Or, if the field of scientific proof is admitted to reach further, the natural sciences—sometimes called "the hard sciences"—still define the paradigm. Since it is impossible to adapt these methodologies so that they can be applied in psychopathology and psychotherapy, the latter two fields are assumed to be doomed to unscientific stagnation.

Much is lost, however, with the withering away of psychopathology and psychotherapy: specifically, a large part of the understanding of mental disorders is forfeited. Moreover, with the loss of this understanding comes a fragmentation and an incoherence in psychiatric conceptualization and treatment. Psychiatrists sometimes deal with this incoherence and fragmentation by claiming that they are "pragmatists": they do "whatever works." This, of course, is only a direct admission that they have little understanding of what they are doing.

Before we entirely despair of the possibility of placing psychopathology and psychotherapy on respectable foundations, we think it wise to reexamine the subject matters of these areas and to try to determine how an understanding of them might be attainable. If the experiential worlds of patients are the subject matter of psychopathology and psychotherapy, then we should note that at least in everyday life we assume that we comprehend the experiential worlds of other people all the time. In my daily interactions with other people I regularly engage in conversations with them, and these conversations often conclude with the two of us believing that we have understood each other sufficiently to be able even to predict more or less what the other person will do. Either one of us may be mistaken, of course, but this only shows that, when we make mistakes in understanding each other, there are ways that those mistakes may be discovered and corrected. In other words, even in daily life our understanding of other people progresses, and not least because false understandings can be proven false and then rectified. It seems to us, therefore, that already in everyday life we find the roots of an evidence-based knowledge of the experiential worlds of other human beings. The evidence is what people do, what they say, and how they act. In the face of this evidence, my beliefs about them and their experience can be confirmed, refuted, or restructured. What we need, then, is further reflection on this everyday, prescientific understanding of other people in order to determine how to render it more rigorous, rational, and testable by confrontation with the given facts.

Around the close of the nineteenth century and into the beginning of the twentieth, a number of German philosophers and social scientists did just this. They were seeking to define and secure a solid methodology for the social sciences (*Geisteswissenschaften*). Today we call that methodology "hermeneutics." The philosophers and social scientists we have in mind are Wilhelm Dilthey (1977), Georg Simmel (1977), Max Weber (1949), and, in psychiatry, Karl Jaspers (1963, 1965, 1968a, 1968b). We shall refer collectively to these thinkers as "hermeneuticians." They noticed the understanding of one person by another in everyday life and sought to sharpen and refine that understanding into a scientific method. We here try to clarify and endorse their efforts. We suggest that this methodology, with some further refinement, can provide a sure foundation for psychopathology and psychotherapy.

HERMENEUTICS AND UNDERSTANDING

At the outset we must introduce a key term, one that the hermeneuticians adopted from everyday speech and turned into a technical methodological term. In everyday speech one speaks — as we have spoken — of one person *understanding* another. We mean by this simply that one person "makes sense" of another person (Taylor 1985: 15). We may pose the question then: *How does* one person make sense of another person, of the other person's experiences and behaviors? We shall follow the hermeneuticians in using this word "understanding" (*Verstehen*) to denote the way in which one person comprehends the experiential world of another person (Dilthey 1977; Simmel 1977, 1980; Weber 1949; Jaspers 1963, 1965, 1968a, 1968b).

The peculiarity of "understanding" as a form of comprehension is that it consists of a way of apprehending something that is not and can never be directly given: namely, the mental life of another person. And yet, this reality that is not and cannot be directly given to me (namely, someone else's mind) is presented by means of something that is directly given (namely, that other person's *expressions*: his or her words, bodily gestures, and facial expressions). In understanding another person, then, I comprehend that person's experiential world via his or her overt expressions of that world (Taylor 1985).

For the German hermeneuticians, the behavior of another person is not simply something I directly observe because, when I directly observe that behavior, I also indirectly apprehend its meaning. The meaning of the behavior is co-presented along with the behavior itself: human behavior and its meaning form a unity, even for me, the external observer. Hermeneuticians thus speak of "meaningful behavior." Understanding is the unified apprehension of directly given behavior and its indirectly presented meaning.

We now illustrate and analyze further the components of this "meaningful behavior" that forms the subject matter of understanding. When I encounter another person and see him smiling, I perceive his smile as expressing an emotion, in most cases the emotion of happiness, amusement, or satisfaction. The observable smile thus performs an expressive function: when I perceive it, I assume the existence of something unperceivable—namely, a particular mental state of the other person. It is this fact that an observable aspect of a person can express an unobservable aspect of the person that led hermeneuticians to speak of "meaningful behavior." If I know more about this other person, I may even assume that I know what he is smiling about. When I see him smiling, I may assume that he is happy about his new job. But how did I learn this "more" about him? This, too, I must have learned through encountering other aspects of his or someone else's meaningful behavior. I may have overheard him tell his wife about his new job, and the tone of his voice and his animated gestures may have expressed his happiness about it. Thus, his smile has the meaning it has for me because other aspects of his behavior have had the meaning they had. Meanings, then, acquire their specific significance from the overall context of meaning within which I encounter them. Hermeneuticians speak, accordingly, of the wider "context, connectedness, or nexus of meaning" that one must comprehend to stand a chance of construing a particular meaning accurately. Meanings depend on one another. Hence if I see a person smiling, but when he speaks his tone of voice evinces depression, I may perceive his smile as forced or feigned, as not expressing happiness after all (Taylor 1985).

From this discussion it can be noted that the term "meaningful behavior" as used by the hermeneuticians is equivocal. We try to surmount this equivocation by explicating the different but interconnected realities to which it refers. The three basic constituents of "meaningful behavior" are as follows:

1. The *subjective (psychological) experience* of the subject: the mental process of the experiencing subject—in our example, the person's happiness.
2. The *expression* of that experience: the "medium" through which the experience is overtly expressed, such as language, facial expression, and bodily movement and gesture—in our example, the man's smile or the words he spoke to his wife.
3. *That which* the subject is experiencing: the phenomenal "object" of the subject's experience—in our example, his new job.

"Meaningful behavior" is therefore a threefold reality composed of experiential process–expression–experienced object. Notice that the expression *expresses* both the experiential process and the experienced object.

We would like to suggest that it is "meaningful behavior" in this three-dimensional sense that forms the subject matter of psychopathology and psychotherapy. It may be noted in passing that it is also "meaningful behavior" in this threefold sense that forms at least part of the subject matter of psychology. Accordingly, the methods of psychopathology, psychotherapy, and psychology must be able to give us access to this threefold reality. Hence, we need to pose our basic methodological question: How does this reality directly present itself to us? In what way is this reality evidentially given?

This turns out to be a question that we have already answered: it is another person's "expression" (item 2 in the preceding list) that is directly given to an observer. It is thus the expressions of others that furnish the evidence we use to understand their behavior and to determine the accuracy of our understanding. In certain situations, the object as experienced by the other person (item 3 in the preceding list) is also directly given to us: for example, when I see my friend smiling about his daughter's painting while the daughter herself is showing me the painting.

When we claim that "meaningful behavior" consists of the three components of experiential process–expression–experienced object, it should be obvious that it is difficult to isolate such a reality in the flow of human experience. It is only through conceptual abstraction that we can analyze experience and find in it these three components. In such an analysis, we abstract from a much fuller human whole whose components are closely interwoven. Therefore, the correlated items, experiential process–expression–experienced object, must be resituated within this human whole. Mental processes occur along with one another and are immediately succeeded by subsequent mental processes. Moreover, the subsequent processes are what they are because they have arisen out of the preceding ones and have been motivated by them. Similarly, expressions, whether words, bodily gestures, or facial expressions, occur simultaneously with one another and succeed one another. Furthermore, expressions derive their meaningfulness from one another; they depend on one another in order to express the meanings they do express. Likewise, the objects that we experience are given not in isolation but, rather, along with many other objects and as standing in manifold relationships with these other objects. In other words, each single mental process is merely a part of a whole mental life; a single expression is only a member of a whole system of expressions; and each experienced object is only part of an experienced world of objects. Moreover, each of these parts derives its meaningfulness and nature from the other parts that constitute the same whole. The hermeneuticians, then, repeatedly emphasize that, through understanding, we are given access to wholes and to relationships (Dilthey 1977). An experiential process becomes understandable only if we understand its relationships to other experiences of the person; a person's bodily gesture becomes understandable only if we understand its relationships to other expressions he or she makes; and we can understand an object that a person experiences only when we understand its meaningful connections to other objects in that person's world. Understanding, then, must contextualize or recontextualize any single item of experience by grasping its meaningful placement within and relatedness to other items that form the same context (Dilthey 1977).

Furthermore, these different contexts or human wholes are shaped by culture.

A smile may mean one thing in one culture and something else in a different culture. Subjective experiences, expressions, and experienced objects are culturally formed. Hence, it is crucial to know the "cultural code" that informs a person's existence in order to hope to understand that person. This, of course, raises the question of what we can do if we do not know the cultural code. The answer to this question is that we can learn a cultural code we do not know only by working to gain an understanding of expressions from that culture. Here, however, we encounter the hermeneutic circle that will occupy us later (Dilthey 1977; Gadamer 1998).

HERMENEUTICS AND PHENOMENOLOGY

To develop an investigative method for psychopathology, the young psychiatrist Karl Jaspers reworked Edmund Husserl's phenomenological procedures so that they incorporated the hermeneutic insights of Dilthey (1977), Simmel (1977, 1980), and Weber (1949). We have explicated Jaspers's reworking of Husserl's method elsewhere (Wiggins et al. 1992, 1997); therefore, in the next section we discuss basic components of Jaspers's methodology of understanding that we have not adequately treated in other publications.

We would like to indicate, however, that the subject matter of understanding as we have explicated it thus far is "intentionality" as Husserl conceived it. We have spoken of experiencing process–expression–experienced object. Recognizing the strict correlation between experiencing (mental) process and experienced (phenomenal) object is precisely what Husserl (1983) meant to capture when he defined intentionality as the correlation between noetic process and noematic object, or simply "noesis" and "noema." By inserting "expression" between experiencing process and experienced object, we have supplemented Husserl's notion in an important way, but it remains crucial to remember that not every intentional correlation between mental process and intended object is expressed. And understanding aims at deciphering unexpressed realities, too. Hence, it is safest to maintain that the subject matter of understanding is intentionality, whether expressed or unexpressed.

Recognizing this prevents us from misconceiving the subject matter of understanding as merely the other person's mind; the subject matter of understanding includes what the other person's mind is *aware of*: namely, intended objects. In psychiatric understanding, in particular, it is crucial to understand the patient's world—that is, the concatenation of realities that the patient is aware of—precisely as the patient is aware of these realities. Hence, we encounter another central Husserlian thesis: manifold mental processes are synthesized in order to constitute the world of objects that we call "reality." It is this world of objects as constituted by the other person's mental life that the method of understanding aims to penetrate.

Moreover, viewing the subject matter of understanding as intentionality prevents mistaking it as solely "texts." Both Hans-Georg Gadamer (1998) and Paul Ricoeur (1970, 1974) tend to restrict the subject matter of interpretation to texts; Ricoeur has even written an essay titled "The Model of the Text: Meaningful Action Considered as a Text," in which he argues that meaningful action—what we called "meaningful behavior"—is so closely analogous to a text that, for purposes of interpretation, it should be treated that way (1981: 197–221). This restriction ultimately leads to the contorted approaches we see so often today in which every reality is deemed a "text" and can therefore be construed as a grouping of "signs." Some writers even go so far as to assert that the reality is *nothing but* an array of signs or "signifiers." Granted, texts do form part of the subject matter of interpretation, but misconceptions abound when it becomes necessary to reconfigure everything as signs in a text.

With this characterization of understanding and its subject matter in hand, we turn now to an important segment of Karl Jaspers's treatment of it in his *General Psychopathology* (1965: 296–99; 1968a: 355–59). Jaspers presents his conception of understanding in six "fundamental laws." The laws as such he formulates very briefly, but he then provides comments on each. After stating each law, we explicate and paraphrase Jaspers's comments on it, sometimes quoting him directly.

Karl Jaspers's "Fundamental Laws of Psychological Understanding and the Understandable"

Jaspers's explication of the "laws of psychological understanding" appears to be motivated, at least in part, by the desire to warn psychiatrists against assuming that one can fully and finally understand a person. Jaspers's "laws" stress how multifarious and open understanding is. And yet these "laws" also point to the limits and testability of understanding. On the one hand, understanding can never reach closure; on the other hand, understanding can be disproven by the given facts. Following are Jaspers's fundamental laws A through F (1965: 296–99; 1968a: 355–59).

A. *Empirical understanding is interpretation*

All understanding is understanding *of something*, and the "something" that we are seeking to understand includes but also transcends the evidence on which we must ground our understanding. What we are seeking to understand is the person and his or her experienced world. What provides the evidence for understanding him or her, Jaspers says, are the "objectively meaningful facts of [his or her] expressions, actions, and works" (1965: 296–97; 1968a: 356). Since the reality we are seeking to understand goes beyond the evidence on which we can base our understanding, the evidence always remains "inadequate," in Husserl's sense; always, more is "meant" in the interpretation than the evidence fully warrants. Hence, the interpretation always remains a "hypothesis," in the dual sense that its truth is not fully demonstrated by the evidence and yet it must always be confronted with and grounded in evidence.

Jaspers points out that interpretations can be very convincing when they take an initially unintelligible set of "expressions, actions, and works" and, by piecing together meaningful relationships among them, make coherent and unified sense of the whole. When such an interpretation emerges, having moved from disparate fragments to integral sense, its truth may even appear "self-evident." But Jaspers cautions that the "truth" for such an interpretation still depends on its empirical foundation: the evidence in the person's "expressions, actions, and works." Thus, regardless of how "convincing" or "self-evident" it may appear as a meaningful whole, the interpretation still remains a mere "hypothesis." Such a strict reliance on the empirically given is necessary if understanding is to qualify as genuinely "scientific" (1965: 297; 1968a: 356).

B. Understanding occurs in a hermeneutic circle

Some experiences are understandable when considered individually; for example, we can understand that a person's body would recoil in fright in the face of a threatening blow. However, when considered in isolation from others, experiences are understood only poorly and vaguely. Moreover, even when considered in isolation, an experience implicitly refers to the whole of the subject's personality. By its very meaning, an experience refers to those other meaningful experiences that compose the whole. Therefore, in order to understand fully, one must move from the individual experience to the whole of the personality. It is only in the context of this whole that the meaning of the individual experience is fully disclosed. What is truly understandable, then, is unisolatable: it is only when an experience is apprehended in its meaningful relationships to the other components of the personality that it makes full sense. Nevertheless, one can develop an understanding of the whole of a personality only by beginning with some of its individual experiences and trying to determine how they are meaningfully related to one another: one must "build up" the whole by gradually piecing together its parts. Understanding thus moves in a circle (*Kreise*). One must start with individual expressions, consider others, and then conceive of their meaningful connections with one another. Once this larger context is pieced together, one can consider other meaningful facts to determine whether they make sense within this context. If they do, then the context is confirmed (or at least not disconfirmed), and one can then proceed to consider further facts. Of course, it is entirely possible that the examination of new experiences will appear unintelligible when situated within the context of meaning. Then the context will have to be reconceived to incorporate the meanings of these new experiences. In this way, both individual experiences and the context within which these experiences attain full meaningfulness undergo modification as the investigator moves through the circle (Jaspers 1965: 297; 1968a: 356–57).

C. Opposites are equally understandable

Having in law B discussed the relationships of parts to wholes, Jaspers warns in law C against a tendency to leap to a conclusion regarding the whole when only some of the parts have been understood. This tendency exists because it seems to "make sense"—be understandable—that if a person has certain characteristics, then he or she would have certain others, too. Jaspers gives an example: "We can understand how a weak and miserable individual would be malicious, disagreeable, envious, and vengeful toward rich, talented, happy, and strong persons, how psychic poverty is related to bitterness." It would be a mistake, however, if the interpreter assumed the malicious, disagreeable, envious, and vengeful attitude on the basis of evidence only for the weakness and the misery. Such a "mental whole" would make sense, but so would others. Jaspers's example continues: "But we can understand equally well how a weak and miserable individual can be honest about himself and his reality; he can be unassuming and love what he himself is not; and in the uprush of this love he can create what he can within his limited possibilities and thereby purge his soul in the school of need and pain" (1965: 297; 1968a: 357). Jaspers is here pointing to the complexity and ambiguity of possible meaningful connections in the human personality, and he draws from it the inference that the interpreter must always consider alternative, even opposite, interpretations of a personality and be sure to test whatever interpretation is considered by demanding that evidence support *all* its parts.

D. *Understanding can never reach closure*

Those meaningful connections that are understandable are conditioned by factors that are inherently not understandable. As a consequence, our efforts to understand a person inevitably run up against unsurpassable limits.

On the one hand, meaningful connections are conditioned by extramental, neurobiological mechanisms. We shall perhaps be able someday to causally explain the workings of these mechanisms, but causal explanation is a different way of rendering something intelligible. Although these mechanisms are not understandable, they condition and shape what is understandable. Hence, at some point in understanding we will have to halt and recognize that further understanding is impossible. On the other hand, the freedom of the person whom one is seeking to understand conditions that understanding. Freedom gives birth to experiences that are understandable, but this source of experiences is not itself understandable (1965, 298; 1968a, 358).

Even with the death of a person, we cannot say that now he or she is fully understandable. As a matter of fact, it is perhaps more accurate to say that now he or she can never be understood. We must at least concede that we have been denied the source of further experiences, expressions, and behavior and that, as a result, we shall obtain no further evidence about that person. The death of our subject prohibits our access to what we need in order to understand him or her.

E. *There is endless interpretability*

Whether it is a question of myths, the contents of dreams, or the contents of psychosis, Jaspers writes, everything turns out to be endlessly interpretable. Almost as soon as one seeks to establish a meaning for something, another possible meaning for it appears. No interpretation, therefore, is ever final. Jaspers writes, "Understanding and that which is understandable is in motion" (1965: 299; 1968a: 358). Even the self-interpretation of one's own life—and even when the external facts of it remain unaltered—can change, thereby changing the *meaning* of external facts that in other respects remain unaltered. Self-interpretation can also move to other depths, and from this deeper level the earlier understanding can appear provisional, partial, and mere foreground.

As a result, understanding should not be oriented by the standards of the natural sciences or the rules of formal logic. Criteria for the truth of understanding lie, for Jaspers, in intuitability, connectedness, depth, and richness (1965: 299; 1968a: 358–59). By "intuitability" Jaspers seems to have in mind an interpretation that penetrates to the innermost heart of the matter. An interpretation is better, then, to the extent that it grasps the unifying core of the person in the light of which his or her manifold behaviors make sense. "Connectedness" may signify relatedness, congruity, and coherence of meaning. An interpretation is better to the degree that its meaningful parts cohere, fit together, and coalesce. "Depth" seems to refer to inclusion of all the various levels of meaning. A "deeper" interpretation might be one that encompasses more of these different layers of meaning. "Richness" might connote the inclusiveness or scope of understanding. An interpretation that encompasses all the objectively meaningful facts and is able to make sense of new ones as they emerge is better than interpretations that cannot.

Thus, while there are ways to judge some interpretations to be better than others, there are no final or conclusive interpretations. As Jaspers writes, "Understanding remains in the sphere of the possible, offering itself constantly as provisional and as a mere proposal" (1965: 299; 1968a: 359).

F. *Understanding is illumination and unmasking*

The process of understanding can proceed in two remarkably different directions. It can often seem malicious when it unmasks deceptions, and it can seem benevolent when, by throwing light on what is truly important in a person, understanding affirms it. Both directions belong intrinsically to understanding.

Jaspers appears to be concerned that the unmasking thrust of understanding had become dominant, at least in his own time. "Whether motivated by skepticism or hate," Jaspers writes, "people seek only to 'see through' everything." For this kind of malicious understanding, truth consists in "seeing through" the universal untruth. Everything that a person does, says, and wants is turned into its opposite. Unmasking psychology debunks and finds "nothing but." To this point it seems that Jaspers has been criticizing the extremist tendencies in the psychology of unmasking. But at this juncture he appears to adopt a more appreciative view of it: he begins to explain how unmasking psychology can serve as a necessary purgation of self-deception so that what is truly essential in the person can come to light. As Jaspers phrases it, "This unmasking psychology is the indispensable purgatory in which a human being must test and prove him- or herself, purify and transform him- or herself." This kind of self-purgation can lead to the positive gains of self-understanding: "illuminating psychology is the mirror in which affirmative self-consciousness and the loving awareness of others becomes possible" (1965: 299; 1968a: 359).

Jurgen Habermas's Conception of Communicative Action

Jurgen Habermas has critically discussed the hermeneutic tradition (1970; Habermas et al. 1971). He develops his own positive conception of "general interpretation" in his examination of Freudian psychoanalysis (Habermas 1971: 246–73). Habermas points out that in the clinical therapeutic situation there exists an interaction between physician and patient that occurs through communication. The understanding of the patient is then different from the interpretation of a text because the patient responds and can always respond further, and the therapist responds to the patient's responses. Hence, understanding here is an ongoing reciprocal process: it takes the form of a dialogue between two living partners.

Granted, this dialogue differs from an ordinary conversation between two people. The physician has a critical and, one may even say, suspicious attitude toward what the patient says. The therapist to some extent objectifies the patient because what the patient says is not "taken at face value." Rather, what the patient says is critically examined for what it might "really" indicate about him or her. The therapist's purpose is to uncover the significance of the patient's statements that remain concealed from the patient him- or herself. But this uncovering process requires that the patient "say more" in response to the therapist's questions and probings. At each step of the way, the physician entertains anticipations (*Vorgriffe*) of what the dialogue will reveal. But these anticipations are held tentatively and self-critically because they must be carefully tested against the evidence that continues to emerge. As Habermas writes, "they too are hypotheses that can prove wrong" (1971: 259). The therapist's understanding thus undergoes repeated restructuring and reformulation as the dialogue unfolds.

We think Habermas's conception of understanding as communicative interaction between two active participants fruitfully extends Jaspers's view. The fact that the subject of interpretation "talks back" and can therefore always reveal more "objectively meaningful facts" about him- or herself imparts a dynamic development to the process of understanding that Jaspers does not adequately appreciate.

HERMENEUTIC PSYCHOPATHOLOGY AND PSYCHOTHERAPY

Jaspers advocates a multiperspectival approach to mental disorders. His criticisms of the various "schools," "orientations," and "theories" in psychiatry usually consist in pointing out their unavoidable one-sidedness. In most cases, he shows appreciation for some of the school's insights, but he also insists on recognizing what it has overlooked. He notes that the school provides useful concepts, but that these concepts constitute merely one perspective among others and hence remain partial in their depiction of reality. Nevertheless, we cannot move beyond one-sided perspectives. There can be no all-inclusive theory of mental disorders: the human reality in which mental disorders are found is too complex and unfathomable. As a result, the comprehension and treatment of mental disorders in the lives of human beings require multiple sets of concepts and treatment modalities (McHugh et al. 1998; Slavney et al. 1987). If Jaspers were writing today, he would no doubt praise the advantages of pharmacotherapy while also specifying its limitations and demonstrating the need to supplement it with other approaches. He would admire the increased knowledge of the brain we have acquired through neurobiology while also insisting on the expanses of our continuing ignorance. Hence, there arises the need for psychopathology and psychotherapy as additional tools for psychiatric conceptualization and practice.

Psychopathology is a science of the *general*. Psychotherapy is a practice-guided investigation of the *individual*. Psychopathology seeks to define the general kinds of pathological mental processes and to delineate their regular relationships with one another. Psychotherapy aims at understanding the life situation of a particular patient sufficiently to treat the patient's mental problems. Psychopathology receives practical application in psychotherapy; psychopathology furnishes concepts by means of which at least some of the patient's difficulties can be understood and therefore more effectively treated.

Both psychopathology and psychotherapy should employ the method of understanding as we have sketched it, following Jaspers and Habermas. This method allows the practitioner to base his or her claims on evidence, but it also explains why this evidence always remains inadequate as proof of the certainty of these claims. The method provides access to the unperceivable reality of the patient's experiential world, and it also shows why this reality admits of manifold alternative interpretations. These features of the method result from the nature of the subject matter that the method is designed to investigate. Attempts to impose other methods on this subject matter — because they are supposedly "more scientific" — would only distort it.

REFERENCES

Dilthey, Wilhelm (1977) *Descriptive Psychology and Historical Understanding*. Translated by R. M. Zaner and K. L. Heiges. The Hague: Martinus Nijhoff.

Gadamer, Hans-Georg (1998) *Truth and Method*. Translated by Joel Weinsheimer and Donald G. Marshall. New York: Continuum.

Habermas, Jurgen (1970). *Zur Logik der Sozialwissenschaften*. Frankfurt am Main: Suhrkamp.

Habermas, Jurgen (1971) *Knowledge and Human Interests.* Translated by Jeremy J. Shapiro. Boston: Beacon Press.

Habermas, Jurgen, Henrich, Dieter, and Luhmann, Niklas (eds.) (1971) *Hermeneutik und Ideologiekritik.* Frankfurt am Main: Suhrkamp.

Husserl, Edmund (1970) *Logical Investigations,* Vol. 2. Translated by J. N. Findlay. New York: Humanities Press.

Husserl, Edmund (1983) *Ideas Pertaining to a Pure Phenomenology and to a Phenomenological Philosophy, First Book.* Translated by F. Kersten. The Hague: Martinus Nijhoff.

Jaspers, Karl (1963) *Gesammelte Schriften zur Psychopathologie.* Berlin: Springer-Verlag.

Jaspers, Karl (1965) *Allgemeine Psychopathologie,* 8th ed. Berlin: Springer-Verlag.

Jaspers, Karl (1968a) *General Psychopathology.* Translated by J. Koenig and Marian W. Hamilton. Chicago: University of Chicago Press.

Jaspers, Karl (1968b) "The Phenomenological Approach in Psychopathology." *British Journal of Psychiatry* 114: 1313–23.

McHugh, Paul R., and Slavney, Phillip R. (1998) *The Perspectives of Psychiatry,* 2nd ed. Baltimore: Johns Hopkins University Press.

Ricoeur, Paul (1970) *Freud and Philosophy: An Essay on Interpretation.* Translated by Denis Savage. New Haven: Yale University Press.

Ricoeur, Paul (1974) *The Conflict of Interpretation: Essays in Hermeneutics.* Edited by Don Ihde. Evanston, IL: Northwestern University Press.

Ricoeur, Paul (1981) *Hermeneutics and the Human Sciences.* Edited and translated by John B. Thompson. Cambridge: Cambridge University Press.

Schwartz, Michael Alan, and Wiggins, Osborne P. (2002) "The Hegemony of the DSMs." In John Z. Sadler (ed.), *Descriptions and Prescriptions: Values, Mental Disorders and the DSMs.* Baltimore: Johns Hopkins University Press, pp. 199–209.

Simmel, Georg (1977) *The Problems of the Philosophy of History: An Epistemological Essay.* Translated by Guy Oakes. New York: Free Press.

Simmel, Georg (1980) *Essays on Interpretation in Social Science.* Translated by Guy Oakes. New York: Free Press.

Slavney, Phillip R., and McHugh, Paul R. (1987) *Psychiatric Polarities: Methodology and Practice.* Baltimore: Johns Hopkins University Press.

Taylor, Charles (1985) "Interpretation and the Sciences of Man." In *Philosophical Papers* 2: *Philosophy and the Human Sciences.* Cambridge: Cambridge University Press, pp. 15–57.

Weber, Max (1949) *The Methodology of the Social Sciences.* Translated by Edward A. Shils and Henry A. Finch. New York: Free Press.

Wiggins, Osborne P., and Schwartz, Michael Alan (1997a) "Commentary on 'Encoding of Meaning.'" *Philosophy, Psychiatry, and Psychology* 4(4): 277–82.

Wiggins, Osborne P., and Schwartz, Michael Alan (1997b) "Edmund Husserl's Influence on Karl Jaspers's Phenomenology." *Philosophy, Psychiatry, and Psychology* 4(1): 15–36.

Wiggins, O. P., Schwartz, M. A., and Spitzer, M. (1992) "Phenomenological/Descriptive Psychiatry: The Methods of Edmund Husserl and Karl Jaspers." In Manfred Spitzer, Friedrich Uehlein, Michael A. Schwartz, and Christoph Mundt (eds.), *Phenomenology, Language and Schizophrenia.* New York: Springer Verlag, pp. 46–59.

CHAPTER 25

NEUROBIOLOGICAL MODELS

An Unnecessary Divide — Neural Models in Psychiatry

ANDREW GARNAR

VALERIE GRAY HARDCASTLE

BIOLOGICAL psychiatry is coming to dominate the treatment of mental illness, because of both the successes of psychopharmacology and its perceived cost-effectiveness by managed health care and government agencies. However, psychiatry as a whole aims at "being physicians for both the mind and the brain" (Andreasen 1997: 593). The strong reductionism present in current biological psychiatry undercuts that goal. Part of what makes this situation all the worse is a rift between biological and psychosocial approaches within psychiatry and the consequent insularity of these wings. As a result, mind and subjectivity are marginalized in psychiatry's neural models.[1] We explore these points by looking at examples of biological approaches to understanding two mental disorders: schizophrenia and addiction.

As we show, biological models in psychiatry depend on an implicit concept referred to as "soma" in what follows. Soma is what holds together biological psychiatry's conception of the body. It is an overarching conception of the kind of thing a body is. As such, it sets the agenda for psychiatric research on bodies: given that the body is such and such kind of thing, psychiatrists expect to find these other kinds of things as part of the body or related to it. For reasons that will become clear, it is our contention that soma functions in a manner analogous to a Sellarsian Given.[2] As a result, it also suffers the problems of the Given. Biological psychiatry would do better to approach soma in a different way, thereby opening a genuine place for the mind in neural explanations.

1. Structure of Neural Models

Neural models in psychiatry rely on the findings and theories of the divergent sciences of molecular biology, neurobiology, neuropharmocology, and psychiatric genetics to create a new brain-based psychiatry. Let us consider Hyman and Nestler's (1993) molecular explanation of psychopathology as an example. Their basic story is relatively simple. One starts with the DNA on the chromosomes. Through mRNA, the information on DNA is used to create proteins. These proteins are involved with the construction and maintenance of neurotransmitters, receptors, and regulatory systems. In turn, these systems influence the phenotype. The proteins also produce transcription factors that regulate gene expression. Environmental inputs influence some proteins and synaptic inputs, which then influence others. Hence, environmental inputs can indirectly transform both the phenotype and the transcription factors. The latter can then influence gene expression, which in turn can alter mRNAs, the proteins, and so forth. Their model is illustrated in Figure 25.1.

We can fill in this model schema in different ways, depending on the psychiatric disorder under discussion. In the cases of schizophrenia and addiction, for example, we must still track down the relevant gene(s). It then becomes a matter of determining how the genetic information is coded to make proteins that influence the individual's behavior. It is also necessary to examine the regulatory region of DNA, to see whether there are problems with the promoters involved. Once these factors have been laid out, we need to trace the connections between the proteins and neural network formation.

On the neural level, we must sketch how environmental factors—things like stress—change the cellular functioning. A given stressor might involve the production of certain hormones and, in turn, proteins, which give rise to different transcription factors. These transcription factors might cause changes in the regulatory region that, after a few more cycles, give rise to the phenotypic expression of the schizophrenic or addict.

One of the principle goals of neural models such as these is to avoid the Cartesian intuition that separates the mind and body. Many see the split between mind and body as one of psychiatry's rather antiquated legacies. Some form of radical reductionism or a modified behaviorism could eliminate the split. However, both

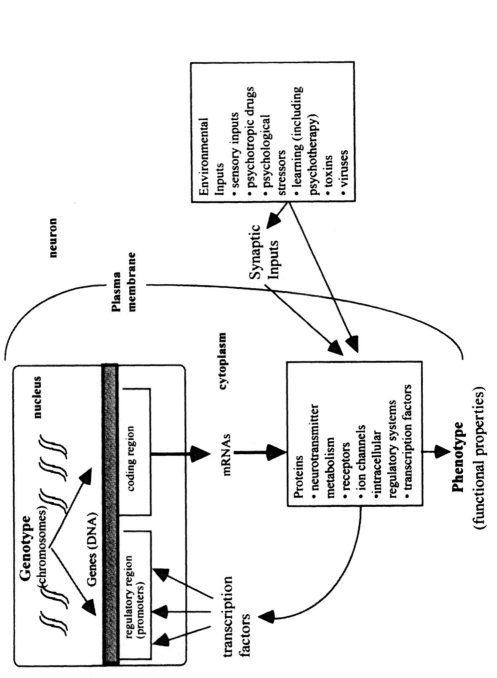

Figure 25.1. Hyman and Nestler's outline for a molecular psychiatry (after Hyman and Nestler 1993: 194)

these routes deny that the mind has any of its own explanatory leverage; the mind ends up being eliminated in favor of biochemical systems or overt behavior. This is not what most psychiatrists want, since they believe the mind should play an important causal role in whatever amalgamation of biological systems psychiatry devises to explain mental disorders and disease.

To avoid the specter of reductionism, Hyman and Nestler propose that causal bridges connect each level of biological system and "that it is a central task of the basic science of psychiatry to elucidate these bridges" (1993: 203). Unfortunately, at this point, we can say little more about the nature of these bridges. Part of what drives the construction of these bridges is practical: "When someone is asked why he hates his mother, an answer based on quantum mechanics or even neural circuitry is likely to be less explanatory than an answer at the psychological level" (203). These various levels have explanatory roles, but which level we turn to for an explanation depends, in part, on what we believe needs explaining. The pragmatics of explanation might not entirely exhaust the concept of causal bridges, however, since it is ambiguous whether these bridges are designed to stave off ontological reductionism (redefining mental entities or episodes in terms of biological entities or episodes), epistemic reductionism (redefining theories of the mind in terms of biological theories), or both.

Let us focus on issues of ontological reduction because it is here that the tensions in biological psychiatry manifest themselves most clearly. On the one hand, neural models propose that there is some sort of causal bridge between the various levels of description. These bridges help prevent reducing all mental phenomena down to the lowest biological level. While there are deep interconnections among genetic material, proteins, the environment, and phenotypes, they each also keep a life of their own, so to speak. Each level is related to those above and below it but cannot be fully accounted for in terms of the levels below. (The picture presented here parallels the discussions of multiple realizibility in philosophy of mind.)

On the other hand, there is a peculiarity to psychiatry's rhetoric that runs counter to this ecumenism about explanation. The goal of neural modeling in psychiatry is to systematize psychiatry in such a way that the work in molecular biology and neuroscience plays a foundational role. While psychological and environmental factors are factors in the account, the biological or molecular level is key. While biological psychiatric inquiry may not start with the brain, the assumption is that there is nonetheless something ontologically and epistemically foundational about it.

This neural or biological foundation is what we refer to as "soma." Within biological psychiatry, soma is intelligible, calculable, stable, and exists independent of human theorizing or intervention. That is, all its properties are already there, waiting to be mapped, classified, and manipulated. In addition, the systems that constitute the body are also ready for human understanding, assuming researchers ask the right questions of it. They can be understood through a matrix of scientific hypothesis and theories that decompose and reassemble them conceptually.

These systems are unchanging; once classified and properly mapped, their model should not change. And the body bound up with soma is essentially like that of Cartesian matter: dead, without the capacity for thought.

It is this final point that brings together the others. Going back to Descartes, we see matter as intelligible, calculable, and stable. Only minds have the capacity to think. Under a neurobiological approach, psychiatry becomes principally a matter of figuring out the correct way to understand the material world. As a result, mind and the mental become marginalized, perhaps even erased entirely.

Soma functions in two simultaneous, but distinct, ways. The first is transcendental. Soma is an abstraction that subsumes all bodies. It is what makes bodies fundamentally *knowable*. The human body—normal or pathological—is determined by, filtered through, soma. There is something about bodies that allows them to be understood in this way. Further still, this method of understanding is the only way to penetrate the veil of appearance to get at the truth of bodies. Part of the power of Figure 25.1 and all other neural models in psychiatry is their alleged universality. What they represent is something that runs through all living human bodies.

The second function is immanent. While soma might be a quasi-Form (in the Platonic sense), it is also embedded within bodies. It is not enough just to have promise of universality when it comes to this sort of research (i.e., the transcendental soma); soma must also live within the body. This guarantees that particular bodies are, in fact, knowable. Every body (hence, everybody) is a particular example of the specific understanding of the body that soma comprises. For instance, any particular body you choose will be made up of the mechanisms described by Figure 25.1 and will be amenable to this sort of analysis.

Soma is analogous to Sellars's (1991) epistemic Givens. The principal similarity is their role as foundation. Epistemic Givens have traditionally served as the starting point for knowledge.[3] Within biological psychiatry, soma functions as the foundation for any understanding of mental illness. Both epistemic Givens and soma are unquestioned within their respective intellectual frameworks. Descartes never doubts those things discovered by the light of nature, nor does Hume mistrust the absolute importance of impressions. Along the same lines, in the theories deployed and developed by biological psychiatrists, soma's primacy is not challenged. That is to say, biological psychiatrists might question soma's foundational role, but that would occur outside the space of theorizing about mental illness.

Moreover, soma falls into a trap similar to that which stymies the Given. One trouble with the Given in Sellars's account is that it must be both epistemic and nonepistemic simultaneously. Soma involves a similar move: it is both a transcendental abstraction and an immanent particular at the same time. Soma is both within bodies and outside of them. This move is absolutely necessary if soma is to serve as a foundation for biological psychiatry. Yet, it is precisely this move that makes the foundationalist impulse a problem. To create a stable foundation, one must use elements that exist outside or beyond the system. But, to be a foundation for understanding the body, these same elements must be part of the body, as well. Hence, the elements have irreconcilable roles. For this reason, Givens of any sort—be they Humean impressions or soma—should be approached with caution. Ignoring the fact that soma is actually something we created to help us to understand particular bodies and ignoring the fact that soma does not actually correspond to anything in the real world means that the stable foundation for biological psychiatry that many desire will elude them.

Therefore, instead of assuming soma to be some sort of foundational entity that allows bodies to be stable objects of knowledge, we should see soma as an intellectual achievement. Hence, soma is not a "thing" per se but a concept used to explain and make sense of kinds of experience. Clearly, the idea that bodies are stable, intelligible, and calculable has yielded a large amount of very productive research. The mistake is in thinking that such properties are intrinsic to the bodies studied. Instead, these properties are part of concepts we use to explain the functioning of these bodies. They are arrived at through all sorts of interactions with bodies, and, in turn, these interactions establish soma and the biological approaches it buttresses as viable concepts for biological psychiatry.[4]

Like Sellars's concept of mind as depicted in "Empiricism and the Philosophy of Mind," the concept of soma is historical. At a particular point, it came to play a key role in psychiatric research. When this exactly occurs is not relevant here. The important point is that this concept has a story. It was developed, took hold, and became part of the background to biological psychiatry.

2. CASE OF SCHIZOPHRENIA

The psychopharmacology of schizophrenia represents both the possibilities and perils of the general approach argued for by Hyman and Nestler. The focus here is on how biological psychiatrists construe the "subjectivity" of schizophrenics.[5] To set the stage properly, we begin with a brief overview of the history of the drugs used to treat schizophrenia and the models that attempt to explain them. What must be kept in mind with the psychopharmacology of schizophrenia is that it is not simply the case that Delay and Deniker synthesized chlorpromazine in 1951 and then all was made right with the treatment of schizophrenia. Instead, a large number of professional, governmental, and social factors contributed to the biological approach to understanding and treating mental illness.

Before the development of antipsychotic medications, most of the treatments for the severely mentally ill, whether somatic or not, were quite limited and generally ineffective. Somatic treatments included lobotomies, insulin coma therapy, and electroconvulsive therapy (Ackerknecht 1968). Even though these treatments were first received with general approval, after World War II their public support quickly dwindled. It was during this period that researchers determined that the drug chlorpromazine (CPZ) has therapeutic effects on schizophrenics (Gelman 1999; Shorter 1997).

Even though chlorpromazine does diminish auditory hallucinations and other positive symptoms of schizophrenia, it also has serious side effects, and it does not work equally well for all schizophrenics. Soon after the discovery of chlorpromazine, a large number of other drugs were developed. Most of these fall into two classes: phenothiazines and butyrphenones. The first class chemically resembles chlorpromazine, the second haloperidol. The differences among these drugs are small; all are about equally effective in ameliorating the positive symptoms of schizophrenia. The major differences among them concern the dosages patients require and the side effects patients develop (Gelman 1999; Lehmann and Ban 1997).

Widespread acceptance of this approach to treating schizophrenia took some time to be achieved. In particular, there was the complicated conflict between the biological and the psychosocial wings of psychiatry.[6] Especially within the United States, psychosocial approaches dominated the treatment of the severely mentally ill (at least at a theoretical level). Since the turn of the century, biological psychiatry had made few major innovations in treatment. CPZ and other psychopharmaceuticals reinvigorated biological approaches to mental illness. Unlike psychosocial approaches, psychopharmacology now seemed to promise a long-term treatment to mental illness. Regardless of whether CPZ and the other drugs actually effected any cures, they did quiet the mental institutions in a way that psychosocial treatments had never done.

Two other factors contributed to the widespread use of antipsychotics. The first was the National Institutes of Mental Health's (NIMH) endorsement in 1964 of CPZ as a safe and effective treatment for schizophrenia.[7] This was the first time the NIMH had ever officially taken a stand on antipsychotics and, given the institute's prominent place in American psychiatry, this was a significant turning point in the widespread acceptance of antipsychotics. The second was the move throughout the 1960s toward deinstitutionalization. Asylums and the like had developed a very bad reputation by 1960, and, with the promise of effective treatments, the Kennedy administration (coordinating with state governments) undertook the task of reforming the U.S. mental health system. By emptying out the asylums, the deinstitutionalization movement set the stage for the contemporary approach among managed care organizations of trying to minimize mental health expenses.

Chlorpromazine constituted the first major breakthrough in the psychopharmacological treatment of schizophrenia. The other drugs refined this method of treatment but did not greatly alter it.

The next breakthrough happened in the late 1980s and early 1990s with the introduction of clozapine. Though it was discussed by psychiatrists as early as 1966, it was not used in North America until much later because it has severe side effects. In the late 1980s, it was resurrected when researchers found that it was effective in many schizophrenics who resisted other medications. After this announcement, clozapine began to see more frequent use.

Clozapine is referred to as an "atypical antipsychotic" because its chemical structure is quite different from those of either the phenothiazines or the butyrphenones. Soon after the psychiatric community accepted clozapine, a number of other similar drugs followed in its footsteps. The principle strength of the newer atypicals is that they do not have the serious side effects of clozapine while still retaining most of its therapeutic value (Gelman 1999; Lehmann and Ban 1997).

Such is the official history of the treatment of schizophrenia. One can see both how social circumstances influenced the treatment of mental illness (thereby, we believe, altering how schizophrenia was understood and approached scientifically) and how psychopharmaceutical research influenced the place soma held in psychiatry's picture of the mind/brain. The history of the schizophrenic therapy is a history of blatant reductionism in psychiatry.

As a result of an increasingly narrow vision for what is relevant in explaining schizophrenia, important aspects of the schizophrenic's personal experience are left out of this so-called biological psychiatry. In both the older and more recent psychiatric discourse on antipsychotics, the schizophrenic subject all but disappears. Specifically, in psychopharmacological texts there are few references, if any, to the mind or self of the patient. Soma is incorporated into these texts, but only through side effects and discussions of the neurophysiology of the brain. Furthermore, there are only limited discussions about the various social dimensions of schizophrenia. Psychopharmacology approaches addressing the "social" dimensions of the illness only through the related discipline of pharmacoeconomics, which analyzes connections between various levels of government, pharmaceutical companies, and psychiatric treatments.[8]

This strange portrait of the schizophrenic subject can be seen throughout the psychiatric literature. Journal articles in psychopharmacology rarely address questions regarding the experiences of the schizophrenic directly. The focus is on the effects and side effects of the drugs, more than on how they restructure the patient's subjectivity. While discussions of effects and side effects of medication do imply aspects of subjectivity, it is only a very narrow part of the broader conversation. There have been numerous discussions of the modes of action of the drugs in question. These, too, portray part of the schizophrenic's subjectivity, but as only a limited element. Subjectivity arises from complex social and biological interactions. While the neurological discussions do refer to aspects of those biological interactions, they present only a rather tiny slice of the discussion, and these references are generally in terms of an idealized soma. That is, neurological discussions focus on how pharmacological treatments might physically affect the "typical" human.

The situation is much the same in psychiatric textbooks and handbooks. Consider Stephen Stahl's *Essential Psychopharmacology* (1996), a recently published and well-reviewed textbook in psychopharmacology. Stahl takes a great deal of care to lay out the fundamental neuroscience behind psychopharmacology and offers rich depictions of the actions of most major psychopharmaceuticals. While lively, detailed, and very descriptive, this book does not touch at all on the patient's experiences with the drugs discussed (with the exception of side effects). Stahl's focus is on the actions of neurons, chemicals, and the like. He does not address how these might translate into subjective experience.

One finds similar discussions in handbooks. The focus is on the mechanisms of action, side effects, when to use one drug rather than another, and similar topics.

For example, while Ronald Pies's *Essential Handbook of Psychopharmacology* (1998) does have an extensive question and answer section that addresses problems of side effects, suggests ways to encourage compliance by the patient, and presents a set of "vignettes" to test the readers' knowledge of antipsychotics, there is no serious discussion of the effects these drugs have on the patient's overall experiences.

However, it must not be thought that psychiatry writ large has obscured the subject. Psychotherapists rely on a number of theories for interpreting the subjectivity of its patients, the most famous being Freudian psychoanalysis. As mentioned, the trouble is that there exists a division of labor between psychopharmacology and psychotherapy. This division of labor operates on several levels. First, there is a division between psychotherapy and biological psychiatry at the clinical level. While many biological psychiatrists are trained in aspects of psychotherapy because it helps them listen to patients, their clinical treatments emphasize pharmacotherapies, and these are considered to be a sufficient course of treatment (Luhrmann 2000). Nonpsychiatrists generally handle the psychosocial aspects of treatment, such as psychotherapy, family therapy, and occupational training. The concomitant discursive rift between biological psychiatrists and psychotherapists makes this division of labor all the more troublesome.

What makes this division even worse, as Luhrmann describes in detail, and as many editorials in psychiatric journals also bemoan, is that managed care seriously limits the role of psychosocial interventions because they cost so much. Managed care is leading biological psychiatry to triumph over psychotherapy, a victory that neither side really wants. As psychosocial intervention is minimized within the treatment protocols of severe mental illness, subjectivity as a genuine category for investigation loses relevance.

In large part this is a practical problem, but there is also a theoretical dimension to the division, which was made clear in a debate focused on whether psychiatry is becoming either "mindless or brainless."[9] The "mindless" aspect arises principally from biological psychiatry, which does little to address patient subjectivity. The flip side is the "brainless" aspect, which arises from psychotherapists who are not concerned with brain functioning (Eisenberg 1986, 2000; Lipowski 1989; Szasz 1985). Especially within the context of the more severe mental illnesses, like schizophrenia, the "mindless" side of psychiatry dominates recent practice. This "mindlessness" obscures the more personal experiences of patients' with these illnesses, which alarms many psychiatrists. The usual response is to find some middle ground that takes a little from each approach, and this move highlights the need for a psychiatry that integrates more fully both mind and body. Practitioners like Hyman and Nestler are quite explicit in saying that psychiatry needs to throw off its lingering Cartesianism; they see Descartes's mind-body dualism as the historical progenitor of the current problem.

The mindless/brainless debate focuses only implicitly on the subjective experience of patients. What is assumed is that psychotherapy adequately addresses issues of subjectivity and selfhood, while biological psychiatry cannot. This is a mistake. Without raising questions of the adequacy of psychotherapy here, let us note that to frame the issue in this way obscures any nascent "subject-constructive" elements within biological psychiatry, whatever they may be. (Following Foucault's 1975, 1976, 1980 discussions of power/knowledge complexes, "subject-constructive" practices simply means that the knowledge generated by biological psychiatrists and its subsequent use presupposes a certain sort of subject and knowledge of how to transform the subject from having a pathological to a normal subjectivity.) We propose that, even though biological psychiatry might not explicitly deal with questions of subjectivity, following arguments from Foucault, biological psychiatry will nonetheless implicitly deal with and transform a patient's subjectivity.

While this debate seems to have run its course, the theme it brings up still resonates in psychiatric journals. For example, recent articles on the philosophy of psychiatry push the integrationist line we too support (Karlsson and Kamppinen 1995; Stein 1998). At the same time, when radical eliminative positions are brought up, they are immediately shot down as irrelevant. In addition, a number of editorials in journals like the *American Journal of Psychiatry* also endorse the idea of an integrationist position.[10]

One can see that the split between biological psychiatry and psychotherapy is both a theoretical problem and a practical problem. The theoretical problem has to do with how to join biological psychiatry and psychotherapy in a cohesive whole. There is a discursive rift between these two groups that neither wants, yet neither seems capable of mending. The practical problem involves the "divide and conquer" strategy that managed care has used on psychiatry to force psychotherapy out of treating severe mental illness. This reifies the theoretical divisions between psychotherapy and biological psychiatry and hence limits the impact of those conversations that do address the subjectivity of schizophrenics in a more robust manner. Both the intellectual divide and the economic forces at work run counter to psychiatry's claim to be concerned with the whole patient.

3. CASE OF ADDICTION

This divide is recapitulated in the research and treatment of addiction. The emphasis of late has been on the neural underpinnings of addictive behavior, with the implicit assumption that once these are mapped out, we will understand all we need to know about how addiction functions. This reductive approach minimizes the role the larger social and psychological forces play in addiction, to the detriment, we believe, of modeling it successfully.

Here is a brief and admittedly selective overview of what we do know about brain chemistry and addiction. In short, addictive substances like ethanol, the opioids, various stimulants, and nicotine, "commandeer" the brain circuits tied to personal motivation; they commandeer one of our affective tagging systems. These alterations in brain chemistry promote the formation of deeply ingrained and highly emotional memories (Institute of Medicine 1997: 38). As a result, we get people who simultaneously crave the addictive substance and are highly motivated to seek it. This is, quite simply, a recipe for personal disaster.

Since the 1950s, when research in rats first showed that we have discrete areas in the brain keyed to significant stimuli or behaviors (Olds and Milner 1954), we have learned a lot about the structure and function of these areas. We originally characterized these circuits as "pleasure centers" in the brain, but it is probably more apt to describe them as reward centers. When these areas light up or become flooded with the neurotransmitter dopamine, our brains pay significant attention to certain events. These events include not only those things we find pleasurable, like consuming food or having sex, but also those things that predict personal rewards, like smelling dinner cooking or seeing one's lover. Highlighting these events as important allows us to recognize and repeat them (cf. Wickelgren 1997).

But, regardless of whether our dopaminergic systems are tied to pleasure or to attention, they go into overdrive when we anticipate or experience especially salient events. In addition, the specific reward circuit indicted in promoting pleasurable activities, the pathway running from the nucleus accumbens (NAc) to the ventral tegmental area (VTA), is sensitive to the substances of addiction (Cooper et al. 1996). Each addictive substance works on this circuit in a different way. While cocaine directly affects dopamine production, for example, ethanol facilitates our GABA-receptors, which then disinhibit dopamine release in the NAc-VTA stream (Tabakoff and Hoffman 1996).

More important, the NAc-VTA circuit is directly tied to the circuits that underwrite our memories. Hence, drugs of abuse indirectly commandeer the circuits that create and maintain our emotionally laden thoughts (Koob 1996). As is now commonly known, memories of especially salient events are likely to be more vivid, more emotional, and more easily triggered. When addicts return to the sights and sounds of where they typically used drugs, the memory of what they did can literally flood their brains.

It is this connection to emotions and memory that makes addiction so confounding and makes the all-too-popular disease model of addiction inappropriate. First articulated by E. M. Jellinek in 1960, the disease model claims that addiction is a "genetically based progressive disease that results in the inability to control one's consumption of [some substance]" (Singer 1997: 10; see also Jellinek 1960, 1962; Levine 1978; Wallace 1982). Once it reaches an advanced stage, victims are no longer able to regulate their own addictive behaviors. If not treated and treated aggressively, victims will continue to indulge until their eventual death.

It would be nice if addiction were a straightforward bodily affliction, something akin to heart disease or diabetes. In those cases, after diagnosis of the chronic condition, and in addition perhaps to prescribing some medication or operating, doctors recommend that patients alter their lifestyles to help prevent further decline. Sometimes patients find these suggestions difficult to follow, especially if they have been leading unhealthy lifestyles for many decades. Still, with practice and encouragement, most manage to shift what they do to promote their own health.

We feel comfortable assigning patients responsibility for the progress of their diseases. We expect people to be able to control their behaviors such that they at least do not encourage further decline. Our reading of AA and other assorted addiction treatment programs is that they try to shove addictions into this sort of disease model: addiction is like heart disease of the brain. With enough encouragement and support, addicts should be able to alter their behavior to halt their own decline. Indeed, by attending meetings, recognizing their powerlessness in the face of their addiction, and turning their lives over to a higher authority, recovering addicts can emerge better, stronger, and personally more successful than before. And if they can't, well, like severe heart disease that triggers defibrillation, the sickness was simply too far along for anyone to control.

However, time and again, the facts weigh against such easy comparisons. All too often, we try to assign people "responsibility" for their behaviors regarding their addictions and are as a result bitterly disappointed. All you have to do, we say, is stop drinking or stop smoking or stop injecting or whatever. How hard can that be? We don't believe addicted people are mentally incompetent. We see them performing responsibly in all other aspects of their lives. Except for their addiction, they appear competent, sane, and in control. Why can't they manage to regulate their addictive behaviors as well?

It is here that simple brain-based explanations of addiction, habit, and controlled behavior break down (for different arguments for the same conclusion, see Fingarette 1988; Peele 1989; Singer 1997; Thombs 1994). Along many dimensions, addiction goes way beyond simple cravings and the NAc-VTA reward circuit. Smokers can fly across the Atlantic without needing to light up, even though they cannot normally go eight to ten hours without smoking. Patients who receive morphine in a hospital and feel withdrawal upon release will not also crave the drug unless they already understand the cause of their symptoms (cf. Elster 1999). Most alcoholics won't drink if there is a heavy price to pay for doing so, even if the drink is sitting in front of them (Fingarette 1988). And yet more than 75 percent of addicted patients who go through an inpatient rehab program relapse within their first year out, and no method for treating addiction appears to be more successful than no treatment at all (Ouimette et al. 1997). Why is this?

Addiction is not a purely natural phenomenon. There are no cases of animal addiction in the wild, even among the higher primates. It requires our peculiar emotional/cognitive constructions and our peculiar social milieu in order to exist. Even then, addictions and addictive behaviors vary widely across cultures and across time. Bulimia, another addictive behavior, was unheard of in the nineteenth century; it is still unheard of outside the West.

We and we alone are the sorts of creatures who become spontaneously addicted to things. What sets us apart? One suggestion is that the connection between our motivational system and emotionally tainted memories holds the key, because it is these memories and feelings we use to create our selves. Something turns off the normal horror reactions to self-destructive behavior if you are caught in a cycle of addiction. That something is the very normalcy the addictive behaviors not only have for the addict but also give to the addict. (Please see Hardcastle forthcoming for a fuller discussion and description of this way of approaching addiction.) An AA recovery assumes that addicts are motivated to stop using, that they are willing and able to share their life stories with a room full of people, and that being sober is better for the addict than using. None of these assumptions may be true.

Those enamored of brain-based explanations of addiction are quick to point out that understanding the dopamine circuits as aids to learning (instead of as pleasure producers) explains why addicts continue to use[10] even though they are no longer getting any sort of pleasure in the activity.[11] Addicts' brains highlight as salient the events that lead to their getting to use. Their brains also recall in vivid Technicolor detail what using does for them, or did for them, at any rate. The alternative—not using and not feeling as they remember feeling—seems too awful to contemplate.

Our plaint is that these explanations don't go far enough. They don't explain why—even when sober, even when the addicts can experience for themselves the alleged advantages of recovering from their addiction, even when they go out of their way to avoid any triggering stimuli, even when they consciously believe that using does them no good at all any more—they still use. To explain fully the mechanisms of addiction and the constraints we face on self-control, we have to supplement the reductive neuroscientific story with psychosocial approaches.

For example, we might do better to think of addiction as a mental device we use to regulate our behaviors, as some sort of habit. Some habits are simple things like picking our toes or cracking our knuckles, and they don't serve any larger purposes. We do these things because they feel momentarily good or they relieve a momentary urge, but we do them for the most part automatically and we see those behaviors as largely inconsequential. Other habits we use to define our very being. We do these things because they express who we are fundamentally. They might feel good as we do them, but they do much more than scratch a momentary itch. They give us a way to define ourselves, to explain ourselves to others, to locate ourselves in our social and cultural environment. They provide the psychological framing for each of us to live a daily life.

Addictions might be such life-defining habits, habits perhaps encouraged and underlined by particular brain chemistries, but habits nonetheless. In this case, chronic addicts don't stop their addictive behaviors because to do so would mean that they could no longer be who they are. Genuine addictions would tap into and feed off the basic scaffolding of our psychologies. Addicts can't stop because they can't genuinely imagine their lives—their particular lives—without the addiction. To stop means to become someone else, someone unknown. And, for most of us, that is a scary thought.

In a nutshell, then, the problem for addicts isn't abusing a substance; it is sobriety itself. Some addicts can reinvent themselves as someone who is recovering or someone sober. These individuals manufacture entirely new life stories, but some, many, cannot. Becoming someone else is hard to do, and most of us simply can't do it. We can't do it in particular when we feel no kinship with the world of recovery or the world of sobriety, the worlds the rest of us inhabit. Addicts might use because they define themselves as Addict. They regulate their lives in terms of their addictive behaviors. Addiction then provides the background for their life stories, the stories they use to create their sense of self. Addicts remain addicted because they don't know, in a profound and fundamental way, how else to be. They cannot conceptually and emotionally bridge the internal gap between seeing oneself as a user and seeing oneself as not a user. To understand addiction, we need to understand both the brain and the mind of the addict.

More accurately: in order to understand addiction, we are going to need to invert the presumed foundation of biological psychiatry. Biological psychiatry takes the brain, or some portion thereof, as the base upon which psychiatric models are constructed. However, it is also possible to think of our brain circuits themselves as subservient to our personal life narratives. To understand and appreciate how we function qua biological organisms, we need to understand first how we mentally place ourselves in our environment, how we think of ourselves as relating to others, and how we have storied our life events. In short: in order to understand human brain activity and human behavior fully, we have first to understand ourselves *as* human.

At the beginning of this chapter, we alluded to a complex set of issues that currently disturb psychiatry. One of these issues is the lingering ghost of Descartes's mind/body split. This split still haunts psychiatry, leading to rifts (at the levels of both theory and therapy) between psychosocial and biological approaches. These rifts are made worse by the current social, economic, and political climate, to the point where the role of psychosocial approaches is becoming increasingly limited.

The cultural and historical dimensions of soma show that it does not have the objectivity assumed by many both inside and outside psychiatry. While not entirely arbitrary, soma still is a concept that we created. It has not always been there, despite what it might feel like for those who have always had it.[12] If soma were some fact existing out in the world, independent of us, one could not challenge it. But it isn't; it is a concept psychiatrists rely on to make sense of bodies. It is a tool. And, because soma is created, it can be challenged. Solutions to these challenges must in part address the explanatory value of soma. In particular, concepts other than soma might work better for biological psychiatry. It might be possible to develop new concepts that allow for the mind to enter back into the space of biological psychiatry. It is our hope that this happens.

NOTES

The order of the authors' names is alphabetical. Their contributions to this essay are equal.

1. For an excellent anthropological account of this, see Luhrmann (2000).

2. In "Empiricism and the Philosophy of Mind," Sellars takes on traditional epistemology, particularly the sort that owes much to Locke and Hume. He uses the concept of the Given, an epistemic thing that ground and makes possible knowledge (in this context at least), to show its incoherence. Consider Hume's impressions, a Given if ever there was one. Impressions are the starting point of his epistemology, that through which everything must be routed.

3. It is important to note a disanaology between soma and epistemic Givens. According to Sellars, a Given is essentially noninferential; this is not quite the case with soma. The development of theories about biological systems is a rather messy business. For a nonpsychiatric example of this biological messiness, see Han-Jörg Rheinberger's *Towards a History of Epistemic Things* (1997). Since soma is bound up with these theories, soma is also somewhat messy. Yet, the very concept of soma implies some sort of directness. While the precise systems that define soma can be complicated, soma promises to be intelligible, capable of being described through the tools of biology.

4. A second disanalogy between Sellars's subject matter and soma creeps in here. Philosophers and others discuss minds and sensory impressions quite frequently. No one, philosopher or psychiatrist, really discusses this thing we have called soma directly. Instead, it is an element that lies behind psychiatric discourse and structures it.

5. It should be noted that "subjectivity" in this discussion is construed very broadly. It covers both the limited sense of the term as used by philosophers of mind (the "first-personness" of experience) to the broader conceptions that are relied on by pragmatists and some poststructuralists (principally Foucault).

6. For two overviews of this conflict, see Ackerknecht (1968) and Shorter (1997).

7. For more on the significance of the NIMH 1964 paper, see Gelmann (1999: 21–37).

8. See, for example, Zito (1998).

9. Curiously, these are the psychiatrists' terms.

10. Two examples of this are Andreasen (1996) and Hyman (2000).

11. This also would help explain schizophrenia and attention deficit disorder (ADD), both of which are tied to abnormal dopamine production or transmission. People with schizophrenia or ADD become distracted by all sorts of sensory (and internal) stimuli that normal brains generally filter out; hence, they can't pay attention to what is really important or significant in their lives.

12. A similar point can be made regarding the mind. The concept seems totally natural because it has been there all along for virtually everyone. Yet, if Sellars is correct, there is a point in humanity's distant past where individuals did not have minds per se. One can also imagine a case like the one Rorty describes, where humans encounter an alien race for whom the concept of minds is utterly meaningless (1979: 70–127).

REFERENCES

Ackerknecht, E. (1968) *Short History of Psychiatry*, 2nd rev. ed. Translated by S. Wolff. New York: Hafner.

Andreasen, N. C. (1996) "Body and Soul." *American Journal of Psychiatry* 153: 589–90.

Andreasen, N. C. (1997) "What Is Psychiatry?" *American Journal of Psychiatry* 154: 591–93.

Cooper, J. R., Bloom, F. E., and Roth, R. H. (1996) "Cellular Formation of Neuropharmacology." In *The Biochemical Basis of Neuropharmacology*, 7th ed. New York: Oxford University Press, pp. 9–48.

Eisenberg, L. (1986) "Mindlessness and Brainlessness in Psychiatry." *British Journal of Psychiatry* 148: 497–508.

Eisenberg, L. (2000) "Is Psychiatry More Mindful or Brainier Than It Was a Decade Ago?" *British Journal of Psychiatry* 176: 1–5.

Elster, J. (1999) *Strong Feelings: Emotion, Addiction, and Human Behavior.* Cambridge, MA: MIT Press.

Fingarette, H. (1988) *Heavy Drinking: The Myth of Alcoholism as a Disease.* Berkeley: University of California Press.

Foucault, M. (1975) *Discipline and Punish: The Birth of the Prison.* Translated by Alan Sheridan. New York: Vintage.

Foucault, M. (1976) *The History of Sexuality: An Introduction,* Vol. 1. Translated by Robert Hurley. New York: Vintage.

Foucault, M. (1980) *Power/Knowledge: Selected Writings and Other Writings 1972–1977.* Edited by Colin Gordon. New York: Pantheon.

Gelman, S. (1999) *Medicating Schizophrenia: A History.* New Brunswick, NJ: Rutgers University Press.

Hardcastle, V. G. (forthcoming) *Constructing Selves.* Cambridge, MA: MIT Press.

Hyman, S. (2000) "The Millennium of Mind, Brain, and Behavior." *Archive of General Psychiatry* 57: 88–89.

Hyman, S., and Nestler, E. (1993) *The Molecular Foundations of Psychiatry.* Washington, DC: American Psychiatric Press.

Institute of Medicine (1997) *Dispelling the Myths about Addiction.* Washington, DC: National Academy Press.

Jellinek, E. M. (1960) *The Disease Concept of Alcoholism.* New Haven, CT: Hillhouse.

Jellinek, E. M. (1962) "Phases of Alcohol Addictions." In D. J. Pittman and C. R. Snyder (eds.), *Society, Culture, and Drinking Patterns.* New York: Wiley, pp. 356–68.

Karlsson, H., and Kamppinen, M. (1995) "Biological Psychiatry and Reductionism: Empirical Findings and Philosophy." *British Journal of Psychiatry* 167: 434–38.

Koob, G. F. (1996) "Drug Addiction: The Yin and Yang of Hedonistic Homeostasis." *Neuron* 16: 893–96.

Lehmann, H., and Ban, T. (1997) "The History of the Psychopharmacology of Schizophrenia." *Canadian Journal of Psychiatry* 42: 152–63.

Levine, H. G. (1978) "The Discovery of Addiction: Changing Conceptions of Habitual Drunkenness in America. *Journal of Studies in Alcohol* 39: 143–74.

Lipowski, Z. J. (1989) "Psychiatry: Mindless or Brainless, Both or Neither?" *Canadian Journal of Psychiatry* 34: 249–54.

Luhrmann, T. M. (2000) *Of Two Minds: The Growing Disorder in American Psychiatry.* New York: Knopf.

Olds, M. E., and Milner, P. (1954) "Positive Reinforcement Produced by Electrical Stimulation of Septal Area and Other Regions of the Rat Brain." *Journal of Comparative and Physiological Psychology* 47: 419–27.

Ouimette, P. C., Finney, J. W., and Moos, R. (1997) "Twelve Step and Cognitive-Behavioral Treatment for Substance Abuse: A Comparison of Treatment Effectiveness." *Journal of Counseling and Clinical Psychology* 65: 230–40.

Peele, S. (1989) *Diseasing of America: Addiction Treatment out of Control.* Boston: Houghton Mifflin.

Pies, R. W. (1998) *Handbook of Essential Psychopharmacology.* Washington, DC: American Psychiatric Press.

Rheinberger, H-J. (1997) *Towards a History of Epistemic Things: Synthesizing Proteins in the Test Tube.* Stanford; Stanford University Press.

Rorty, R. (1979) *Philosophy and the Mirror of Nature*. Princeton: Princeton University Press.

Sellars, W. (1991) *Science, Perception and Reality*. Atascadero, CA: Ridgeview.

Shorter, E. (1997) A *History of Psychiatry: From the Era of the Asylum to the Age of Prozac*. New York: Wiley.

Singer, J. A. (1997) *Message in a Bottle: Stories of Men and Addiction*. New York: Free Press.

Stahl, S. (1996) *Essential Psychopharmacology: Neuroscientific Basic and Practical Application*. New York: Cambridge University Press.

Stein, D. (1998) "Philosophy of Psychopharmacology." *Perspectives in Biology and Medicine* 41: 200–11.

Szasz, T. (1985) "Psychiatry: Rhetoric and Reality." *Lancet* 2: 711–12.

Tabakoff, B., and Hoffman, P. L. (1996) "Alcohol Addiction: An Enigma among Us." *Neuron* 16: 909–12.

Thombs, D. L. (1994) *Introduction to Addictive Behaviors*. New York: Guilford.

Wallace, J. (1982) "Alcoholism from the Inside Out: A Phenomenological Analysis." In N. J. Estes and M. E. Heinemann (eds.), *Alcoholism: Development, Consequences, and Interventions*. St. Louis, MO: Mosby.

Wickelgren, I. (1997) "Getting the Brain's Attention. *Science* 278: 35–38.

Zito, J. M. (1998) "Pharmacoeconomics of the New Antipsychotics for the Treatment of Scizophrenia." *Psychiatric Clinics of North America* 21(1): 181–202.

CHAPTER 26

COGNITIVE-BEHAVIORAL MODELS

Cognitive-Behavior Therapy

EDWARD ERWIN

PART I: HISTORY

WHEN behavior therapy was developed in the late 1950s and 1960s, most of the leading figures in the field, including Joseph Wolpe, Hans Eysenck, and B. F. Skinner, were willing to describe their theoretical position as "behaviorist." In addition, behavior therapy was widely believed to be based on behaviorist foundations. What this meant, in part, was that the behavior therapies were derived from, or their workings could be explained by, conditioning principles, especially principles of classical and operant conditioning. Finally, many spoke of a "behavior therapy paradigm," said to include a commitment to certain philosophical principles, such as logical or methodological behaviorism, the requirement that theoretical concepts be operationally defined, and the demand for experimental testing of both theoretical and outcome hypotheses.

Even in the early period, however, there were disagreements about whether, or to what degree, behavior therapy was based on behavioristic principles and whether the refusal to postulate cognitive or emotional causes was unduly restricting the field. Some, for example, argued that the use of imagery in Wolpe's systematic desensitization technique disqualified it as a behaviorist-based therapy (Breger and McGaugh

1965; Locke 1971). Michael Mahoney published a book (1974) in which he argued for a cognitivist point of view, and, perhaps most important, one of the most influential behavior therapists, Albert Bandura, broke ranks with the behaviorists (1974).

Most of the critics of a behaviorist approach relied primarily on empirical arguments—that is, arguments that contain premises that make reference to observational data. In contrast, Erwin (1978), which Franks (1997: 392) describes as virtually the only single-authored book to deal exclusively with scientific, conceptual, and ethical issues in behavior therapy, argued that empirical arguments had to be combined with philosophical ones to make a serious dent in the behaviorist position. The reason is that, when confronted with empirical objections to their position, many behaviorists fell back on various philosophical principles that, if they were correct, would refute the objection. For example, Gewirtz (1971: 303) objects to Bandura's use of a cognitive concept if it is not operationally defined in terms of independent empirical operations and suggests that its use is pointless if it is so defined. Davison and Neale (1974: 475) make the same sort of objection to Carl Roger's use of the concept of self-actualization.

When confronted with the obvious point that Wolpe was forced to use the concept of mental imagery in his description of systematic desensitization, Eysenck (1979) replied that the critics overlooked the fact that talk of mental imagery was simply shorthand for talk about behavior. When Bandura and his colleagues (Bandura and Adams 1977) presented compelling experimental evidence that cognitive factors and not counterconditioning, as alleged by Wolpe, explained how systematic desensitization works, behaviorists responded by appealing to operationism or, more often, to some principle of methodological behaviorism. In brief, the various principles that underlay methodological behaviorism, operationism, and logical behaviorism were used to shield a behaviorist model against empirical criticisms. To make merely empirical objections without undermining the philosophical and methodological principles accepted by various behaviorists was regarded as question-begging. As MacCorquodale (1970: 84) argued in his defense of Skinner, the Chomsky-Skinner dispute cannot be settled by appeal to "directly relevant facts"; the disagreement between the two, he claimed, is primarily epistemological.

Erwin (1978: ch. 2) challenges the behaviorist position by first arguing that all of the arguments for methodological behaviorism, 12 in all, lack cogency and that the principles of logical behaviorism and operationism are false. The result is that the attempt to shield behavioristic theories from empirical criticisms eventually fails. Once the protective philosophical and methodological principles are stripped away, the empirical data show that behavioristic conditioning principles are, with one important exception, either false, unwarranted, or too narrow in scope to serve as a foundation for behavior therapy (see Brewer's 1974 discussion of the disassociative design experiments and the reply to criticisms of these experiments in Erwin 1978: 109–13). The main exception is Skinner's most important principle of learning, the Principle of Positive Reinforcement, also known as the Law of Effect. No empirical data refute it, or could refute it, because the principle is a mere tautology and hence has no predictive or explanatory power. Once "reinforcer" is defined as *that which increases the probability of a response*, the principle that a reinforcing event increases the probability of a response says no more than "an event that increases the probability of a response increases the probability of a response." There are also nontautological versions of the principle, but they are either trivial or false (see Erwin 1978: 97–103).

What have been the responses to these arguments? Some, perhaps many, behavior therapists have agreed with them, or at least with the main conclusions about the failure of behavioristic conditioning principles and the need to postulate cognitive causes; one writer claims that Erwin (1978) was the first to demonstrate clearly that behavior therapy was not really behavioristic (Rotgers 1988: 187). Hans Eysenck (1979), in contrast, claimed that my arguments refuted the Skinnerian position but did not tell against his own conditioning theory. I agree with Eysenck, but his theory is not behavioristic in that it allows for the causal role of cognitive factors even if it downgrades their importance, and it explains, at most, the etiology of a few clinical disorders, such as phobias, and fails to explain the workings of most behavior therapy techniques (Erwin 1997: 117–18). Some who have been more sympathetic to operant conditioning theory than to Pavlovian conditioning have either been unacquainted with the arguments of Erwin (1978) or have not been convinced. They still hold to a behaviorist position, although today it goes by various names.

By the 1980s, behavior therapists began to talk of a "paradigm shift" from behaviorism to cognitivism (see Fishman et al. 1988). It was reported during this period that about 75 percent of the members of the Association for the Advancement of Behavior Therapy now described their position as cognitivist, rather than behaviorist. This change in position of so many behavior therapists was probably the result of many factors, but I would conjecture that one important development was the demonstrable failure of therapies heavily influenced by conditioning theories, including token economy programs, the use of electric shock in treating alcoholism and sexual problems, and various Skinnerian-based behavior modification techniques for treating smoking and obesity. Another important influence, perhaps the most important, was the experimental work and arguments of Albert Bandura and his colleagues (see the references and arguments in Bandura 1995, 1997). Whatever the reason, behavior therapy became known as "cognitive-behavior therapy," although not everyone is pleased with this usage. Some, especially those who advocate what they call a "behavioral" position, continue to use the term "behavior therapy" (or sometimes "behavior modification"), and even some nonbehaviorists try to distinguish between cognitive and behavior therapy.

In the past 15 years or so, many of the old disputes have vanished or been submerged. It is hard to find many disagreements now about operationism or logical behaviorism; yet, deep disagreements persist about the alleged causal role of cognitive factors (see, for example, the special issue on cognition, behavior, and causality in the *Journal of Behavior Therapy and Experimental Psychiatry* [1995], and the special issue of *Behavior Therapy* [1997], "Thirty Years of Behavior Therapy: Promises Kept, Promises Unfulfilled"). As in an earlier period, the issues are neither entirely empirical nor entirely philosophical but a combination of both.

PART II: CURRENT ISSUES

Because many critics of a cognitivist paradigm in the field of behavior therapy refer to their position as "contextualist" or "applied behavior analyst," in what follows I sometimes do the same.

Cognitive Causation

Bandura (1995) makes a powerful argument for the causal role of human thought and, in particular, for the contributions of self-efficacy beliefs in explaining how much anxiety and depression people experience in coping with stressors and in explaining various sorts of behavior of interest to behavior therapists (but see the replies of his critics, including Catania 1995; Dougher 1995; Lee 1995). Because most behaviorists object to the use of *any* cognitivist theory in explaining behavior therapy phenomena, rather than merely to Bandura's particular theory, I focus on this broader issue.

Catania (1995) makes several points. One is that reinforcement is not a theory but, contrary to what Bandura claims, a phenomenon, one that can more easily be observed than evolution and one that can be routinely demonstrated to humans (192). Of course, Catania is partly right. The theory of reinforcement is a theory, whereas reinforcement is a phenomenon; in the paper Catania criticizes, Bandura nowhere misses this obvious point. But, can reinforcement be easily observed, as Catania claims? Catania gives no example, but consider one that Skinner liked to use: someone plays a slot machine and is rewarded with a monetary payoff enough times so that the person continues to play until he runs out of money. We observe the playing, but are we observing reinforcement? No, we are not, at least if the concept of reinforcement is defined causally as Skinner does. In order to know that reinforcement occurred, we would have to know whether the contiguous event, winning a payoff, combined with the person's history of reinforcement, caused the later responses. That is not something we can tell just by looking at what occurs. For all we know, the player believes that he has a "lucky machine" or that his initial success makes it likely that he will win again, and it is his belief, not merely the external events, that makes the difference as to whether he continues playing. The dissociative design experiments referred to earlier addressed this very issue and almost always, if not in every case, favored a cognitive explanation over one that appealed to conditioning.

One could use the term "reinforcement" so that it merely means *reward*; in that case, we can correctly say that we have observed the responses of the slot machine player being reinforced, but then we are leaving it entirely open whether mental events rather than environmental ones are causing the responses. Some writers use "conditioning" so that even if cognitive factors play the main causal role, conditioning may still have occurred. For example, Martin (1987: 453) points out that contemporary conditioning research has been expanded to encompass cognitive representations and information processing that involves learning about the causal structure of the world. However, if the slot machine player acts because he believes that there is a causal connection between playing and eventually winning, than his response of pulling the slot machine handle is neither automatic nor unmediated by thinking. One can use the term "conditioning" to cover such cases, but conditioning explanations of this sort are really cognitive explanations.

Catania (1995: 195) also makes the point that both Skinner and he allow that private events, such as mental multiplication (his example), can be causes—something long denied by most behaviorists (see, for example, Reitman 1997: 342), including Skinner himself—but they cannot be "initiating causes." Any argument that private events are initiating causes, Catania notes, is a variety of creationism, because it denies that these events themselves have prior causes; if we carry the causes back far enough, he points out, we must eventually get to events outside the organism. However, neither Bandura nor any cognitivist that I know of believes that mental events are "initiating causes" if one defines this concept so that an initiating cause is one that has no prior cause. Cognitions, such as are involved in doing mental arithmetic, make a difference to how we act; they are, consequently, causally relevant to human action. If we trace the causal chain backward, say from the utterance "14 + 13 + 7 = 34" to the mental acts involved in doing the sum, to what caused the agent's thinking, we will eventually be led outside the organism. The same is true if we postulate a brain injury as a cause of violent behavior, but that is no reason to say that neither the mental theorizing nor the brain injury affected the behavior. To say that mental events and neurological events are sometimes causes of behavior and must be appealed to in a correct explanation of the events they cause does not imply that such events are "initiating causes."

Dougher (1995: 215) claims that the disagreement between Bandura and his critics is really a conflict between equally legitimate but incompatible worldviews. The issue, Dougher contends, cannot be resolved by empirical data. I agree with part of what Dougher claims, but only a small part. He objects to Bandura's claim that, because behavior analysts now include internal surrogates in their explanatory schemes, the theoretical issue comes down to whose internal determinants have the greater explanatory and predictive power. Dougher's objection is that behavior analysts do not appeal to inner determinants. However, he ignores Bandura's point: given the evidence that behavior is often unaffected by immediate antecedents and consequences, proponents of the contingency model of causation (i.e., the behavior analysts who appeal to Skinnerian functionalism) increasingly place the explanatory burden on a conjectured internal surrogate—namely, the residue of the history of reinforcement.

If Skinnerians do not appeal to any such inner determinants, then how, on their theory, can the history of reinforcement affect current behavior? Suppose that the slot machine player had previously engaged in behavior that resembles his current behavior and that he was rewarded for his earlier behavior—let us grant that it was reinforced—but that he has no memory of this and that the earlier events have left no impact on his unconscious mind or his brain or his central nervous system. In that case, how can the earlier events now influence his current behavior? The earlier events are no more; they are gone. So, it looks as if Skinnerians have to appeal to some sort of inner residue of the earlier events to explain the impact of reinforcement histories. Perhaps some behavior analysts will refuse to take that step, but then their theory leaves it a total mystery how reinforcement is supposed to work.

Dougher tries to answer this objection by contending that behavior analysts adopt a "selectionist" view of causation, one that quite easily encompasses causal action over temporal distance (1995: 218). Adopting such a view does nothing to eliminate the mystery, however. The slot machine player, let us stipulate, won at cards five years before playing slot machines. But how can the early event affect the later event if during the intervening years there was no causal linkage? How can one event cease to occur and yet affect much later events with no connecting causal chain? Saying that causes can jump over temporal distances does not answer these questions.

I agree with Dougher's key contention that appeal to empirical data alone does not resolve the issues about cognitive causation. As argued in Erwin (1978), some of the key issues are philosophical. Where we disagree is on the question of whether the worldviews of cognitivists and contextualists (or behaviorists) are equally legitimate. Behavior analysts who call themselves "contextualists" have increasingly invoked this idea of different worldviews, appealing to the ideas of the philosopher Stephen Pepper (1942) to argue that the differences between cognitivists and behavior analysts cannot be rationally adjudicated (see Hayes et al. 1988). I believe that this is a deep mistake, one likely to lead contextualists into an intellectual dead end (see Erwin 1997: 87–94).

Dougher (1995: 215–17) makes no appeal to Pepper's writings, but he does claim that Bandura and his opponents have "equally legitimate but incompatible" worldviews. He further claims that cognitivists and behavior analysts have different scientific objectives and that there is no basis for arguing the superiority of one objective over another. The primary scientific goal of behavior analysis is prediction and control. In the very next sentence, Dougher speaks of a third goal—explanation—but he contends that adopting the first two goals necessarily places some constraints on the kinds of statements that can serve as an adequate explanation. Thus, he points out, explanations that appeal to inner determinants are considered inadequate by behavior analysts with respect to their goal of control.

As a sheer empirical statement about what some behavior analysts consider inadequate, Dougher is right, but as a defense of the claim that their view is legitimate, which is the important issue, he is mistaken. If our goal is control, it is really too bad if, in fact, what causes autistic children to injure themselves is not the reinforcement patterns of nurses and parents, as behaviorists used to claim, but instead is some malfunction of the brain or central nervous system. The environmental events would have been so much easier to control, but legitimate science requires that we explain the world that is, not the one that fits best with our desires. If autistic behavior is caused primarily by genetic and neural events, then any causal explanation that refuses to appeal to these events is false. One can refuse to give causal explanations, although behavior analysts seldom go that far, but one's goals cannot determine the truth about what causes behavior.

It is also part of the worldview of behavior analysts, according to Dougher (1995: 217), that they use a different unit of analysis from cognitivists. The cognitivists use a process or event that is not directly observable (such as thinking or believing some-thing), whereas for behavior analysts, the unit of analysis is the relation between behavior and the context in which it occurs. This is correct, but it is not clear why Dougher believes that the choice does not raise an empirical issue. If contexts are restricted to environmental contexts, with no appeal to inner determinants, then the behavior analysts are right if inner determinants never cause behavior, but their choice is wrong otherwise. Empirical evidence, not the choice of a worldview, is what must decide the issue about which units of analysis are useful.

Dougher also quotes with approval Skinner's claim that selection is a fact, but there is no disagreement with this claim except by those who object to Darwin's theory. Yet, to make the claim that something is selected is to make a causal claim. In the case of, say, mosquitoes, one might say that a trait was selected by a changing environment, meaning in part that the trait came into existence as the result of mechanical and automatic environmental influences, with no conscious help from the mosquito. Is it true, however, that the behavior of humans is typically caused by the mechanical and automatic workings of the environment and that conscious thought processes make no difference? To assume that this is a fact is just to assume without argument that Skinner's account of these matters is correct. One can, of course, argue for the position, but to say, as Skinner does, that selection is not a metaphor but a fact adds nothing of substance to the argument.

Dougher (1995: 218) closes by pointing out that behavior analysts require of an explanation of behavior that it describe the functional relations between the phenom-enon to be explained and its *manipulable* determinants. This point is related to the issue of scientific objectives dealt with earlier. The environmental events surrounding the head banging of an autistic child may be manipulable: we can tell the nurse and the parents to stop rewarding the child's actions. Yet, if the environmental events are not the cause of the head banging, then trying to explain the behavior by appealing to them is to incorrectly specify the cause of the behavior. If genetic and neural events are the cause, then they are the cause *whether or not* they are manipulable. Manipulability may serve as a criterion of what one is interested in, but not as a criterion of what makes a difference to human action.

There is another way to describe what some behavior analysts seek. Suppose that a stroke victim can speak only haltingly and that the cause is an insult to the brain. A psychologist might take the position that the brain injury cannot be manipulated but the environment of the stroke victim can, possibly in beneficial ways. From the point of view of applied psychology, one might argue, what is important is not the cause of the speech problem but the events that can be altered: the environmental events. Taking this point of view obviously does not require the adoption of a non-standard view of causation or the denial of inner causes, whether they are cognitive or neurological.

Reightman and Drabman try to some degree to reconcile the views of radical behaviorists and cognitivists, but they cannot reconcile logically incompatible views on the issue of cognitive causation. On this issue, they make the point that radical behaviorists adopt a framework that a priori places all causal events outside the organism itself (Reightman and Drabman 1997: 421). Many radical behaviorists do attempt to do this, but, as argued in Erwin (1978: ch. 2), they cannot possibly succeed. The proposition that some causes of behavior lie within the organism is not self-contradictory, nor is it false in all possible worlds. Consequently, one cannot know a priori that it is false. What causes human behavior of any sort is an empirical question that can be justifiably answered only through empirical inquiry. It cannot be answered through armchair a priori theorizing.

Reightman and Drabman also make the point that, in contrast, to cognitivists, contextualists adopt a "successful working" account of truth. Some do (e.g., Hayes 1993), but this view of truth is demonstrably mistaken (see Erwin 1997: 90–92). The authors also contend that cognitivists "respect empiricism and treatment outcome" and, therefore, operate by the same pragmatic truth criterion as the radical behaviorists (Reightman and Drabman 1997: 423). This does not follow. Both sides agree with the need for empirical evidence in assessing treatment outcome, but cognitivists generally do not advocate a pragmatic theory of truth.

Most of Reightman and Drabman's additional points, about causation, units of analysis, and explanation, depend on the arguments of Doughy (1995), arguments just shown to be unsound.

Lee (1995: 259) makes the point, as have others, that cognitive models implicitly assume a dualist view: that there exists a nonmaterial mental realm that has the capacity to act on the material world. The critics of a cognitive model, she notes, frequently argue from an epiphenomenalist position. I believe, however, that this is only partly right. The thesis that thinking and believing affect human action does not logically imply or presuppose dualism. There is a range of positions on the mind-body problem that is consistent with a cognitivist model. A cognitivist could reject Cartesian dualism and adopt property dualism: the view that the only substances in the world are physical substances but that there are mental events or states that have irreducible mental properties. Or, a cognitivist could reject all kinds of dualism and adopt a materialist view: two leading contemporary materialist views are functionalism and a form of the identity theory that identifies mental states and events in humans with brain states and events. Lee is quite right, however, that the cognitivist, to be consistent, must reject epiphenomenalism, the view that mental events and states have no causal efficacy. The obvious basis for the rejection is whatever empirical evidence we have that thinking, believing, wishing, and feeling make a difference to how we act. Despite this evidence, in recent years, philosophers have once again begun taking epiphenomenalism seriously (Kim 1998; Chalmers 1996).

The "new" epiphenomenalism does not favor a behaviorist view that locates all causation of human behavior in the environment, for it postulates inner determinants of behavior. The basic idea is that on certain metaphysical views, such as property dualism or Donald Davidson's anomalous monism, mental events supervene on brain events; that being true, it is, on these views, the brain events that ultimately cause behavior. The mental events are all causally impotent. Although the new epiphenomenalism does not support typical behaviorist views, it is obviously incompatible with cognitivism. The issues are too complicated to discuss in any detail here, but there is a strategy that cognitivists can adopt to combat the new arguments.

So far, the philosophers who are taking epiphenomenalism seriously are not endorsing the view. Rather, they are arguing for a hypothetical proposition: if a certain view of the mind is correct, such as property dualism or anomalous monism, then epiphenomenalism is true. Call this hypothetical proposition S_1 and the propositions that make up property dualism and anomalous monism S_2 and S_3, respectively. Is there credible empirical evidence for S_1 or S_2 or S_3? There is not. The grounds typically offered for these propositions consist of metaphysical arguments. If that is granted, it is reasonable to ask which has more credible support—the conjunction of the hypothetical proposition S_1 with one of the other two propositions, or the view that what humans believe, think, and feel sometimes makes a difference to human behavior? Assuming that it is the latter, given not merely the results from so many well-designed psychological experiments but also the observations from everyday experience, then there is good reason to reject the new arguments for epiphenomenalism.

One could change the epiphenomenalist's argument by replacing property dualism and anomalous monism with a third view of the mind-body relation, but the resulting argument would be vulnerable to the same type of objection. A cognitivist need not say that it is impossible in principle for metaphysical arguments to override observational evidence; it is just that, in this case, the observational evidence appears to be so much more powerful than the metaphysical grounds for epiphenomenalism. If this reply is too facile, if a case can eventually be made for epiphenomenalism, then trouble lies ahead for cognitivism—and, indeed, for all of psychology. Whether this is likely, I leave open.

Some contextualists and other radical behaviorists have tried to defend a behaviorist position by relying in part on controversial theories of truth, logic, and justification. For example, Stephen Hayes (1993) endorses a pragmatic account of truth, which he explains in terms of "successful working." Houts and Haddock (1992) try to shore up the behaviorist position by explaining the normative force of principles of logic in terms of operant conditioning theory. Leigland (1993) tries to analyze the concept of justification by giving behavioristic translations of justificatory statements. All of these views, however, have serious problems (for details, see Erwin 1997: 90–94).

Identity of Behavior Therapy and Cognitive Therapy

Some behaviorists claim that once behavior therapy and cognitive therapy are grouped together in a single category, "cognitive-behavior therapy," both kinds of therapy lose their identity. We are then unable to say what these therapies have in common that justifies calling them by the hyphenated name. I believe that the behaviorists have a sound point here, but the question is: What is to be done?

David Barlow, as far back as 1978, raised the issue of whether behavior therapy was not likely to lose its own identity and become the basis for a broader, more integrated approach to behavior problems (Barlow 1978: xi). One could try to identify behavior therapies in terms of the epistemological commitments of those who use them: behavior therapists study and change behavior by drawing on the methods used by experimental psychologists in their study of normal behavior (Davison and Neale 1974: 485). However, as I pointed out earlier (Erwin 1978: ch. 1), this account does not pick out a kind of *therapy*. Those who use the cognitive therapies of Albert Ellis and Aaron Beck accept the commitment to use experimental methods, as do some who practice psychodynamic therapy, but that does not mean that all of these different kinds of therapy are of a single kind. I suggested (Erwin 1978) a stop-gap, atheoretical account: behavior therapy is a nonbiological form of therapy developed largely out of learning theory that is normally applied directly, incrementally, and experimentally in the treatment of specific maladaptive behavior patterns (for an explanation of what these terms mean, see Erwin 1978: 39–44). However, I also suggested that, as new behavior therapy techniques were developed, we might have to conclude that there was a behavior therapy paradigm but no behavior *therapies*. I believe that this has now come to pass.

In the *Dictionary of Behavior Therapy Techniques* (Bellack and Hersen 1985), there are listed approximately 158 separate techniques. If we add to these what used to be called the "cognitive therapies," including Beck's therapy and Ellis's Rational Emotive Behavior Therapy, and classify them all as "cognitive-behavior therapy," what characteristics do they have in common that justify the use of a single classification? It is hard to find any such characteristics. The remedy of some behaviorists is to delete the cognitive therapies and use the older category, "behavior therapy." However, that hardly solves the problem. As argued in Erwin (1978), even the relatively few therapies that were then called behavior therapies were not based on modern learning theory, as many had claimed, or on conditioning principles or on behavioristic principles. Once that is agreed to, it becomes quite difficult, I believe impossible (see Erwin 1997: 116–19), to specify any interesting common properties shared by all 158 so-called behavior therapies. One could say that the behavior therapies are just those that are *called* "behavior therapies" (Sweet and Loizeau 1991: 161), but one could also say that the cognitive-behavior therapies are exactly those that go by the name "cognitive-behavior therapy." For certain purposes, this is enough, but that does not mean that either "behavior therapy" or "cognitive-behavior therapy" picks out a kind of therapy.

REFERENCES

Bandura, A. (1974) "Behavior Theory and the Models of Man." *American Psychologist* 28: 859–69.

Bandura, A. (1995) "Comments on the Crusade against the Causal Efficacy of Human Thought." *Journal of Behavior Therapy and Experimental Psychiatry* 26: 179–90.

Bandura, A. (1997) *Self-Efficacy: The Exercise of Control.* New York: W. H. Freeman.

Bandura, A., and Adams, N. (1977) "Analysis of Self-Efficacy Theory of Behavioral Change." *Cognitive Therapy and Research* 1: 287–310.

Barlow, D. (1978) Foreword to E. Erwin, *Behavior Therapy: Scientific, Philosophical and Moral Foundations.* New York: Cambridge University Press.

Bellack, A., and Hersen, M. (eds.) (1985) *Dictionary of Behavior-Therapy Techniques.* New York: Pergamon Press.

Breger, L., and McGaugh, J. (1965) "A Reformulation of 'Learning Theory' Approaches to Psychotherapy and Neurosis." *Psychological Bulletin* 63: 335–58.

Brewer, W. (1974) "There Is No Convincing Evidence for Operant or Classical Conditioning in Adult Humans." In W. Weimer and D. Palermo (eds.), *Cognition and the Symbolic Processes.* Hillsdale, NJ: Lawrence Erlbaum Associates.

Catania, A. C. (1995) "Higher-Order Behavior Classes: Contingencies, Beliefs, and Verbal Behavior." *Journal of Behavior Therapy and Experimental Psychiatry* 26: 191–200.

Chalmers, D. (1996) *The Conscious Mind: In Search of a Fundamental Theory.* New York: Oxford University Press.

Davison, G., and Neale, J. (1974). *Abnormal Psychology: An Experimental Clinical Approach.* New York: Wiley.

Dougher, M. (1995) "A Bigger Picture: Cause and Cognition in Relation to Differing Scientific Frameworks." *Journal of Behavior Therapy and Experimental Psychiatry* 26: 215–19.

Erwin, E. (1978) *Behavior Therapy: Scientific, Philosophical and Moral Foundations.* New York: Cambridge University Press.

Erwin, E. (1997) *Philosophy and Psychotherapy: Razing the Troubles of the Brain.* London: Sage.

Eysenck, H. J. (1979) "Behavior Therapy and the Philosophers." *Behavior Research and Therapy* 17: 511–14.

Fishman, D., Rotgers, F., and Franks, C. (1988) "Paradigms in Wonderland: Fundamental Issues in Behavior Therapy." In D. Fishman, F. Rotgers, and C. Franks (eds.), *Paradigms in Behavior Therapy: Present and Promise.* New York: Springer, pp. 109–40.

Franks, C. (1997) "It Was the Best of Times, It Was the Worst of Times." *Behavior Therapy* 28: 389–96.

Gewirtz, J. (1971) "The Roles of Overt Responding and Extrinsic Reinforcement in 'Self' and 'Vicarious Reinforcement' Phenomena and in 'Observational Learning' and Imitation." In R. Glaser (ed.), *The Nature of Reinforcement.* New York: Academic Press.

Hayes, S. (1993) "Analytic Goals and the Varieties of Scientific Contextualism." In S. Hayes, L. Hayes, H. Reese, and T. Sarbin (eds.), *Varieties of Scientific Contextualism.* Reno, NV: Context Press, pp. 11–27.

Hayes, S., Hayes, L., and Reese, H. (1988) "Finding the Philosophical Core: A review of Stephen Pepper's *World Hypotheses.*" *Journal of the Experimental Analysis of Behavior* 50: 119–37.

Houts, A., and Haddock, C. (1992) "Answers to Philosophical and Sociological Uses of Psychologism in Science Studies: A Behavioral Psychology of Science." In R. Giere (ed.), *Cognitive Models of Science*. Minnesota Studies in the Philosophy of Science, 15. Minneapolis: University of Minnesota Press, pp. 367–400.

Kim, J. (1998) *Mind in a Physical World: An Essay on the Mind-Body Problem and Causation*. Cambridge, MA: MIT Press.

Lee, C. (1995) "Comparing the Incommensurable: Where Science and Politics Collide." *Journal of Behavior Therapy and Experimental Psychiatry* 26: 259–63.

Leigland, S. (1993) "Scientific Goals and the Context of Justification." In S. Hayes, L. Hayes, H. Reese, and T. Sarbin (eds.), *Varieties of Scientific Contextualism*. Reno, NV: Context Press, pp. 28–33.

Locke, E. (1971) "Is Behavior Therapy Behavioristic?" *Psychological Bulletin* 76: 318–27.

MacCorquodale, K. (1970) "Chomsky's Review of Verbal Behavior." *Journal of the Experimental Analysis of Behavior* 13: 83–99.

Mahoney, M. (1974) *Cognitive Behavior Modification*. Cambridge: Ballinger.

Martin, I. (1987) "Concluding Comments on Theoretical Foundations and Requirements in Behavior Therapy." In H. J. Eysenck and I. Martin (eds.), *Theoretical Foundations of Behavior Therapy*. New York: Plenum Press, pp. 451–64.

Pepper, S. (1942) *World Hypotheses: A Study in Evidence*. Berkeley: University of California Press.

Reitman, D. (1997) "The Relation between Cognitive and Behavioral Therapies: Commentary on 'Extending the Goals of Behavior Therapy and of Cognitive Behavior Therapy.'" *Behavior Therapy* 28: 341–45.

Reitman, D., and Drabman, R. (1997) "The Value of Recognizing Our Differences and Promoting Healthy Competition: The Cognitive Behavioral Debate." *Behavior Therapy* 28: 419–29.

Rotgers, F. (1988) "Social Learning Theory, Philosophy of Science, and the Identity of Behavior Therapy." In D. Fishman, F. Rotgers, and C. Franks (eds.), *Paradigms in Behavior Therapy: Present and Promise*. New York: Springer, pp. 187–210.

Sweet, A., and Loizeaux, A. (1991) "Behavioral and Cognitive Treatment Methods: A Critical Comparative Review." *Journal of Behavior Therapy and Experimental Psychiatry* 22: 159–85.

CHAPTER 27

SOCIAL CONSTRUCTIONIST MODELS

Making Order out of Disorder — On the Social Construction of Madness

JENNIFER CHURCH

CONTEMPORARY enthusiasm for social constructivist accounts — of almost everything — is both exciting and exasperating. On the one hand, very concretely, it has greatly increased our understanding of the ways that social values and priorities have affected the history of medicine, music, marriage, and much else; it has been remarkably effective in undermining pernicious notions of gender, race, and intelligence, for example. On the other hand, more abstractly, it has encouraged the view that social values and priorities are the sole historical determinants of medicine, music, and marriage, and it has helped create a culture in which the distinction between what is real and what is contrived, or between how things are and how things are thought to be, threatens to disappear entirely. This tension between the promise and the dangers of social constructivism is especially sharp in the case of mental disorders or madness, where disclosing the social agendas that often guide diagnoses can lead to more self-searching, case-specific interventions while also fueling the conviction that there is nothing "really" wrong with those who are mentally ill—that madness is nothing more (and nothing less) than what we make of it.

Social construction in general is not particularly popular among psychiatrists, but it is certainly the dominant theoretical framework within the broad field of work now known as "cultural studies."[1] And social constructivism about madness, in particular, has attracted a steady following ever since the early work of Michel Foucault and Thomas Szasz became popular in the 1960s.[2] I do not attempt a history of this movement, but I do attempt to answer the following three questions:

1. What does it mean for a mental disorder to be socially constructed?
2. How can we decide whether or not a mental disorder is socially constructed?
3. What are the practical implications of deciding that a mental disorder is socially constructed?

These might be called the metaphysical, epistemological, and ethical questions, respectively; as we shall see, though, the traditional separation and ordering of these categories is part of what social constructivists seek to challenge.

METAPHYSICS OF SOCIAL CONSTRUCTION

The notion of social construction emphasizes the importance of societal conditions as opposed to individual beliefs and desires on the one hand and as opposed to physical forces on the other.[3] Societies are composed of individuals, and individuals are composed of physical parts, of course, but these facts do not require that a society's condition be explained in terms of individual beliefs and desires or that an individual's beliefs and desires be explained in terms of physical forces. Depressive disorders, for example, may involve individual beliefs and desires and may involve physiological changes without being explained by these things if the underlying causes are primarily social: the breakdown of family ties, the loss of meaningful work, the decline of religion, and so on.[4] Similarly, certain neuroses, manifest in an individual's beliefs and desires, might be viewed as psychic irruptions of social practices that have been repressed.[5]

Of course, the idea that various instances of madness can be *caused* by one's social surroundings is not new, and is not particularly controversial. Betrayal by one's friends and family can cause psychotic rage, the loss of one's home can cause profound depression, and membership in an obsessive profession can cause one to develop an obsessive personality. Fiction as well as life is full of instances of madness brought on by such circumstances: Clytemestra's murderous rage in the face of Agamemnon's betrayal, Werther's depression upon losing the woman he loved, Judith's obsessiveness in response to that of Bluebeard. And the psychological literature that identifies social factors that contribute to mental illness is enormous. But the notion of construction is somewhat different from that of cause. Construction implies the emergence of some new structure, in which various items or various features, previously separate, are brought together to form a new whole. In a very literal case of construction, such as the construction of an anthill by a colony of ants, bits of dirt and food and bodily secretions that were previously separate are combined and re-arranged to form a structure that sustains the life of that colony. In the case of a socially constructed mental disorder, an assortment of behaviors and experiences are brought together and ordered in some new way that plays a role in the life of that society. In just what sense, though, can social conditions bring different experiences and behaviors together into a new whole? We cannot simply pick them up and carry them, antlike, to their newly assigned locations next to one another.

There are two basic possibilities: first, social conditions may create lawlike regularities between experiences and behaviors that were previously disparate or non-existent (whether or not we recognize or conceptualize these new regularities); second, social conditions may create the *belief* that there are lawlike regularities between experiences and behaviors where there are, in fact, none (with the further possibility that these beliefs will actually produce the regularities in question). Anorexia appears to be an instance of the first sort: a refusal to eat, perfectionist tendencies, delayed psychosexual development, and a distorted body image began to co-occur regularly in America, in the late twentieth century, in response to some very specific social forces (and the concept of anorexia followed the reality of this convergence of symptoms). Borderline personality disorder appears to be an instance of the second sort: the idea of an identity disturbance, of manipulative social relations, of affective instability, and of self-destructive behavior are brought together under a single concept without there being (or prior to there being) any lawlike relations that link these experiences.[6] This second possibility, in which psychological regularities are posited when there are, in fact, none, is of particular interest to those who believe that the whole point of a mental disorder is its refusal to adhere to lawlike regularities, as well as to those who believe that there is no order in the world apart from the order that we project onto it.[7] Whether or not there is such a thing as a natural order, though, a social disorder that is socially constructed is not something that already exists as a unity within that natural order.[8]

Bringing disparate features together under a new concept and believing that these features belong together (the second possibility) may, of course, produce lawlike connections among those features (the first possibility). We are highly suggestible beings, especially in therapeutic contexts, and others' expectations about what behaviors and experiences belong together are often made true by our responsiveness to those expectations. Predicting auditory hallucinations in someone who has been called schizophrenic, or supposing that childhood abuse will result in a multiple personality disorder, may indeed bring about the expected outcome (by offering a novel interpretation of what might otherwise be experienced as merely talking to oneself, or by suggesting an effective way of escaping from one's pain).[9] This is particularly true of so-called personality disorders — paranoid, schizoid, antisocial, borderline, narcissistic, dependent, obsessive-compulsive, or passive-aggressive personalities—insofar as our self-definitions are particularly responsive to social expectations.[10] (Judgments about the sort of person one is operate at a more theoretical level than judgments about what one feels, what one remembers, or how one will behave in a particular situation; for this reason, we are more dependent on the judgments of others when it comes to deciding personality types.)

Succumbing to the power of suggestion may or may not involve the activation of a common cause for the relevant behaviors and experiences. Deciding that we are depressed may actually alter our serotonin uptake profile (an instance of what Hacking calls "biolooping"[11]), or it may simply encourage us to behave in the ways we are expected to behave and to interpret our experiences—sensations of numbness, sleeplessness, lack of concentration, and so on—as signs of depression, with the result that the occurrence of one symptom makes an occurrence of the others more likely (what Hacking calls "classificatory looping"[12]). It would be wrong, however, to assume that alterations of the first sort create "real" instances of depression while alterations of the second sort create only "imaginary" depression. In either case, there is a lawlike regularity that links certain defining symptoms; while the presence of an underlying disease may affect the treatment of a mental disorder, it doesn't affect its reality.

In addition to there being two basic ways in which social construction can occur, there are several levels at which a societal construction can occur. At the most general level, a society might be said to construct mental states as disorders, insofar as that society creates the rules of rationality or mental "order" against which aberrant experiences and behaviors get grouped together (in thought or in reality) into disorders.[13] This is the level at which it is easiest for social constructivists to make their case, for there is no question that different societies have drawn the line between normalcy and madness in different ways and that disparate experiences and behaviors that are deemed mad come to be correlated with one another—both in thought and in reality.[14] (For this reason, if no other, the DSM's insistence that "conflicts that are primarily between the individual and society" are not mental disorders is unconvincing to many.)[15]

At a somewhat less general level, the social constructionist may claim that a society is responsible for creating the particular groupings of syndromes that constitute disorders such as hysteria, depression, paranoia, attention deficit disorder, anorexia, borderline personality disorder, schizophrenia, and so on. In our society, various experiences of inner voices may be grouped together and may reinforce one another to create the syndrome of schizophrenia, while, in another society, they may be treated as unrelated instances of daydreaming, remembering conversations, listening to the gods, or communing with one's ancestors—with the result that various experiences of inner voices do not tend to reinforce one another and support lawlike generalizations. Likewise, a range of behaviors that counts as unrelated cases of investigating, organizing, or planning in our society may add up to obsessive-compulsive behavior in another society. To establish the social constructivist thesis at this level, it is not enough to show that some societies do not have the concept of "paranoia," for example (since the reality may exist without the concept) or do not treat those who imagine they are being persecuted as mad (since the relevant syndrome may exist without being considered abnormal or insane); one must show, rather, that the experiences and behavior that we define as paranoid do not regularly co-occur in these other cultures (and perhaps not even in our own).

Finally, at a still more detailed level, a society may construct the very behaviors and experiences in terms of which mental disorders are defined: flat affect, delusions, confusion about identity, antisocial behavior, disordered thought, and so on. Experiences that we group together as instances of flat affect may be variously thought of as instances of mature, considered, restrained, or subtle feeling within another society.[16] Or what we group together as delusions may be viewed as unrelated instances fantasy, visions of an afterlife, and normal misperceptions within another society.[17] To be a social constructivist at this level is to be a social constructivist about the very experiences and behaviors that make up a disorder. And, again, this second possibility is of particular interest to those who believe that there is no preexisting structure in the world—no such thing as a "natural" order of things. ("It's turtles all the way down.")

Because I find social constructivism concerning the broad category of madness (or mental disorder, or mental illness) uncontroversial, and I find social constructivism about such experiential categories as flat affect and delusions implausible (I say a bit more about this later), the discussion in this chapter is focused mainly on social constructivism about diagnostic categories such as schizophrenia, depression, and borderline personality disorder.

Before we consider the sorts of evidence that are relevant to establishing social constructivism at this level, it is worth noting the range of social conditions that might contribute to the construction of a mental disorder. In the case of anorexia, relevant social factors seem to include advertising's promotion of thinness, an explosion in the achievements (and hence the expectations) of women, and economic conditions that cast a pall over the future. In the case of borderline personality disorder, relevant social factors seem to include the fact that insurance companies demand labels for the disorders whose treatment they are willing to cover and the fact that the introduction of medical jargon is one way to counteract a patient's manipulativeness. The resulting disorders may not be intended, of course (our higher expectations of girls are not intended to make them sick, and the "borderline" label is not intended to increase the convergence of difficult behaviors), but the results may be socially useful, nonetheless. Social constructivists about hysteria, for example, have argued that hysteria provides a safe outlet for the frustrations of women who are systematically silenced or discounted in society at large—an outlet that does not challenge the existing power structure and, indeed, may help to rationalize it.[18] Or, to take a very different sort of example, a diagnosis of neurasthenia, whatever its intent, often functioned to excuse various sorts of laziness and self-indulgence and sexual nonconformity on the part of wealthy young men in nineteenth-century Europe.[19]

The societal usefulness of such disorders often depends on society's ability to disguise its own role in their creation, to foster the illusion of a natural rather than an imposed convergence of symptoms. It is easier not to assign responsibility, easier (and more profitable) to pursue individual cures rather than systematic prevention, easier to distance oneself from the afflicted and accept a certain amount of madness as inevitable. (I say more about this in the last section.) But it is also a fact about the nature of perception and thought that we are better able to hold things together in our minds to the extent that we can "see" or assume that they have an underlying "nature." So even if we can trace the social conditions that led to the regular co-occurrence of confusions about identity, manipulative social relations, affective instability, and self-destructive tendencies, it is extremely tempting, when we are actually confronted with this syndrome (so-called borderline personality disorder), to suppose that there is an underlying disease after all. Given the potential deceptiveness of this supposition, though, it is important to consider just how we can know whether or not a particular disorder is socially constructed.

EPISTEMOLOGY OF SOCIAL CONSTRUCTION

There are several types of evidence that, taken together, can support the claim that a mental disorder is socially constructed: evidence that there is no one biological or chemical condition responsible for the relevant array of symptoms, evidence that instances of the disorder (or alleged instances of the disorder) are closely correlated with specific societal conditions and interests, and evidence that alternative taxonomies are equally plausible. I consider each of these types of evidence in turn, indicating some of the difficulties involved.

If the symptoms that we use to define a given disorder can be traced to a single biological or chemical condition — to a genetic abnormality in the case of schizophrenia or to excessive serotonin uptake levels in the case of depression, for example — then it is reasonable to suppose that both the disorder and our concept of the disorder should be explained by natural facts as opposed to social facts. Social factors might explain the distress that leads to certain genetic disorders, and social factors might explain our interest in certain syndromes rather than others, but the disorder itself will not be socially constructed since, in such cases, it will be nature, not society, that is responsible for the relevant convergence of symptoms. (If one objects that the categories of genetics and chemistry are themselves socially constructed, we may ask: Socially constructed as opposed to what? And socially constructed out of what? Being a social constructivist about everything seems incoherent — for much the same reason that being an antirealist about everything seems incoherent, but that argument is outside the scope of this essay.)[20]

We do not have unified biological explanations for most mental disorders, however, and in many cases there is good reason to think that different instances of a disorder are correlated with quite different biological and chemical conditions. In the case of depression, for example, some instances of depression seem correlated with low levels of serotonin between synapses, while other instances are clearly not. And in the case of schizophrenia, some sufferers have a family history that suggests a genetic component, while others do not.[21] The most recent diagnostic manual of the American Psychiatric Association announces a rather conflicted position according to which, on the one hand, many diagnoses depend on ruling out organic factors (stipulating that if amphetamines are held to be responsible for one's delusions, the diagnosis should be "organic delusional disorder" rather than schizophrenia, and if a brain tumor is responsible for one's low mood, the diagnosis should be "organic mood disorder" rather than depression); on the other hand, we are assured that in the future "we may be able to identify specific organic factors that are responsible for initiating and maintaining these disorders."[22] The guiding thought, presumably, is that it is only "abnormal" organic causes of the disorder that have been identified and that the normal organic cause is yet to be found—but the more varied the identified causes turn out to be, the more one must doubt the existence of a more unified "normal" cause.

If there is no one biological condition that underlies all (or most all) instances of a mental disorder, then it may well be that the disorder is a social construct—a set of symptoms that has been brought together (in thought or in reality, or both) by a variety of social forces. But that is not the only possibility. Accounts of mental disorders that emphasize individual beliefs and desires (psychoanalytic explanations of depression that appeal to one's anger at what has been lost and one's narcissistic tendency to overidentify with what one loves, for example) are not social constructivist accounts insofar as they locate the relevant causal factors within the individual, rather than within the society at large. The distinction between individual factors and societal factors can be a difficult one, of course. Is it individuals who make their society narcissist or a society that makes its individuals narcissists? Do family dynamics (such as the Oedipal triangle) count as social dynamics, and are they the cause or the effect of larger cultural practices (concerning gender, for example)? But the social constructivist is committed to social explanations in contrast to both biological explanations and individual (psychological) explanations. So, evidence against a biological basis for a given mental disorder is not yet evidence for a social basis.

This is where a second, historical type of evidence becomes important—evidence of a correlation between certain social conditions and reported instances of the disorder in question. Hysteria, it seems, flourished in late-nineteenth- and early-twentieth-century Europe, especially among women. Charcot's hospital in Paris housed hundreds of (alleged) hysterics in the 1880s, yet now the diagnosis has practically disappeared. More recently, thousands of cases of multiple personality disorder were documented after the case of Sybil became famous in the 1960s, yet now the numbers seem to be diminishing. And there has been a virtual epidemic of attention deficit disorder among children in the United States, especially boys, since the 1980s. Whether these patterns reflect the rise and fall of actual syndromes or merely imagined syndromes (or syndromes that become actual because they are imagined), the absence of a common biological basis, together with a strong correlation with specific historical conditions, does suggest that these disorders are syndromes that have been created by societal conditions. And it is not hard to speculate on what some of these factors might be: the growing aspirations of women alongside the systematic repression of their sexuality, in the case of hysteria; a growing fascination with altered states of consciousness together with increased social service inquiries into childhood sexual abuse, in the case of multiple personality disorder; growing pressure to excel in school plus greater exposure to frantically paced media entertainment, in the case of attention deficit disorder.

It is of course possible that the symptoms of hysteria, of multiple personality disorder, and of attention deficit disorder converge with pretty much the same frequency in all societies; they may only be noticed more in some societies. It is hard to eliminate this possibility, given the difficulty of accessing the relevant data in historical cases and the difficulty of being an unbiased observer in cross-cultural cases. It would be unusual, though, for the prevailing diagnoses in a society to have no effect on the frequency of the syndromes in question (through the power of suggestion); more important, given the enormous number of regularities that *might* be noticed, society's focus on one set rather than another may itself be thought of as a kind of "construction"—a case of bringing some patterns rather than others into focus (much as a sculptor might bring out one preexisting form rather than another from a piece of marble).

The existence of equally plausible alternatives to the way we categorize mental disorders is, then, another type of evidence in favor of social constructivist accounts of those categories. For if two or more theories have equal empirical support, the choice between them must be made on other grounds, and social considerations provide one way to tip the balance in favor of one categorization rather than the other. (The balance might also be tipped with a coin toss, or on the basis of the idiosyncratic aesthetic preferences of an influential individual, but these are less likely options.) It is not easy to produce alternative taxonomies that have equal empirical support, however.[23] It is not just a matter of inventing an amusing encyclopedia entry that divides animals into those that belong to the emperorversus those that are embalmed, those that are tame versus those that are sucking pigs, those that are drawn with a very fine camelhair brush versus those that from a long way off look like flies, and so forth.[24] To have equal empirical support, an alternative scheme must group things in ways that do, in fact, hang together in the sense that they tend to support lawlike generalizations and predictions. Animals that belong to the emperor do not tend to look alike, do not behave in any special way, and are not necessarily capable of producing offspring with one another; surely there are more lawlike similarities between a pig that belongs to the emperor and a sucking pig than between a pig that belongs to the emperor and a bird that belongs to the emperor.

Radical social constructionists are likely to respond that it all depends on what sorts of laws you are interested in. If the laws surrounding the handling of the emperor's estate are more important to you than the laws surrounding the reproductive potential of various animal pairings, then the divisions as described will reflect more relevant lawlike generalizations; if not, not—and there is no interest-neutral way to compare the two. (This is where the traditional distinction among metaphysics, epistemology, and ethics can be seen to break down; rather than reality determining what we can know and what we hold valuable, what we hold valuable determines what we can know and what constitutes reality.) If this is right, though, then the alleged alternatives are not really alternatives after all; they are self-sustaining worlds that remain incommensurable.[25] And that means that they can no longer be used to provide evidence for the social constructivist thesis, for they no longer demonstrate the need for social factors to break an empirical impasse.

Less radical social constructionists, on the other hand, may prefer to argue for the empirical equivalence of different taxonomies simply by asking whether we are demonstrably better at predicting or curing mental disorders now than we were 100 years ago (when the prevailing taxonomy was quite different), or whether the categories and cures of contemporary American psychiatry have any better track record than those of traditional Chinese medicine.

ETHICS OF SOCIAL CONSTRUCTION

I turn, finally, to the practical implications of believing that mental disorders are socially constructed. What difference does it make whether paranoia or schizophrenia, depression or anorexia, obsessive-compulsive disorder or borderline personality disorder are created by society, rather than by individuals or by biology?

Ian Hacking suggests that the crucial thing about a socially constructed category as opposed to a natural category is that it is not inevitable; it can be changed.[26] Change would be more or less difficult, though, depending on the sort of construction at issue. Insofar as it is the mere concept of a syndrome that has been constructed, that concept can probably be abandoned pretty much at will. (We might simply quit using the concept of "borderline personality disorder," for example.) But insofar as an actual syndrome has been constructed by social conditions, those conditions would have to be altered for the syndrome to be eliminated. (Gender relations, advertising practices, and economic trends would need to change before anorexia disappears.) Social conditions can be changed, of course, but social change is not necessarily easier than biological change. Delusions caused by brain tumors are more easily eliminated than delusions caused by childhood neglect, attention deficit disorder is more easily cured with Ritalin than by systematic changes in the education and entertainment industries, and it is certainly easier to take Prozac than to change the conditions that make one depressed. So, knowing that a mental disorder is socially constructed may actually make it seem more rather than less inevitable.

Is it even desirable to eliminate socially constructed categories of mental illness? Surely we can't assume that all socially constructed syndromes are undesirable, any more than we can assume that all naturally occurring syndromes are desirable. One can even imagine cases in which a socially constructed syndrome helps one deal with a more debilitating natural syndrome—where obsessive-compulsive personality types counter the worst effects of a biologically based tendency toward depression, for example.[27] As with all medical or psychological interventions, the desirability of certain social interventions depends on what would be gained and what would be lost if a certain disorder were eliminated, and just what the alternatives are.

Should we at least abandon the mental disorder concepts that do not reflect lawlike regularities—concepts that group disconnected experiences and behaviors together to produce the illusion of a syndrome? Again, it depends on the costs and benefits, and it depends on the alternatives. The concept of borderline personality disorder, for example, may be very useful for indicating a diverse set of experiences and behaviors that psychiatrists have trouble understanding—especially if some such label is crucial for receiving insurance benefits; abandoning it, in the absence of better alternatives, would probably be a mistake.

Still, recognizing the socially constructed character of a particular syndrome or concept does help to dispel the illusion of naturalness, and dispelling the illusion of naturalness should encourage us to at least consider the social factors involved and the alternatives they suggest. Might an alternative school environment and restrictions on television entertainment be a better alternative than Ritalin? Might immersion in a new project or profession be an alternative to Prozac? And so on. Simply considering such alternatives will tend to make us less passive in our dealings with disorder: less willing to turn decisions over to medical or psychiatric authorities, more willing to imagine radical alternatives, and more attentive to our own contributions to the problem.[28]

Finally, it has been suggested—rightly, I think—that social constructivism about mental disorders results in a tendency to abandon any attempt to reach a consensus about which diagnostic categories to use.[29] If there is no objective ordering of experience and behavior for our categories to capture, then there is no more reason for us to agree about how to categorize mental disorders than there is for us to agree about how to categorize contemporary art or how to categorize different types of beauty. This does not mean that anything goes; some ways of categorizing will be more useful for some purposes, others for other purposes. But, if a category is socially constructed, there is no reason for people with different interests to try to achieve consensus about which scheme of categories to use.

Is abandoning the attempt at consensus a good or a bad thing? It is a bad thing if it discourages scientific research and debate that would lead to the discovery of the underlying "natures" of various mental disorders, but such a complaint clearly begs the question: we can expect to discover the underlying nature of a mental disorder only if we expect that it has one—which is precisely the assumption that the social constructionist rejects. It might also be a bad thing if it leads to types of disagreement and strife that cause those who suffer to suffer even more—because their troubles fail to be recognized as such by doctors, or in courts, for example. Or it may be a good thing insofar as it encourages sufferers to greater participation in their own diagnoses and cures.[30] Whatever the trade-offs, however, they will be purely pragmatic trade-offs if social constructivism is correct—if there is no independent reality to get right.

In conclusion, then, there is no reason to suppose that a socially constructed mental disorder is easier to change than a naturally constituted mental disorder; and until one considers the situation-specific alternatives, there is no reason to suppose that change is even desirable. There is, however, reason to think that believing that a mental disorder is socially constructed will tend to elicit more imaginative and more responsible responses from us and that it will make us less inclined to seek consensus.

NOTES

1. Just how popular it has become is made vivid in the opening pages of Ian Hacking (1999), where he lists a wide range of book titles describing things as socially constructed.

2. Michel Foucault's *Histoire de la folie* was published in France in 1961, a year after Thomas Szasz's paper "The Myth of Mental Illness" was presented to the American Psychological Association. Subsequently, Foucault's book was translated into English as *Madness and Civilization* (1965), and Szasz published his book *The Manufacture of Madness* (1970).

3. Evolutionary accounts of madness may also emphasize the importance of social factors, but only insofar as such factors have managed to modify our genetic makeup (over many centuries). The social constructivist focuses on more variable societal forces, acting on us in the present.

4. There is a continuing controversy, within philosophy and within the social sciences more generally, over whether social causes must ultimately reduce to psychological causes and whether psychological causes must ultimately reduce to physical causes. This controversy turns, in part, on whether the causes in question admit of multiple "realizations": Can the same social problem be realized by individuals with quite different psychologies, and can the same psychological problem be realized by quite different neurologies? It also turns on the question of whether multiple realizability stands in the way of reductions. (The recent work of Jaegwon Kim is particularly useful on this topic.) Social constructivists, though, are committed antireductionists.

5. This is a central theme in Peter Stallybrass and Allon White's influential book *The Politics and Poetics of Transgression* (1987).

6. The listed experiences and behaviors are the main indicators of anorexia and of borderline personality disorder according to the most recent edition of the American Psychiatric Association's *Diagnostic and Statistical Manual of Mental Disorders* (DSM-III-R; 1987).

7. Foucault, for example, uses Borges's list of things that fall under a single Chinese term to suggest that there is no such thing as a natural grouping of properties, only groupings that seem natural within some cultural or linguistic context—and unnatural within another (opening page of the preface to *The Order of Things: An Archeology of the Human Sciences* [1970]). I question the ultimate coherence of this view in the next section.

8. Preexisting unities include natural kinds (in which a variety of experiences and behaviors have a single underlying cause) and natural conglomerates (in which there is no single underlying cause—a physiological imbalance, for example—but in which there are reliable causal connections between the symptoms (e.g., anxiety tends to cause obsessiveness, and obsessiveness tends to cause anxiety). Within medicine, and within contemporary psychiatry, the first is usually called a disease, the second a mere syndrome. If the relevant behaviors form a preexisting unity of either sort, they are not socially constructed.

9. According to Ofshe and Watters (1994), multiple personalities emerge, on average, seven years into therapy!

10. This is a list of personality disorders cited in DSM-III-R (1987).

11. Hacking (1999: 109).

12. Ibid., 110.

13. As both Foucault and Szasz are fond of pointing out, mental disorders have been variously treated as instances of demonic possession, as indications of inspired madness, and as forms of medical illness. The different associations that characterize each of these conceptualizations are part of what make them different social constructions.

14. The opponent of social construction at this level must argue that there is an objective basis for drawing the line between normalcy and madness one way rather than another—on the basis of natural functions, perhaps. (There was a lively discussion of this possibility in several contributions to the journal *Philosophy, Psychiatry, and Psychology*, vol. 5, 1998.) But if the critical functions are social functions, and if what is functional in society varies greatly among societies, it is hard to resist the conclusion that madness as such is socially constructed.

15. Introduction to DSM-III-R: xxii.

16. This is one way to interpret the observations reported by anthropologist Jean L. Briggs (1970).

17. Anthony David (1999), for example, argues that the concept of a delusion is really just a societal marker for whatever assortment of beliefs and images are discredited in that society. K. W. M. Fulford (1994) also details various difficulties in determining what counts as a delusion.

18. Recent books that explore analyses along these lines include Bernheimer and Kahane (1985), Micale (1995), and Showalter (1997).

19. Note that this is a case of mental disorder but not of madness or insanity—a disorder that is valued (as conducive to artistic sensitivity and creativity), rather than disvalued.

20. Paul Boghossian has published a number of articles that address these problems, especially "Who's Afraid of Social Construction?" (2001).

21. The fact that no single drug works dependably to relieve symptoms of depression or schizophrenia is also indirect evidence against a unified biological basis for either.

22. DSM-III-R: 23.

23. It is not individual diagnoses but the taxonomy of a field that is at issue here. The fact that it is sometimes just as plausible to categorize someone as paranoid as to categorize her as schizophrenic only indicates fuzzy boundaries; it does not show that there are equally plausible alternatives to the prevailing categorical scheme.

24. The list is that of Michel Foucault (following Borges) at the opening of his preface to *The Order of Things* (1970).

25. Thus, Nelson Goodman's willingness to embrace the existence of many different worlds, in *Ways of Worldmaking* (1978).

26. Hacking (1999: 6). In this and other passages of his book, Ian Hacking seems to treat causation by individual beliefs and desires as a case of social construction. At least

within psychology and psychiatry, however, it is important to distinguish the two; otherwise, psychoanalysis, for example, will turn out to be a form of social constructivism.

27. If all categories are socially constructed, this contrast doesn't even make sense, of course, but I shall continue to assume that it does.

28. Thomas Szasz has long argued that mental illness is a myth designed to disguise the social origins of various "problems of living" and their various "solutions." And this myth, he argues, has allowed us both to deprive people of liberty when they are guilty of no crime and to excuse people of responsibility when they are guilty of crimes. (See, most recently, Szasz 1998.) Should a social constructivist about mental disorders, then, object to involuntary incarceration and to insanity pleas in criminal court? This conclusion, I think, confuses social responsibility with individual responsibility; if societal forces are responsible for making an individual delusional, then society may also be responsible for minimizing the ill effects of those delusions and for accepting responsibility for the ill effects that do occur.

29. Eric Gillett (1998), for example, complains that "constructivist relativism undermines the search for consensus achieved through scientific debate."

30. The importance of self-determination within a liberal society is discussed in connection with multiple personality disorders, by Jennifer Radden (1996), esp. pp. 220–26.

REFERENCES

American Psychiatric Association (1987) *Diagnostic and Statistical Manual of Mental Disorders* (DSM-III-R) Washington, DC: American Psychiatric Association.

Bernheimer, Charles, and Kahane, Claire (eds.) (1985) *In Dora's Case: Freud-Hysteria-Feminism*. New York: Columbia University Press.

Boghossian, Paul (2001) "What Is Social Construction?" *Times Literary Supplement*.

Briggs, Jean L. (1970) *Never in Anger: Portrait of an Eskimo Family*. Cambridge, MA: Harvard University Press.

David, Anthony (1999) "On the Impossibility of Defining Delusions." *Philosophy, Psychiatry, and Psychology* 6(1): 17–20.

Foucault, Michel (1965) *Madness and Civilization*. New York: Random House.

Foucault, Michel (1970) *The Order of Things: An Archeology of the Human Sciences*. New York: Random House.

Fulford, K. W. M. (1994) "Value, Illness, and Failure of Action: Framework for a Philosophical Psychopathology of Delusion." In George Graham and G. Lynn Stephens (eds.), *Philosophical Psychopathology*. Cambridge, MA: MIT Press.

Gillett, Eric (1998) "Relativism and the Social Constructivist Paradigm." *Philosophy, Psychiatry, and Psychology* 5(1): 37–48.

Goodman, Nelson (1978) *Ways of Worldmaking*. Indianapolis: Hackett.

Hacking, Ian (1999) *The Social Construction of What?* Cambridge, MA: Harvard University Press.

Micale, Mark S. (1995) *Approaching Hysteria*. Princeton, NJ: Princeton University Press.

Ofshe, Richard, and Watters, Ethan (1994) *Making Monsters*. Berkeley: University of California Press.

Radden, Jennifer (1996) *Divided Minds and Successive Selves*. Cambridge, MA: MIT Press.

Showalter, Elaine (1997) *Hystories*. New York: Columbia University Press.

Stallybrass, Peter, and White, Allon (1987) *The Politics and Poetics of Transgression*. Ithaca, NY: Cornell University Press.

Szasz, Thomas (1960) "The Myth of Mental Illness." *American Psychologist* 15(2): 113–18.

Szasz, Thomas (1970) *The Manufacture of Madness*. New York: Harper and Row.

Szasz, Thomas (1998) "Commentary on 'Aristotle's Function Argument and the Concept of Mental Illness,'" *Philosophy, Psychiatry, and Psychology* 5(3): 203–7.

PART V

CIRCUMSCRIBING
MENTAL DISORDER

CHAPTER 28

SETTING BENCHMARKS FOR PSYCHIATRIC CONCEPTS

ROM HARRÉ

How do we know that someone is properly to be brought before a medically qualified person and diagnosed? When fragments of bone are sticking through someone's flesh, or when a body is covered in suppurating sores and there is a raging temperature, the question answers itself. Despite, or maybe as some might say, because of the widespread use of DSM in whatever happens to be its current format, the application of psychiatric concepts is "essentially contested." I have recently been a consultant to a research group organized by Richard Sykes, of Westcare, that had the task of locating the now familiar complaints of those who suffer from debilitating and persistent tiredness within the domain of "troubles" (Sykes and Campion 2003). This experience encouraged some general reflections on the "benchmark problem." Along what dimensions ought one to consider "troubles," and where, on any one of those dimensions, do we pass from the scope of the ordinary to the domain of the extraordinary?

In the "medical model," the medical expert sets the benchmark for diagnosis, as well as the subsequent regime to restore the human organism to the locally determined condition of "health." For the most part the assertion "I feel ill" is accepted as a basis for making the effort to diagnosis—as in "You have an abscess in that tooth"—and the initiation of the subsequent procedure. The concept of "hypochondria" fills the gap between the benchmark beliefs of the client and the beliefs of the professional. "Feeling ill" and "being ill" are distinct concepts for physical diseases. In the domain of problems that end up in the psychiatrist's consulting room, however, the distinction is blurred and contested. The conceptual problem of chronic fatigue syndrome (CFS) began when declarations of "feeling ill" did not routinely lead to diagnoses of "being ill" but, rather, to assertions of malingering. The social construction dimension is also involved. For example, if a client confesses to Oliver Sacks that she believes she is controlled by aliens, the good doctor does not believe that she is. This is not a way to be. When a shaman declares that he has been on a journey through the spirit world, the rest of the villagers do believe him. In rural Mexico, it is a way to be. If a client complains of being tired all the time, that is a culturally acceptable way to be. How can we find a place into which to fit CFS as a problem—that is, as not a culturally acceptable way to be? Cognitive psychotherapy aimed at changing the beliefs of the client in such a way that she no longer believes that she is subject to extraterrestrial control makes sense in our culture, though it would be inappropriate to deal with a shaman's declarations in the same way. Does it make sense to try to persuade a client that he is not really exhausted? Clearly not.

THE BENCHMARK PROBLEM

This brief discussion highlights some aspects of the contrast between schizophrenia and chronic fatigue syndrome (CFS) in reflecting on the benchmark problem. The meta-narrative of schizophrenia has turned once again on the question of where to set the benchmark beyond which the actions and talk of someone merit a diagnosis. There seems to be some anecdotal evidence that fewer patients are currently being diagnosed as "schizophrenic" than was the case a decade ago. If this is correct, it raises questions about diagnostic criteria that are even more problematic in CFS. That there should be a question as to whether CFS should be assimilated to clinical depression or to malingering or to neither throws light, I believe, on the meta-discourse of schizophrenia. This discussion shows that CFS brings out very sharply the role of a benchmark for the concept "mental illness."

The basic principle of a sophisticated approach to physical medicine (Herzlich 1973) can be formulated as "All illnesses have both personal aspects (private experiential) and social aspects (public observable)." These aspects are associated with characteristic transformations in social relations and bodily states from some locally valid benchmark. Herzlich's studies showed how differently the benchmarks were set in Paris and in the French countryside. Country people ignored symptoms of common diseases such as colds and arthritis to a degree that Parisians used to ground their taking up the "sick role." This principle is "grammatical" in Wittgenstein's sense. In each distinctive milieu it fixes the sense of such remarks as "I'm sick," "She was ill last week," and so on.

There are exceptions to the principle that claims to be ill follow directly from experienced abnormal bodily states:

1. There are bodily malfunctions and abnormalities that are not accompanied by experiential distress or other abnormalities (e.g., high blood pressure). One comes to know that one is ill from being told a diagnosis.
2. There are experiential abnormalities that are not accompanied by discernible physical abnormalities (e.g. fibromyalgia and CFS).

Applying the basic principle to item 2 on the good inductive grounds that, in schizophrenia, the benchmark conditions in physical abnormalities have been found suggests that indiscernible physical abnormalities are implicated in CFS. The situation is very clear in the case of Alzheimer's disease. Postmortem studies of the brains of those whose word-finding problems deteriorate into dementia reveal a distinctive abnormality of the neural structures. Ways of dealing with people with these troubles can do much to improve the quality of life, yet the material basis is untreatable (Sabat 2002). With schizophrenia and Alzheimer's, the one-time contestable phenomenological and behavioral benchmarks are now more or less settled. The problem with CFS is not just the absence of lesions but the setting of a benchmark for what level of tiredness it is proper to feel.

DIAGNOSIS AS A COGNITIVE PRACTICE

Benchmark conditions have a role in the patterning of cognition that leads to "diagnosis" in contestable cases. Diagnosis involves two phases:

1. *Naming*: From an emerging gestalt of experiential matters derived from the patients' story and from that patient's discernible demeanor, the psychiatrist arrives at a categorization of the patient's situation as a known condition. The sequence of DSM publications fixes the benchmarks pro tem as thereby socially constructed.
2. *Aetiology*: From existing bodies of knowledge, the psychiatrist constructs a hypothesis as to the causes (origins) of the condition. It is in phase 2 that the benchmark condition subtly dominates the diagnostic narrative. It is a general principle in psychology that the identification of a brain state or process as being psychologically relevant is "top-down." The neural taxonomy is driven by a shifting combination of socially determined phenomenological and behavioral systems of classification of thoughts, feelings, and actions.

In physical medicine the physician usually collapses these phases into one cognitive act. Thus, a treatment plan follows unproblematically from the elided diagnostic phases. In schizophrenia, the two phases were once separable, since the physical aspect was unknown. Currently, in the case of CFS, the diagnostic phases are separable. It follows that there are two routes open for the setting up of a treatment plan:

> *Route* 1: Based on the hypothesis that the experiential aspects of CFS can be tackled directly, a psychological treatment plan is proposed. This corresponds to the narrative of schizophrenia in the Laing (1962) era, in which social construction was declared to be the sole aetiological pathway.
>
> *Route* 2: Based on the hypothesis that the indiscernible physical aspects of CFS as some subtle structural abnormality in the nervous system can be tackled indirectly, a physical treatment plan is proposed. Now the narrative of schizophrenia as it is currently understood serves as a benchmark, defining the story line. Pharmacology is called in to assist.

The possible medical responses to a phase 1 diagnosis—that is, a classification as a state beyond the locally fixed level of the ordinary—can be crude:

1. Whatever it is, it is only a physical disease: that is, it has physical causes only. Though this move cannot delete the experiential character of diagnostic phase 1, the medical response can ignore it and move on to physical treatment regimes. So the treatment is assimilated to a condition with a known physical cause and a known pharmacology. For some time, CFS was treated as if it were a form of clinical depression.

2. Since the physical causes of the alleged condition are indiscernible and therefore whatever it is is only a psychological disease, it has psychosocial causes only. Whatever treatment plan emerges from this move, the strong possibility exists that the patient is offended, since the lay concept of "mental illness" is pejorative and demeaning.

Medical responses can be nuanced. There are many aspects involved in diagnostic phases of any abnormal condition, including CFS, fibromyalgia, and other "imaginary" illnesses, so an overall treatment plan should involve both route 1 and route 2 procedures and regimes in principle. Any treatment plan involves personal management in several dimensions.

EXTENDING THE BENCHMARK RANGE
OF ABNORMALITIES

Here we encounter a principle, enunciated by Fulford (1989). A decision to emphasize the psychological aspects in developing a predominantly psychological treatment regime must be based on positive evidence that there are psychological abnormalities in the life of the patient, and not on the mere absence of discernible physical causes. This offers an alternative benchmark and a different meta-narrative from that derived by using schizophrenia as the exemplary case. We can briefly present the story of Tourette's syndrome (Hamilton 2000) as offering a different benchmark condition from schizophrenia and reflect on how that would affect the metanarratives we have been exploring.

Giles de Tourette described a pattern of involuntary but unacceptable public behavior. Currently such behavior ranges from bodily tics and cries to obscene shouting. Hamilton's work follows the transformation of the meaning of "Tourette's" as it passes through the diagnostic phases described earlier. The need to find a neurological abnormality matches the need to find a physical cause for CFS, avoiding the stigma of "mental illness." Once that has been found, another social force becomes operative — "support." Just as the fibromyalgia sufferers have formed support groups to counter medical skepticism and indifference (Harré 1991), so too have the Tourette's sufferers. Hamilton (2000) has demonstrated how these support groups have opened up a new social dimension in which the diagnosis of Tourette's is something to be sought. Tying this in with medical insurance enlarges the domain of the condition still further. It seems that the neural condition that leads to the range of involuntary behavior characteristic of Tourette's may be inherited. Now the possibility of achieving an advantageous diagnosis of "Tourette's" expands to include the relatives of sufferers who may harbor the gene without its having any overt expression.

A similar pattern emerges in the social dimension of CFS. That there is a real though unobservable biological malfunction that is responsible for the condition not only leads away from the socially undesirable diagnoses of malingering and/or mental illness and toward a respectable physical abnormality but also triggers financial support from the National Health Service, in the form of "home helps." This is denied to those whose problems are mental.

Conclusion

The interplay between unpleasant experiences and unacceptable conduct and medical intervention is complicated by the complex ways that "benchmarks" for normality and tolerability are set and reset. The most problematic situations arise where there are experiential benchmarks unattended by discernible physically abnormal states. On close examination, diagnosis and treatment regimes turn out to be at the intersection of phenomenological, social, physical, and even political dimensions.

REFERENCES

Fulford, W. (1989) *Moral Theory and Medical Practice*. Cambridge: Cambridge University Press.

Hamilton, S. (2000) "Tourette's Syndrome and the Social Conditioning of Illness." Ph.D. dissertation, Georgetown University, Washington, DC.

Harré, R. (1991) *Physical Being*. Oxford: Blackwell.

Herzlich, C. (1973) *Health and Illness*. Translated by J. Graham. London: Academic Press.

Laing, R. D. (1962) *The Divided Self*. London: Penguin Press.

Sabat, S. (2002) *The Experience of Alzheimer's*. Oxford: Blackwell.

Sykes, R., and Campion, P. (2003) *The Physical and the Mental in Chronic Fatigue Syndrome*. Bristol: Westcare UK.

CHAPTER 29

DEFINING MENTAL DISORDER

BERNARD GERT
CHARLES M. CULVER

DSM-IV DEFINITION OF MENTAL DISORDERS

A worthwhile philosophical discussion of the concept of mental disorders should be a discussion of what is used as a definition by those who treat mental disorders, such as the official definition of mental disorders, presented in the *Diagnostic and Statistical Manual of Mental Disorders* (DSM).[1] Although this definition is not accepted by all psychiatrists, it is accepted by most and has been used to revise the account of some of the conditions that count as mental disorders.[2] Of course, there is much more agreement on what count as the paradigm cases of mental disorders (schizophrenia, bipolar disorder, phobias, and compulsions) than on the general definition, but this definition of a mental disorder does include all of the clear cases of mental disorders and excludes all of the clear cases of conditions that are not mental disorders. DSM is such an official, accepted account of mental disorders that for psychiatrists to be reimbursed by an insurance company or the government for treating a patient, they must classify the patient's mental disorder by listing the number assigned to that disorder by DSM-IV.

Although psychiatrists are properly wary of definitions, it is significant that, even with a change in editors, the definition of mental disorder in DSM-IV (1994) is essentially the same as the definition in DSM-IIIR (1987).[3] The definition in DSM-III-R made some important philosophical changes to the definition in DSM-III, but its primary practical significance is that it made absolutely clear that deviation from a social norm by itself is never a sufficient condition for having a mental disorder. Mental disorders must involve the suffering of a nontrivial harm or a significantly increased risk of suffering such a harm.

The qualifications that are mentioned in DSM-IV prior to the definition being presented show that psychiatrists do not take the definition to be the final word on what a mental disorder is. These preliminary remarks make clear that mental disorders are viewed as a somewhat imprecise subclass of disorders or diseases, which differ from physical disorders primarily in their dominant symptoms. Thus, the definition of mental disorder, like most definitions of terms that are commonly used, must not be taken to provide a precise set of necessary and sufficient conditions for a condition of a person to be classified as having a mental disorder. This is made clear by the remark in DSM prior to the presentation of the definition:

> Although this volume is titled the *Diagnostic and Statistical Manual of Mental Disorders*, the term *mental disorder* unfortunately implies a distinction between "mental" disorders and "physical" disorders that is a reductionistic anachronism of mind/body dualism. A compelling literature documents that there is much "physical" in "mental disorders" and much "mental" in "physical disorders. . . .
>
> Moreover, although this manual provides a classification of mental disorders, it must be admitted that no definition adequately specifies precise boundaries for the concept of "mental disorder." The concept of mental disorder, like many other concepts in medicine and science, lacks a consistent operational definition that covers all situations. . . . Despite these caveats, the definition of *mental disorder* that was included in DSM-III and DSM-IIIR is presented here because it is as useful as any other available definition and has helped to guide decisions regarding what conditions on the boundary between normality and pathology should be included in DSM-IV. In DSM-IV each of the mental disorders is conceptualized as a clinically significant behavioral or psychological syndrome or pattern that occurs in a person and that is associated with present distress (a painful symptom) or disability (impairment in one or more important areas of functioning) or with a significantly increased risk of suffering death, pain, disability, or an important loss of freedom. In addition, this syndrome or pattern must not be merely an expectable and culturally sanctioned response to a particular event, for example, the death of a loved one. Whatever its original cause, it must currently be considered a manifestation of a behavioral, psychological, or biological dysfunction in the person. Neither deviant behavior (e.g., political, religious, or sexual) nor conflicts that are primarily between the individual and society are mental disorders unless the deviance or conflict is a symptom of a dysfunction in the person, as described above.[4]

The first sentence of the definition provides the essential features of mental disorders. The first part of this sentence makes clear that mental disorders involve behavioral or psychological features, rather than the physical features of the person. This demonstrates that a disorder is classified as a mental disorder rather than a physical disorder on the basis of its symptoms, not its cause or etiology. Like many physical disorders, the treatments for many mental disorders should include, as they increasingly do include, drugs, rather than some kind of cognitive psychotherapy. This fact reinforces what the preliminary remarks suggest, that, apart from their primary symptoms, there is no essential difference between mental and physical disorders.

Scientists are now even discovering genetic causes and structural neurological abnormalities that accompany some paradigm cases of mental disorders, such as schizophrenia and bipolar disorder. These discoveries have rendered irrelevant Thomas Szasz's claim that mental disorders are a myth because they are not related to any identifiable malfunction of the body. The discovery that at least some cases of bipolar disorder have a genetic cause does not affect at all whether bipolar disorder is classified as a mental disorder. Regardless of its etiology, bipolar disorder is a mental disorder because it involves "a clinically significant behavioral or psychological syndrome or pattern" that involves suffering death, pain, disability, or an important loss of freedom, or a significantly increased risk of suffering these harms.[5] However, many disorders, for example, dementia, have both behavioral or psychological symptoms and physical symptoms. It is often arbitrary whether these disorders are classified as mental or physical, and most often the classification depends on historical precedent.

Contrary to the views of many philosophers, cognitive disorders make up only a small fraction of mental disorders. There are mood disorders, anxiety disorders, sexual disorders, sleeping disorders, and impulse control disorders, and although these sometimes involve false views about oneself or the world, they often do not. Mental disorders may include desires to kill oneself, cause oneself pain, disable oneself, or cause oneself an important loss of freedom or pleasure; they may also include the extreme dread of some situation, and these desires and fears need not be based on false beliefs or any lack of information.

Both mental disorders and physical disorders must be associated with either "present distress (a painful symptom) or disability (impairment in one or more important areas of functioning) or a significantly increased risk of suffering death, pain, disability, or an important loss of freedom." Arthritis is a physical disorder that involves both present distress and disability. High blood pressure is a physical disorder that may involve no present distress or disability but does involve a significantly increased risk of death. Specific phobias are mental disorders that are associated with both present distress and disability.[6] Anorexia nervosa is associated with a significantly increased risk of death.[7] Nothing counts as a disorder, either mental or physical, unless it is associated with either present distress or disability or significantly increased risk of death, pain, disability, or an important loss of freedom or pleasure. The DSM-IV definition is an improvement over most definitions of disorders because it provides a list of universally acknowledged harms, rather than simply talking about harm in general. This acceptance of specific objective harms is incompatible with the relativist view that what counts as a harm is determined by particular societies. As is discussed in more detail later in this chapter, rejecting the relativist view is essential for maintaining the objective nature of the concept of disorder, while at the same time incorporating values into the concept of a disorder.

CRITICISMS OF THE DSM DEFINITION
OF MENTAL DISORDER

The kind of definition of mental disorder offered by DSM-IV is in conflict with two quite distinct and opposing views. The first kind of definition, whose most prominent exponent is Christopher Boorse, provides an objective account of mental disorders solely in value-free scientific terms. The second kind of definition, which is represented by Tristam H. Engelhardt and Peter Sedgwick, defines mental disorder solely in society-based value terms. R. E. Kendell is talking about these two opposing views when he says the following: "The most fundamental issue, and also the most contentious one, is whether disease and illness are normative concepts based on value judgments, or whether they are value-free scientific terms; in other words, whether they are biomedical terms or sociopolitical ones."[8] Thus, Kendell, in a paradigm of the fallacy of assumed equivalence, accepts the view that biomedical terms are value-free scientific terms and that normative concepts based on value judgments are sociopolitical terms. That some biomedical terms such as "disease" or "mental disorder" are objective value terms is not even considered as a possibility.

Jerome Wakefield, while agreeing with Kendell that value terms are sociopolitical, attempts to provide an account that reconciles the two opposing views of mental disorder that Kendell mentions. Against these two extreme accounts, Wakefield says: "I argue that disorder lies on the boundary between the given natural world and the constructed social world; a disorder exists when the failure of a person's internal mechanisms to perform their functions as designed by nature impinges harmfully on the person's well-being as defined by social values and meaning."[9] Wakefield defines a disorder as "a harmful dysfunction, wherein harmful is a value term based on social norms, and dysfunction is a scientific term referring to the failure of a mental mechanism to perform a natural function for which it was designed by evolution."[10] It is useful to examine Wakefield's attempt at compromise in some detail as it illustrates the problems with both of the views that he is attempting to bring together.

The first problem involves the claim that a dysfunction is "the failure of a person's internal mechanisms to perform their functions as designed by nature."[11] This view is reminiscent of Kant, who says: "In the natural constitution of an organized being, let us take it as a principle that in such a being no organ is to be found for any end unless it be the most fit and the best adapted for that end."[12] Kant simply assumes a teleological account of nature, derived from the view that God designed the best possible world. Wakefield's account of dysfunctions as failures "of a person's internal mechanisms to perform their functions as designed by nature" has the same characteristic. There is no reason to believe that *every* dysfunction is a failure of nature's design. Evolution may not be quite as perfect as Wakefield takes it to be. A person is suffering from a dysfunction when she is suffering one of the harms mentioned in the definition of mental disorder in DSM-III-R and DSM-IV, and there is no sustaining cause distinct from the person responsible for her suffering that harm. This is what DSM means by saying "Whatever its original cause, it must currently be considered a manifestation of a behavioral, psychological, or biological dysfunction in the person." This would have been clearer if the DSM definition had explicitly used the concept of a distinct sustaining cause.

CONCEPT OF A DISTINCT SUSTAINING CAUSE

The concept of a distinct sustaining cause is a crucial concept in defining a malady, disease, or disorder, including a mental disorder. A sustaining cause is a cause that not only brings about an effect, as a tree falling on a person's leg causes it to break, but whose removal results in the removal of the effect. A person's broken leg is not cured when the tree is removed. Being locked up in a cell causes a loss of freedom, but unlocking the cell restores that freedom, so being locked in a cell is a distinct sustaining cause of the locked-up person's loss of freedom In definitions of malady or mental disorder, a distinct sustaining cause is a sustaining cause of the harm or increased risk of harm that the person is suffering that is distinct from the person. A person in a car with no brakes going down a steep hill is suffering from anxiety and an increased risk of death, pain, and disability. However, he has no malady or mental disorder, because the harms and increased risk of harms he is suffering result from his being in the car, not from some internal condition.

Determining whether there is a distinct sustaining cause is often a difficult matter. Sometimes lack of something, such as food, water, or oxygen, can be a distinct sustaining cause. If providing the food, water, or oxygen, immediately or almost so, removes the distress or disability and any significantly increased risk of other harms, then the lack was a distinct sustaining cause. If the harms and increased risk persist for some time after the food, water, or oxygen has been supplied, then the lack of food, water, or oxygen may have caused some disorder, but their lack is no longer a distinct sustaining cause. The same is true of lack of education. If a person cannot read because he has not been taught to read, but with normal teaching the person gains the ability to read, the lack of the ability to read should be regarded as an inability rather than the kind of disability that constitutes a disorder. If the inability persists despite education, then it is a disability, and he suffers from a disorder.

Allergies and phobias are examples of maladies where it is important to make clear exactly what harms the person is suffering that do not have a distinct sustaining cause. Otherwise, there can be some difficulty in determining whether there is a distinct sustaining cause for the distress or disability or increased risk of harm. In these kinds of cases, the norm for the species is used to determine whether there is a distinct sustaining cause. If most people are not at increased risk of distress when exposed to a specific food or pollen or to a small enclosed space, then those people who are have a disorder. The food and small enclosed space may be distinct sustaining causes for any actual distress, but neither one is a distinct sustaining cause for the person's being at significantly increased risk of suffering distress in the presence of that food or small enclosed space.[13]

If the substance to which a person is allergic is not present, the person will not suffer any symptoms. Similarly, if the person who has a phobia is not confronted with that about which he has a phobia, he will not feel distress. It might be thought that the person with the allergy and the person with the phobia must have a current increased risk of suffering the harms associated with their malady. However, this may not be the case as they may have arranged their lives (e.g., moved to Arizona) so that they will not be in contact with that which brings on their symptoms. But they still suffer from a disability or loss of freedom. Unlike most people, they are not able to come into contact with the symptom-causing items without suffering some distress. Being confronted with what does not bother most people causes them to suffer some distress. For adults, comparison with all human beings in their prime, not merely a comparison with people in their own society, is what determines whether a person has a disability or a significantly increased risk of harm or suffers from a loss of freedom.[14]

Although Wakefield claims that there is a dysfunction only if there is a "failure of a person's internal mechanisms to perform their functions as designed by nature," he actually relies on the lack of a distinct sustaining cause to diagnose a dysfunction. He says: "The fact that in PTSD [posttraumatic stress disorder] the person's coping mechanisms often fail to bring the person back to functional equilibrium months and even years after the danger is gone, and that PTSD reactions are dramatically out of proportion to the actual posttraumatic danger, suggests that the response is indeed independent of any environmental maintaining cause and therefore is a dysfunction."[15] It is from the fact that there is no "environmental maintaining cause" that he infers that the person's distress is the result of a dysfunction. He does not and cannot know directly that there is a "failure of a person's internal mechanisms to perform their functions as designed by nature." The claim that a dysfunction is a failure of nature's design is often unverifiable. Perhaps nature designed people to deteriorate and die to allow for the species to develop. Regardless of nature's design, if a person is suffering or at a significantly increased risk of suffering death, pain, disability, or an important loss of freedom or pleasure, and there is no distinct sustaining cause, he has a dysfunction. It is significant that Wakefield never mentions conditions that significantly increase the risk of suffering a harm, such as very high blood pressure, as disorders, for, on his view, until there is a failure of nature's design, there is no dysfunction.[16]

VALUES AS DETERMINED BY PARTICULAR
SOCIETIES VERSUS VALUES AS UNIVERSAL

Wakefield's second problem is his acceptance of the common view of social scientists that values are constructed by particular societies. By accepting this account, he opens the door to the kind of relativity that the definitions of mental disorder in DSM-III-R and DSM-IV were designed to close. He does not seem to realize that if harms are determined primarily by social norms, then this opens the door to the criticism that psychiatry primarily enforces social norms. Wakefield claims, "The requirement that there be harm also accounts for why albinism, reversal of heart position, and fused toes are not considered disorders even though each results from a breakdown in the way some mechanism is designed to function."[17] Since Wakefield claims that albinism is a failure of nature's design, if a particular society negatively evaluates albinism, then it is a disorder in that society, but not a disorder in a society that does not negatively evaluate it. A person can cease to have a disorder simply by moving from one society to the other.

Also, if homosexuality and sexual deviations are taken as involving a breakdown in the way some mechanism is designed to function, homosexuality and other sexual deviations would be mental disorders in those societies where they are negatively evaluated and not in those societies where they are not so evaluated. His suggested definition would reverse the progress that was made in DSM-III-R and especially in DSM-IV, when "conflicts that are primarily between the individual and society" were explicitly ruled out as a criterion of mental disorder. Only traits that would result in conflict with any society count as a dysfunction in the person. This is the way in which the additional criterion that was added to the list of criteria for the paraphilias in DSM-IV — "The fantasies, sexual urges, or behaviors cause clinically significant distress or impairment in social, occupational, or other important areas of functioning" — should be understood.[18]

Wakefield's acceptance of the common view of social scientists that values are constructed by particular societies is what leads him to think that harm cannot be defined in universal terms. However, it is universally true that, in the absence of reasons to hold otherwise, every society regards death, pain, disability, and loss of freedom or pleasure as harms. No person who is considered rational wants to suffer any of these harms unless he has some belief that he or someone else will avoid what is considered by a significant number of persons to be either a greater harm or a compensating benefit, such as greater consciousness, ability, freedom, or pleasure. The universality of these harms is shown by the fact that nothing counts as a disorder unless it involves one of these harms or a significantly increased risk of suffering them, and nothing counts as a punishment unless it involves the infliction of one of these harms.[19]

The agreement of rational persons in all societies about the universality of the basic harms is extremely important, for it establishes the objectivity of the concept of a disorder. Disorders, mental or physical, are conditions that are associated with suffering distress or disability or a significantly increased risk of suffering death, pain, disability, or an important loss of freedom or pleasure. Mental disorders, properly understood, like physical disorders, are not merely labels for conditions that some culture or society has arbitrarily picked out for special treatment.[20] Mental disorders are conditions that no rational person in any society wants himself, or anyone he cares for, to suffer, unless there is some compensating benefit. There are times when a person might want to suffer a minor disorder in order to gain some advantage (e.g., mild asthma may result in a deferment from a wartime draft). But, as this example indicates, although society can arrange things to make it advantageous to have a disorder, mental or physical, having a disorder still involves at least an increased risk of suffering some harm. The disorder does not cease to exist merely because in that society, on balance, it is advantageous to have it.[21]

A disorder is a condition of a person, not of his environment. Activities that are not themselves symptoms of disorders may in time cause a person to have a disorder in which these same activities are symptoms of a disorder (e.g., smoking, drinking, or taking various recreational drugs may result in a person's coming to have a substance abuse disorder, which significantly increases his risks of death, pain, and so on).[22] The mental disorders of substance abuse, like high blood pressure, undoubtedly often involve genetic predispositions, which reinforces the view that what distinguishes mental disorders from physical disorders is primarily their symptoms, not their etiology.

It is not a symptom of a mental disorder to be distressed on discovering that one has a physical disorder, such as cancer, because the physical disorder counts as an event in the world, just as one's distress over the death of a loved one is an expectable and culturally sanctioned response. However, if the distress goes beyond an expectable and culturally sanctioned response to a particular situation, then one may be suffering a mental disorder that the physical disorder, just like other unfortunate events in the world, may have played a significant role in causing. What counts as an expectable and culturally sanctioned response to a particular event often differs from society to society and from culture to culture within large, multicultural societies like the United States. But, suffering distress or disability or having a significantly increased risk of death, pain, disability, or an important loss of freedom is a necessary feature of any disorder, mental or physical.

The fact that it is primarily on the basis of their symptoms that mental disorders differ from physical disorders makes it clear that "neither deviant behavior (e.g., political, religious, or sexual) nor conflicts that are primarily between the individual and society are mental disorders unless the deviance or conflict is a symptom of a dysfunction in the person." However, if the conflicts between a person and society are such that they would occur in any society, this is a symptom of a dysfunction in the person. Although deviance, by itself, is not sufficient to count as a disorder, some deviance seems to be so closely related to distress or disability or to a significantly increased risk of suffering death, pain, disability, or an important loss of freedom or pleasure that it is often classified as a disorder. Thus, having a third eye in one's head might actually give one greater visual abilities than those who have the normal number of eyes. Nonetheless, normal human responses to this kind of deviance may so regularly involve either pain or an important loss of freedom or pleasure that the deviance itself is regarded as a physical disorder. Similarly, normal human responses to some deviant behavior (e.g., sexual intercourse with corpses) may normally call forth such a universal negative human response that the behavior itself is regarded as a symptom of a mental disorder. However, for the reactions of others to any deviance, either physical or mental, to make a deviant condition count as a disorder, the reactions must be universal human responses, not merely the response of those in a particular society.

Although the DSM-IV definition of mental disorder can be improved, it is far superior to any of the alternatives, including Wakefield's, that have been proposed to replace it. Its major achievement is its acceptance of universal values, so that values can be included in the definition of a mental disorder without thereby making a disorder relative to each individual society. That is a significant achievement.

NOTES

1. Published by the American Psychiatric Association. "Those preparing ICD-10 and DSM-IV have worked closely to coordinate their efforts, resulting in much mutual influence" (DSM-IV: xxi). ICD-10 is the tenth edition of the *International Statistical Classification of Diseases and Related Health Problems* and was developed by the World Health Organization (WHO). This shows that the DSM-IV account of mental disorders is not merely some American idiosyncrasy.

2. In DSM-III-R, there was an inconsistency between the criteria for the paraphilias and the definition of mental disorder. In DSM-IV, this inconsistency was eliminated by changing the criteria for the paraphilias. See Gert (1992).

3. The only difference between the definition presented in DSM-III-R and DSM-IV is the addition of three words, "and culturally sanctioned," so that "expectable response" is now "expectable and culturally sanctioned response." This expresses more clearly what was meant in the DSM-III-R definition and so is an improvement.

4. DSM-IV: xxi.

5. "A significant loss of pleasure" should be added to this list to account for various sexual dysfunctions, as well as other psychological problems.

6. DSM-IV: 405–11.

7. DSM-IV: 539–45.

8. "What Are Mental Disorders?" in Freedman et al. (1986).

9. Ibid. Wakefield, like the editor of DSM-IV, regards the definition of mental disorder in DSM-III as "essentially the same as DSM-III-R's" (1992a: 380). Partly, this may be the result of his not knowing that Spitzer responded to conceptual criticisms of the definition of mental disorder in DSM-III in Culver and Gert (1982: 201) by inviting one of us to revise the definition to make it compatible with the definition of malady that we provided in that book. See Wakefield (1992b).

10. Wakefield (1992a: 373). This quotation is from the abstract that precedes the paper. Wakefield's view is listed as a mixed model by Christian Perring in his article "Mental Ill-

ness" for the Stanford online *Encyclopedia of Philosophy* (Perring 2002). We have benefited from reading this article and from comments by Perring on an earlier draft of this article. However, we do not agree with Perring on several points.

11. It seems that on this account of dysfunction, dyslexia is not a disorder because it is unlikely that nature designed an internal mechanism to perform the function of distinguishing between *b*'s and *d*'s.

12. Kant (1949), *Grounding for the Metaphysics of Morals*, first section, 395.

13. For a fuller account of the definition of malady, disorder, or disease and for an account of disabilities, including volitional disabilities, see chapter 5, "Malady," in Gert et al. (1997). For a fuller account of volitional disabilities, see "Free Will as the Ability to Will," in Gert and Duggan (1979), reprinted in *Moral Responsibility*, edited by John Martin Fisher (1986).

14. See Gert et al. (1997), chapter 5, "Malady."

15. Wakefield (1992b: 239).

16. See ibid.: 233, where there is no mention of increased risk of suffering the universal harms.

17. Ibid.: 384.

18. American Psychiatric Association (1994: 523–32). In DSM-III-R, this criterion was not included, and so there was an inconsistency between the criteria for the paraphilias and the definition of mental disorder. See Gert (1992: 155–71).

19. See Gert (1998), chapter 4, "Goods and Evils."

20. Appendix I of DSM-IV (844–49) contains a "Glossary of Culture Bound Syndromes," but all of these that are considered disorders also involve distress or disability or a significantly increased risk of suffering death, pain, disability, or an important loss of freedom. Wakefield (1992a: 380) says that "this list might be considered to be an operationalized approximation to the requirement that there must be harm." That he does not realize that this is a list of universal harms, not merely negative evaluations that depend on the judgments of particular societies, is confirmed by his statement on the following page: "Although a typology of harms such as that provided by DSM-III-R is useful, it should not be forgotten that . . . the underlying reason these effects are relevant to disorder is that they are negative and this evaluative element is fundamental to our judgments about disorder."

21. However, if what would otherwise clearly be a disorder, such as pregnancy, has advantages built into its very nature, it is generally not regarded as a disorder.

22. See DSM-IV, "Substance Abuse Disorders," pp. 182–83.

REFERENCES

American Psychiatric Association (1987) *Diagnostic and Statistical Manual of Mental Disorders*, 3rd ed., rev. [DSM-III-R]. Washington, DC: American Psychiatric Association.

American Psychiatric Association (1994) *Diagnostic and Statistical Manual of Mental Disorders*, 4th ed. [DSM-IV]. Washington, DC: American Psychiatric Association.

Culver, C. M., and Gert, B. (1982) *Philosophy in Medicine: Conceptual and Ethical Issues in Medicine and Psychiatry*. New York: Oxford University Press.

Fisher, J., (ed.) (1986) *Moral Responsibility*. Ithaca, NY: Cornell University Press.

Gert, B. (1992) "A Sex Caused Inconsistency in DSM-III-R: The Definition of Mental Disorder and the Definition of Paraphilias." *Journal of Medicine and Philosophy* 17(2): 155–71.

Gert, B. (1998) *Morality: Its Nature and Justification*. New York: Oxford University Press.

Gert, B., and Duggan, T. (1979) "Free Will as the Ability to Will." *Nous* 13(2): 197–217.

Gert, B., Culver, C. M., and Clouser, K. D. (1997). *Bioethics: A Return to Fundamentals.* New York: Oxford University Press.

Kant, E. (1949) *Grounding for the Metaphysics of Morals.* New York: Liberal Arts Press.

Kendell, R. E. (1986) "What Are Mental Disorders?" In A. M. Freedman, R. Brotman, I. Silverman, and D. Hutson (eds.), *Science, Practice, and Social Policy.* New York: Human Sciences Press.

Perring, C. (2002) "Mental Illness." In Edward Zalta (ed.), *Stanford Online Encyclopedia of Philosophy.* Available at http://plato.stanford.edu/archives/sum2002/entries/mental-illness

Wakefield, J. (1992a) "The Concept of Mental Disorder: On the Boundary between Biological Facts and Social Values." *American Psychologist* 47(3): 373–80.

Wakefield, J. (1992b) "Disorder as Harmful Dysfunction: A Conceptual Critique of DSM-III-R's Definition of Mental Disorder." *Psychological Review* 99(2): 23–39.

World Health Organization (1992) *International Statistical Classification of Diseases and Related Health Problem,* 10th ed. Washington, DC: World Health Organization.

CHAPTER 30

MENTAL ILLNESS AND
ITS LIMITS

CARL ELLIOTT

IF the studies are to be believed, we are in the midst of an epidemic of psychopathology. These newly popular pathologies range widely, not just in their incidence but in their presentation: social anxiety disorder, panic disorder, posttraumatic stress disorder, obsessive-compulsive disorder, generalized anxiety disorder, anorexia nervosa, bulimia, body dysmorphic disorder, depression, attention deficit hyperactivity disorder, multiple personality disorder (or dissociative identity disorder), gender identity disorder, and apotemnophilia, among others. Alongside these commonly accepted disorders have also arisen a number of new conditions whose very status as mental disorders is hotly disputed, such as fibromyalgia, chronic fatigue syndrome, and repetitive stress injury. Many of these disorders did not even exist a few decades ago, and others, now common, were once seen as very rare.[1]

Just as notable as the frequency with which these new disorders are being diagnosed is the controversy that surrounds them. Many physicians see the rise in psychopathology as the natural result of more astute diagnosis and greater public awareness.[2] Skeptics, in contrast, see phony disorders created by pharmaceutical manufacturers, the insurance industry, and the mental health profession in order to maximize profits.[3] A growing biological orthodoxy in psychiatry insists that all mental disorders are potentially explainable by neurochemistry,[4] while academic critics insist that mental disorders are socially constructed entities that have emerged to prop up existing power structures. Third-party payers resist paying for psychotherapy and long-term hospital stays, while pharmaceutical companies advertise new disorders and their newly approved psychoactive treatments on television. Analytic philosophers survey this therapeutic landscape and see conceptual confusion. If only philosophers could merely devise commonly accepted definitions as to what counts as a proper mental disorder, they suggest, then the confusion could be sorted out.[5]

Where some see confusion, however, others see the need for interpretation. What exactly is going on here? Why these particular ways of describing and expressing psychological suffering? Psychological suffering may well be universal, but our particular ways of organizing it are not. Many mental disorders have emerged only in particular historical periods and cultures, and others have taken different shapes under different social circumstances. Perhaps the question to be asked is not the one typically asked by analytic philosophers—"How can we refine and codify our currently confused definitions of various mental disorders?"—but, rather, "How have these mental disorders, in all their various permutations, become such widely used, common-sense ways of understanding psychological distress?"

Ian Hacking has compared the place held by a psychopathology in a particular culture to an "ecological niche." In the same way that a biologist might use the concept of an ecological niche to explain how a dragonfly is adapted to the southern swamplands or an antelope to the African savannah, Hacking uses it as a way of explaining how particular mental disorders emerge and thrive in particular places and ages. What cultural conditions accounted for the epidemic of multiple personality disorder in the United States in the 1970s and 1980s? Why hysterical paralysis in nineteenth-century Vienna and *taijin kyofusho* in twentieth-century Japan? To ask this question is not to suggest that mental disorders do not have identifiable physiological mechanisms. It is only to point out that every culture and age has its own ways of understanding illness and psychological suffering. To understand why particular disorders become widespread, we must look not just at their pathophysiology, not just at genetics and neurochemistry, but also at the social and historical context in which these disorder have arisen.[6]

Different disorders demand different explanations, of course. It would be simplistic to suggest that all currently popular disorders have similar causes or even that all the social conditions that shape mental disorders emerge could be briefly described. Different mental disorders occur in different populations, under different conditions, for different reasons. Anorexia nervosa, posttraumatic stress disorder, and multiple personality disorder are, in many ways, the products of very different social currents. Even so, the question remains: why such a recent upsurge of mental disorder? I want to suggest that there are at least four factors at work.

The first is the background to the upsurge: the ascendancy of biomedicine as the dominant way of understanding and explaining psychological distress. Until the end of the nineteenth century, the domain of psychiatry was almost exclusively seen to be madness, or what is now called psychosis. Psychiatric patients were asylum inmates. If ordinary people wanted help with personal problems, they went to family and friends or to the clergy. But this changed with the rise of psychoanalysis and psychodynamic theory. Psychodynamic explanations of mental life blurred the lines between psychopathology and more ordinary varieties of unhappiness and thus dramatically expanded the range of people considered possible candidates for psychiatric treatment. By the early decade of the twentieth century, the domain of psychiatry was no longer limited to the asylum. It had expanded to include problems in living.[7]

While psychodynamic theory greatly expanded the jurisdiction of the psychiatric profession, it did not suggest that psychic distress should be carved up into discrete units called "mental disorders." That came with a number of other social and institutional changes that entrenched the disease model of psychopathology. Some of these were internal to the psychiatric profession, such as the popularity of Emil Kraepelin's categorical, disease-based model of psychopathology and its eventual influence over the development of the American Psychiatric Association's *Diagnostic and Statistical Manual*, especially the third revision in 1980 (DSM-III).[8] The DSM-III formally classified psychopathology into distinct medical entities identifiable by lists of signs and symptoms.

But American psychiatry itself got a tremendous boost from larger social developments, such as the founding of the National Institute of Mental Health in 1946, as well as the 1951 and 1962 amendments to the 1938 Federal Food, Drug and Cosmetics Act. In the earlier part of the twentieth century, most drugs were available to patients without a prescription. But in 1951, the Humphrey-Durham amendment gave the FDA the power to decide which drugs were available only with a prescription. This gave tremendous power to doctors by making them the gatekeepers to drugs, including the psychoactive drugs developed in the 1950s, such as chlorpromazine (Thorazine) and meprobamate (Miltown). The biomedical model of illness was given a further boost in 1962 when the U.S Congress passed the Kefauver-Harris amendments in response to the thalidomide disaster. The 1962 amendments expanded the mandate of the FDA to include over-the-counter drugs, endorsed randomized clinical trials, and encouraged companies to develop drugs for specific diseases.[9] Drugs that once might have been thought of as tonics, pick-me-ups, or energy boosters were now thought of as treatments for psychological illnesses.

By the end of the twentieth century, the biomedical model of understanding psychic distress had become thoroughly entrenched in the American health-care system and elsewhere. Reimbursement codes for third-party payers, diagnostic instruments, specialty associations and specialty clinics, randomized clinical trials, formal research papers, pharmaceutical marketing campaigns, medical conference symposia—all are now organized around a biomedical model of illness that says that psychological distress can be categorized into discrete, diagnosable conditions, to be diagnosed and treated by mental health professionals working in the health-care system.

Yet, even as our social institutions have entrenched discrete categories of mental disorders, the boundaries of these disorders have remained fluid and flexible. Not only are the pathophysiological mechanisms behind most mental disorders unknown, but also most disorders are not characterized by any objective findings on physical examination, medical imaging devices, or laboratory tests. Instead, clinicians diagnose and categorize most mental disorders solely by virtue of the patient's thought and behavior (e.g., guilt, hallucinations, delusions, compulsions, sleep loss). This aspect of diagnosis makes the boundaries of mental disorders unavoidably flexible, despite the profession's attempts to draw clear lines between psychopathology and eccentricity or between unhappiness and other forms of psychological suffering. Social anxiety disorder blends into shyness; attention deficit hyperactivity disorder into distractibility; depression into sadness, loneliness, or alienation.

A second broad reason for the upsurge in mental illness, paradoxically, is the success of biomedicine in treating it. Medical treatments do not simply cure or control medical conditions; they also create them. Once a method of remedying a particular condition is developed and placed in the hands of medical practitioners, that condition tends to become reconceptualized as a medical problem. This phenomenon is not limited to psychiatry. The inability of some people to have children, for example, was reconceptualized as the medical problem of infertility only after the development of new reproductive technologies such as sperm donation and in vitro fertilization.[10] But psychiatry provides the best examples of this phenomenon. When the new disorder of "neurasthenia" arose in the nineteenth century, it was accompanied by the new treatment of the "rest cure" in private clinics.[11] When the new disorder of "gender dysphoria" arose in the mid-twentieth century, it was accompanied by new surgical techniques for sex reassignment.[12] When anxiety disorders became widespread in the 1950s and 1960s, they were accompanied by the development of "minor tranquilizers" such as meprobamate (Miltown) and the benzodiazepines (such as Valium and Librium).[13] And when the concept of "hyperactivity" (soon renamed "attention deficit disorder") became widespread in the 1970s, it was accompanied by an upsurge in prescriptions for methylphenidate (Ritalin).[14]

Such developments help explain the upsurge in at least some of the recently popular mental disorders. Twenty years ago, social anxiety disorder—an extreme fear of being embarrassed or humiliated in public—was thought to be a rare disorder, if it was thought about at all; it was not even listed in the third edition of the American Psychiatric Association's *Diagnostic and Statistical Manual* (DSM-III), in 1980. In the mid-1980s, however, studies began to be published indicating that social anxiety disorder (then called social phobia) could be treated with the antidepressant phenelzine (Nardil).[15] In the mid-1980s, social phobia was added to DSM-III-R. Later came evidence that it responded to the SSRI (selective serotinin reuptake inhibitors) antidepressants, such as Paxil (paroxetine).[16] Today, it is often described as the third most common mental disorder in the United States, affecting more than 13 percent of the population.[17]

A similar story could be told for other disorders. The diagnosis of panic disorder did not become common until the anxiolytic drug alprazolam (Xanax) began to be widely prescribed in the 1980s.[18] By 1998, panic disorder had become so widely diagnosed that the National Institute of Mental Health reported that it affected 2.4 million adults between the ages of 17 and 54.[19] Obsessive-compulsive disorder was considered very rare in the years before the FDA approved clomiprimine (Anafranil) as a treatment in 1990. Today, obsessive-compulsive disorder is said to affect 3 percent of the population.[20] Such patterns do not necessarily mean that psychoactive drugs are being overprescribed. In fact, it is usually because these drugs show some measure of success that they become popular. Rather, these patterns indicate just how flexible the boundaries of mental disorders are and how they can expand or contract in response to the demands of clinical practice.

A third factor in the upsurge of mental disorder has come from patients themselves. As many mental disorders have become more widely diagnosed and treated, they have also been accompanied by the growth of support and advocacy groups.[21] Some of these groups provide emotional support for patients who suffer from the disorder in question. Many groups have a prominent presence on the Internet, and some are quite large. A number of advocacy groups have aims that are explicitly political, and these groups lobby professional and governmental authorities for funding and legislative change.[22]

These groups help build communities around mental disorders. They give sufferers a shared vocabulary with which to describe their problems, a shared set of behaviors, and, often, a sense of solidarity. By communicating with a group of like-minded people, potential sufferers of a disorder learn what psychological symptoms are important, where to seek help, what treatments to ask for, who and how to lobby for political change. This community-building aspect of support and advocacy groups has taken on even greater importance with the rise of the Internet, which allows people with uncommon and often stigmatized problems to communicate easily and anonymously with one another over great distances.[23] Some support and advocacy groups have been loosely allied with broader political movements, such as eating disorders with the women's movement, or posttraumatic stress disorder with the Vietnam veteran's movement.[24]

Stigma plays an interesting role in sustaining many of these groups.[25] For at least some support and advocacy groups, one explicit purpose is to combat the stigma associated with a particular condition — by providing sufferers with a sense of solidarity, by conducting public awareness campaigns, by encouraging sufferers to feel that they do not have to hide their conditions, and so on. One way of combating the stigma of a condition is to reconceptualize it in the public mind as a medical problem — in the way, for instance, that attempts have been made to reconceptualize the vice of "drunkenness" into the medical problem of "alcoholism" or "substance abuse disorder." Medicalizing a condition typically removes some of its stigma by taking the condition from the realm of personal responsibility (which makes it a vice, a sin, or a crime) and placing it in the realm of misfortune. For this reason, many support and advocacy groups are strong advocates of biomedical models of psychopathology, arguing that depression, social anxiety disorder, panic disorder, attention deficit hyperactivity disorder, and so on are bona fide medical problems and that sufferers should be seen in the same light as sufferers of physical illnesses such as cancer, heart disease, and diabetes.[26] In some cases, these groups have lobbied successfully for access to the social advantages of illness, such as coverage by health insurance and admission to the vocational and educational exceptions due to people with physical illnesses or disabilities.[27] The very use of the term "mental illness" (rather than, say, "neurosis," "insanity," "nervous breakdown," or other euphemisms) can be seen as an effort to move certain kinds of psychological distress into the biomedical realm.

Yet, even as sufferers of some kinds of psychological distress are trying to get into the DSM, others are trying to get out. For instance, people who wished to have sex reassignment surgery were once willing to be diagnosed as having the mental disorder "gender dysphoria" if such a diagnosis would gain them access to surgery. Yet, today, some groups of transgendered people resist the concepts of gender dysphoria or gender identity disorder, arguing that their condition should be seen as normal human variation.[28] For different reasons, support groups for sufferers of controversial conditions such as chronic fatigue syndrome, fibromyalgia, multiple chemical sensitivity disorder, repetitive stress injury, and chronic Lyme disease have fiercely resisted the suggestion that their problems might have psychological roots, arguing that their symptoms, even if they are currently mysterious, will ultimately be shown to have physical causes.[29] Unlike some transgendered people who resist the suggestion that they are in any way ill, sufferers of these controversial conditions argue that they are ill—but not *mentally* ill. Their reasons are quite understandable. Despite efforts to compare "mental illness" to physical illness, the two are still widely seen as different. It is still less stigmatizing to have one's condition seen as a physical illness or as normal human variation than as a mental illness.

A fourth factor behind the upsurge in the diagnosis and treatment of psychopathology is commercial. Many of the newly popular psychopathologies are currently treatable (and widely treated) with psychoactive medication, and most of these medications have been developed and marketed by the pharmaceutical industry. Unlike most commodities in a market economy, however, medications must be marketed not just to the patients who will take them but also to the doctors who must prescribe them. This is not simply a matter of convincing doctors that the medication is safe and effective. It is also a matter of convincing doctors that the medication treats a proper illness. Prozac must not merely lift a person's mood; it must treat a patient's depression. Ritalin must not merely improve a person's attention span; it must treat a patient's attention deficit hyperactivity disorder. Thus, the pharmaceutical industry is not just in the position of selling psychoactive medications. It must also sell psychopathology.

In order to market a drug, the industry must (in the words of a writer for *Pharmaceutical Marketing* magazine) "reinforce the actual existence of a disease," especially to doctors.[30] This kind of marketing goes beyond mere advertisements in medical journals and even beyond the 83,000 "drug representatives" the U.S. industry employed in 1999 to visit physicians and dispense nearly $8 billion worth of free drug samples.[31] The pharmaceutical industry also sponsors academic conference sessions, special journal symposia, educational sessions for medical residents, and continuing medical education for practicing physicians. It distributes reprints of favorable journal articles and popular books about psychiatric disorders. It donates money to patient support and advocacy groups and to professional associations such as the American Psychiatric Association, and it sponsors events to promote public awareness of mental disorders.[32] It pays ghostwriters to write editorials for scientific journals and then pays prominent researchers to sign their names to the editorials.[33] The industry recruits

and pays community physicians to conduct postmarketing or "seeding trials" in order
to make physicians more familiar with recently approved medications and the illnesses these medications treat.[34] In efforts such as these, marketing merges with medical education and research to widen the scope and reach of psychiatric diagnosis.[35]

Until recently, such marketing efforts were aimed mainly at physicians. But, in
1997, the U.S. Food and Drug Administration relaxed its restrictions on direct-to-
consumer advertising of prescription drugs. As a result, pharmaceutical companies
now advertise psychiatric medications with television commercials, ads in glossy mag-
azines, and, in the case of Prozac Weekly, cut-out newspaper coupons and unsolicited
drug mailings directly to potential patients.[36] In 2000, the U.S. pharmaceutical industry spent $2.4 billion on direct-to-consumer advertising, a tenfold increase since
1996.[37] Direct-to-consumer advertising has been especially effective for antidepressants, whose use has expanded beyond the treatment of depression to encompass
disorders such as social anxiety disorder, posttraumatic stress disorder, obsessive-
compulsive disorder, generalized anxiety disorder, anorexia nervosa, and premenstrual
dysphoric disorder, among others. Antidepressants are now the best-selling category
of drugs in the United States. From 1999 to 2000, antidepressant prescriptions increased by 20.9 percent, generating $10.4 billion in sales. In 2000, Prozac was Amer-
ica's fourth most prescribed drug; Zoloft was the seventh most prescribed drug, and
Paxil was the eighth.[38]

Some skeptics point to social factors such as marketing as evidence that many
newly emerging mental disorders are not real and that healthy people are being gulled
into believing they are sick. But a condition cannot simply be medicalized at the
wish of a pharmaceutical company. The marketing of a mental disorder would not
be effective without a social background against which the notion of such a disorder
makes sense, and the marketing of a psychoactive drug would not be effective if the
drug did not work. If shyness can be medicalized into social anxiety disorder or
distractibility into attention deficit hyperactivity disorder, it is because we live in a
society in which such disorders and their explanations sound plausible.

Psychological distress is shaped in ways much more complicated than mere marketing. It is influenced not just by what we feel happening in our own bodies or
minds but by the social context that shapes our experience of the world. From this
social context we learn a vocabulary to describe and express our psychological distress,
a set of theoretical structures with which to interpret it, and the socially sanctioned
behaviors that go along with it. By participating in a linguistic community, we learn
the meanings of words such as "social phobia" and "anorexia nervosa" and "gender
dysphoria," as well as the experiences and behaviors that go along with them. In turn,
the meanings of these words change in response to the experiences and behaviors of
those people the words describe. As the language and theoretical apparatus of biomedicine begins to dominate our social institutions, from diagnostic manuals and
reimbursement codes to television advertisements and public awareness campaigns,
it is reasonable to expect they will also influence the way we describe our mental
lives.

NOTES

1. For an excellent, well-documented sociological and historical overview of these developments, see Horwitz (2002).

2. See, for example, the report of an AMA task force on ADHD: Goldman et al. (1998).

3. Kutchins and Kirk (1997).

4. Guze (1989).

5. Reznek (1991); Daniels and Sabin (1998).

6. See especially Hacking (1998) and (1995).

7. Abbott (1988): 280–314.

8. See Horwitz (2002); also Healy (2000).

9. Healy (1997): 23, 27 and (2002): 367–68.

10. Gaylin (1993).

11. Shorter (1997): 129–30.

12. Gilman (1999): 258–88.

13. Smith (1985): 69–74.

14. Conrad and Potter (2000).

15. Liebowitz et al. (1986) and (1988).

16. Stein et al. (1998); Baldwin et al. (1999).

17. Kessler et al. (1994); Lamberg (1998): 685–86.

18. See Shorter (1997): 320.

19. Narrow et al. (1998).

20. Kaplan et al. (1994): 599.

21. Sabshin (1990).

22. Valenstein (1998).

23. Elliott (2000).

24. See Conrad and Potter (2000); also Young (1995).

25. Goffman (1963/1986).

26. Valenstein (1998): 177.

27. See, for example, Diller (1998): 149–50.

28. Nelson (1998).

29. Groopman (2000); Aronowitz (1998): esp. 19–38, 57–83.

30. Cited in Moynihan et al. (2002).

31. National Institute for Health Care Management, "Prescription Drugs and Mass Media Drug Advertising 2000."

32. Koerner (2002): 58–63, 81; Valenstein (1998): 180–82.

33. Bosely (2002).

34. La Puma and Kraut (1994).

35. Angell and Relman (2001); Stolberg (2001); Appleby (2001).

36. Davis (2001); Neergard (2002).

37. National Institute for Health Care Management, "Prescription Drugs and Mass Media Drug Advertising 2000."

38. Figures taken from "Prescription Drug Expenditures in 2000: The Upward Trend Continues," a report by the National Institute for Health Care Management. See especially pp. 17 and 19.

REFERENCES

Abbott, A. (1988) *The System of Professions*. Chicago: University of Chicago Press.
Angell, M., and Relman, A. S. (2001) "Prescription for Profit." *Washington Post*, June 20.
Appleby, J. (2001) "Sales Pitch: Drug Firms Use Perks to Push Pills." *USA Today*, May 16.
Aronowitz, R. (1998) *Making Sense of Illness*. Cambridge: Cambridge University Press.
Baldwin, D., Bobes, J., Stein, D. J., Scharwachter, I., and Faure, M. (1999) "Paroxetine in Social Phobia/Social Anxiety Disorder: Randomised, Double-Blind, Placebo-Controlled Study." Paroxetine Study Group. *British Journal of Psychiatry* 175: 120–26.
Bosely, S. (2002) "Scandal of Scientists Who Take Money for Papers Ghostwritten by Drug Companies." *Guardian* (U.K.), February 7, 2002.
Conrad, P., and Potter, D. (2000) "From Hyperactive Children to ADHD Adults: Observations on the Expansion of Medical Categories." *Social Problems* 47(4): 559–82.
Daniels, N., and Sabin, J. E. (1998) "Last Chance Therapies and Managed Care: Pluralism, Fair Procedures, and Legitimacy." *Hastings Center Report* 28(2): 27–41.
Davis, R. (2001) "Lilly Seeks a Lift with Weekly Prozac." *USA Today*, June 6.
Diller, L. (1998) *Running on Ritalin*. New York: Bantam Books.
Elliott, C. (2000) "A New Way to Be Mad?" *Atlantic Monthly*, December, pp. 72–84.
Gaylin, W. (1993) "Faulty Diagnosis," *Harper's*, October, pp. 57–64.
Gilman, S. (1999) *Making the Body Beautiful: A Cultural History of Aesthetic Surgery*. Princeton, NJ: Princeton University Press.
Goffman, I. (1963/1986) *Stigma: Notes on the Management of a Spoiled Identity*. New York: Simon and Schuster.
Goldman, L. S., Genel, M., Benzman, R. J., and Slanetz, P. J. (1989) "Diagnosis and Treatment of Attention-Deficit/Hyperactivity Disorder in Children and Adolescents." *Journal of the American Medical Association* 279(14): 1100–7.
Groopman, J. (2000) "Hurting All Over." *New Yorker*, November 13, pp. 78–79.
Guze, S. B. (1989) "Biological Psychiatry: Is There Any Other Kind?" *Psychological Medicine* 19: 315–23.
Hacking, I. (1995) *Rewriting the Soul: Multiple Personality and the Sciences of Memory*. Princeton: Princeton University Press.
Hacking, I. (1998) *Mad Travelers: Reflections on the Reality of Transient Mental Illness*. Charlottesville: University Press of Virginia.
Healy, D. (1997) *The Antidepressant Era*. Cambridge, MA: Harvard University Press.
Healy, D. (2000) "Good Science or Good Business?" *Hastings Center Report* 30(2): 19–22.
Healy, D. (2002) *The Creation of Psychopharmacology*. Cambridge, MA: Harvard University Press.
Horwitz, A. V. (2002). *Creating Mental Illness*. Chicago: Chicago University Press.
Kaplan, H. I., Sadock, B., and Grebb, J. (1994) *Kaplan and Sadock's Synopsis of Psychiatry*, 7th ed. New York: Williams and Wilkins.
Kessler, R. C., McGonagle, K. A., et al. (1994) "Lifetime and 12-Month Prevalence of DSM-III-R Psychiatric Disorders in the United States: Results from the National Comorbidity Survey." *Archives of General Psychiatry* 51(1): 8–19.
Koerner, B. I. (2002) "Disorders, Made to Order." *Mother Jones*, July/August, pp. 58–63, 81.
Kutchins, H., and Kirk, S. A. (1997) *Making Us Crazy: DSM—The Psychiatric Bible and the Creation of Mental Disorders*. New York: Free Press.
Lamberg, L. (1998) "Social Phobia: Not Just Another Name for Shyness." *JAMA* 280(8): 685–86.

La Puma, J., and Kraut, J. (1994) " 'How Much Do You Get Paid If I Volunteer?' Suggested Institutional Policy on Reward, Consent, and Research." *Hospital and Health Services Administration* 39(2): 193–203.

Liebowitz, M. R., Fyer, A. J., Gorman, J. M., Campeas, R., and Levin, A. (1986) "Phenelzine in Social Phobia." *Journal of Clinical Psychopharmacology* 6(2): 93–98.

Liebowitz, M. R., Gorman, J. M., Fyer, A. J., Campeas, R., Levin, A. P., Sandberg, D., et al. (1988) "Pharmacotherapy of Social Phobia: An Interim Report of a Placebo-Controlled Comparison of Phenelzine and Atenolol." *Journal of Clinical Psychiatry* 49(7): 252–57.

Moynihan, R., Heath, I., and Henry, D. (2002) "Selling Sickness: The Pharmaceutical Industry and Disease-Mongering." *British Medical Journal* 324: 886–91.

Narrow, W. E., Rae, D. S., Regier, D. A. (1998) "NIMH Epidemiology Note: Prevalence of Anxiety Disorders. One-year Prevalence Best Estimates Calculated from ECA and NCS Data. Population Estimates Based on U.S. Census Estimated Residential Population Age 18 to 54 on July 1, 1998." Unpublished. Information provided by NIMH Public Inquiries, 6001 Executive Boulevard, Rm. 8184, MSC 9663, Bethesda, MD 20892–9663 U.S.A. Available at http://www.nimh.nih.gov/publicat/numbers.cfm#12

National Institute for Health Care Management (2001a) "Prescription Drugs and Mass Media Drug Advertising 2000." Information provided by NIHCM Foundation, 1225 19th St. NW, Suite 710, Washington, DC 20036. Available at www.nihcm.org

National Institute for Health Care Management (2001b) "Prescription Drug Expenditures in 2000: The Upward Trend Continues." Information provided by NIHCM Foundation, 1225 19th St. NW, Suite 710, Washington, DC 20036. Available at www.nihcm.org

National Institute of Mental Health (NIMH) (2001) Data available at http://www.nimh.nih .gov/publicat/numbers.cfm#12

Neergard, L. (2002) "Floridians Get Prozac Samples in the Mail." *New York Times*, July 4.

Nelson, J. L. (1998) "The Silence of the Bioethicists: Ethical and Political Aspects of Managing Gender Dysphoria." *GLQ: A Journal of Lesbian and Gay Studies* 4(2): 213–30

Reznek, L. (1991) *A Philosophical Defense of Psychiatry.* New York: Routledge.

Sabshin, M. (1990) "Turning Points in Twentieth Century American Psychiatry." *American Journal of Psychiatry* 147: 1267–74.

Shorter, E. (1997) *A History of Psychiatry: From the Era of the Asylum to the Age of Prozac.* New York: Wiley.

Smith, M. (1985) *Small Comfort: A History of Minor Tranquilizers.* New York: Praeger.

Stein, M. B., Liebowitz, M. R., Lydiard, R. B., Pitts, C. D., Bushnell, W., and Gergel, I. (1998) "Paroxetine Treatment of Generalized Social Phobia (Social Anxiety Disorder): A Randomized Controlled Trial." *JAMA* 280(8): 708–13.

Stolberg, S. (2001) "Scientists Often Mum about Ties to Industry." *New York Times*, April 25.

Valenstein, E. (1998) *Blaming the Brain: The Truth about Drugs and Mental Health.* New York: Free Press.

Young, I. (1995) *The Harmony of Illusions: Inventing Post-Traumatic Stress Disorder.* Princeton: Princeton University Press.

INDEX

....

abnormality, 305, 412–13
accessibility assumption, 109
action, 78–88
actus reus, 297
adaptation, 331, 333–34
addiction, 80, 81–85, 373–77
adolescents
   ethical issues in treatment of, 148–52
   female, 239–40
   mental disorder in, 155–56
advance directives, 139–40
advocacy, 289–90
advocacy groups, 430
affectivity, 36–53
African Americans. *See* blacks
agoraphobia, 80
AHS. *See* Alien Hand Syndrome
Ainslie, George, 82–85
akratic action, 79–81
Algeria, 250
Alien Hand Syndrome (AHS), 123–24, 127–
   28, 129nn.10–11
Allen, Clifford, 54
amnesia, 109, 110
Analytic Freud, The (Levine), 339
Anarchic Hand Syndrome, 124, 128
anorexia nervosa, 122–23, 125, 127, 395,
   417, 427
antidepressants, 48–49, 148, 432
antidiagnosis, 163–79
antipsychotics, 369–71
antireductionism, 191–204
antisocial personality disorder, 334,
   335
anxiety, 331–32
Apel, Karl-Otto, 185
appreciation, 260
a priori scientific principles, 31–32

Ardal, Pall, 42
Aristotle, 41, 187n.1, 302
artistic genius, 38
attention, 27–30, 33
attentional disorder, 25–26
attention deficit disorder, 378n.11, 399,
   400, 401, 429
Austin, J.L., 219
autism, 127, 153
autonomy, 283–85, 293

Bandura, Albert, 382, 383, 385, 386
Barlow, David, 390
Beck, Aaron, 50n.2, 390
behavior therapies, 381–83, 389–90
   See also cognitive-behavioral models
Bentham, Jeremy, 42, 303
berdache, 238
Binswanger, Ludwig, 342, 345
bioethics, 218, 222, 225
biological function, 195, 200
biopower, 248
bipolar mood disorders, 138
bisexuality, 342
Black Rage (Grier and Cobbs), 247
blacks, 246, 247, 250
blame, 245, 297, 304
Bleuler, Eugen, 317
blindsight, 103n.1
body, 118–32, 368–69
body image, 119–20, 123
body schema, 119–20, 123, 125
Boorse, Christopher, 418
Boothby, Richard, 339
borderline personality disorder, 395, 397
Bordo, Susan, 122, 123
Bracton, Henri de, 297
Bradley Ctr., Inc. v. Wessner, 274

brain
    and addiction, 373–74, 376
    chemistry, 373–74
    and criminal responsibility, 307
    parallel processing, 99–100
    split-brain behavior, 124
"brain pain," 34
Brentano, Franz, 338, 340–41, 343
Breuer, Josef, 341
Brindle, David, 288
Browning, Don, 313
Butler, Judith, 47–48
Butler-Sloss, Dame Elizabeth, 269n.2
butyrphenones, 370
Byron, Lord, 50

Cade, John, 214
Campbell, J., 31–32
capability assumption, 108
capacities, 108
Cartesian parallelism, 344
Cartwright, Nancy, 202, 203
Catania, A.C., 384, 385
causal bridges, 367
CFS. See chronic fatigue syndrome
character, 64–77
characterization
    diagnosis as, 166–67
    identity, 142–43
character theory, 306
Charcot, Jean-Martin, 338, 341, 345, 399
children
    disorders of, 147–60
    ethical issues in treatment of, 148–52
    medication for, 148–49
    sexual abuse of, 241
    theories of development and
        psychopathology, 153–54
chlorpromazine, 369–70, 428
choice, 269n.8
chronic fatigue syndrome (CFS), 410–11,
        412, 413, 431
clang associations, 24
Clark, Lee Ann, 65
clinical decision making, 208–9
clinical depression. See depression
closure, 359

clozapine, 370
Cobbs, P.M., 247
cognition, 21–34
cognitive-behavioral models, 381–92
    cognitive causation, 384–89
    current issues, 384–90
    history, 381–83
    identity of behavior therapy and
        cognitive therapy, 389–90
collusion, 245, 246
communication skills, 223–24, 225
communicative action, 361
communitarianism, 293–94
community care, 287–89
community treatment orders (CTOs),
        289
compelled action, 80–81
competence, 258–70, 285
    as ability to make rational decision,
        265–67
    inadequacy of pure understand and
        appreciate definition, 261–62
    irrational patient decision, 262–63
    logic of, 259
    modifying understand and appreciate
        definition, 263–64
    symmetry and asymmetry of consents
        and refusals, 265
    understand and appreciate definition,
        260–61
confidentiality, 320
confusion, 33, 34
connectedness, 360
Connecticut, 278
conscious denial, 110
consciousness, 322, 341
conversation, 28
Copernican Revolution, 344–45, 346
corpus callosum, 124
countervailing influences, 276
criminal responsibility, 296–311
    antirealist approach, 303–4
    legal evolution of, 297–99
    psychiatric/pragmatic approach,
        304–8
    realist approach, 301–2
    thought experiments, 300–308

Cross Cultural Psychiatry (Herrera et al.), 246

CR principle. *See* principle of compositional reversibility

CTOs. *See* community treatment orders

cultural genius, 41

culture, 244–57, 341, 355–56, 427

dangerousness, 271–81

Darwinian models, 329–37

Davidson, Donald, 388

deafferentation, 122, 127

de Beauvoir, Simone, 154

decision making, 208–9, 224–26

delusions, 21–22
 cause of, 401
 of control, 126
 Cotard, 122, 123, 125, 127
 and criminal responsibility, 306
 phenomenology of, 229n.11
 thought insertion, 90

dementia, 417

democracy, 230n.14

denial, 110

depersonalization disorder, 122, 123, 125, 127

depression, 36–53, 396, 398
 depressive realism, 37–44
 Elliott on, 40
 and gender, 47–49
 melancholic modernity, 45–47
 poetry and prose of, 38–40
 psychopharmacological Calvinism, 38, 43–44
 social/political analysis of, 44–49

depth, 360

Descartes, René, 368

descriptivism, 229n.11

desire(s)
 irresistible, 79–82
 paraphilia and distress in DSM-IV, 54–63

determinism, 301

development, 147–60

deviance, 56

diagnosis, 163–79, 186–87
 benchmarks for, 409
 as characterization, 166–67
 as cognitive practice, 411–12
 decision making on, 208
 definition of, 166
 as disclosure, 167–68
 as embedded observation, 168
 labeling, 171–72
 medicalization, 172
 as privilege, 169
 and psychiatric power, 173–74
 as rationality, 169–70
 reductionism, 173
 as relevance, 168–69
 as ritual, 170–71
 and values, 174–76

Diagnostic and Statistical Manual of Mental Disorders, 351
 definition of mental disorders, 415–19, 421
 homosexuality in, 54–55, 56, 58, 59, 239
 paraphilias and distress in, 54–63, 423n.2
 personality disorders in, 65–67, 69, 70

DID. *See* dissociative identity disorder

Dilthey, Wilhelm, 180–82, 186, 187n.2

diminished responsibility, 298–99

disclosure, 167–68

discourse, 25–26, 27

discursive naturalism, 25

disease, 185

disjunction problem, 198

dissociation, 106–17
 accessibility assumption, 109
 capability assumption, 108
 definition of, 107–13
 diversification assumption, 108
 nonuniqueness assumption, 108
 ownership assumption, 109

dissociative identity disorder (DID), 106, 108, 109, 110, 115, 136–38, 141

distinct sustaining cause, 419–20

diversification assumption, 108

diversity, 210, 213, 216, 229n.11, 230n.14

DNA (deoxyribonucleic acid), 365–66

dopamine, 374, 376

Dougher, M., 385–87

Down syndrome, 153
Drabman, R., 388
drugs. *See* pharmacology
DSM. *See Diagnostic and Statistical Manual of Mental Disorders*
dualism, 344, 388
due process, 277, 278
Durham Rule, 298

eating disorders, 154, 240
EBM. *See* Evidence-Based Medicine
ECT. *See* electroconvulsive therapy
ego-dystonic homosexuality, 55, 58, 59
ego-impairment index, 29
electroconvulsive therapy (ECT), 287
Eli Lilly (co.), 42
Elliott, Carl, 40, 68–69, 78, 81, 86
Ellison, Ralph, 252
embodiment, 118–32
    disorders, 121–24
    phenomenological distinctions, 119–21
    problems in comprehensive disorders, 124–27
Engelhardt, Tristam H., 418
environment, 330, 331–32, 334
epiphenomenalism, 388–89
epistemic Givens, 368, 378nn.2–3
Erwin, E., 382, 383
Essential Handbook of Psychopharmacology (Pies), 372
Essential Psychopharmacology (Stahl), 371
ethics
    and clinical decision making, 208
    communitarianism, 293–94
    of psychiatry and religion, 320–21
    quasi-legal, 219, 222, 225–26, 230n.14
    in research, 290–92
    of social construction, 401–3
    training, 223
    of treatment, 285–90
    in treatment of children and youth, 148–52
Evidence-Based Medicine (EBM), 205, 207, 214–16
Evison, Ian, 313
evolutionarily stable strategy, 335
evolutionary theory, 199, 329–37

exclusivity position, 112–13
experience, 153, 188n.4, 354–55
explanation, 180–90
expression, 354, 355
Eysenck, Hans, 381, 383

Fair Sex, Savage Dreams: Race, Psychoanalysis, Sexual Difference (Walton), 246
false beliefs. *See* delusions
Fanon, Frantz, 249–51, 254
FDA. *See* Food and Drug Administration
Fechner, G.W., 341
Feinberg, Joel, 79
femaleness, 238, 239
Ficino, Marsilio, 41
filtering, 108
Fischer, John, 80, 81
Fliess, Wilhelm, 342
flight of ideas, 24
Fodor, Jerry, 197–98, 201
folk psychology, 153
Food and Drug Administration (FDA), 428, 432
Forensic Psychiatry, Race and Culture (Fernando et al.), 246
Foucault, Michel, 248–49, 301, 303, 373, 394
Fourteenth Amendment (U.S. Constitution), 277, 278
Fox, George, 314
free will, 301
Freud, Sigmund
    critique of philosophy of passions, 345–47
    debt to Kant, 343–45
    debt to philosophy, 338–50
    on melancholia, 40, 45
    and psychoanalysis, 185, 340–43
    psychosexual theories, 154
    and religion, 317, 319
    and self-reflexive judgment, 26
Freudian Marxism, 251
Frith, Christopher, 98–99
Fromm, Erich, 251
Fulford, Bill, 69, 164, 194
Fulford, K.W.M., 313, 315, 316, 322

Gadamer, Hans-Georg, 187, 357
Galenic medicine, 43
Gardner, Sebastian, 339
gender, 47–49, 237–43, 345–47
gender assignment, 237
gender attribution, 237
gender dysphoria, 431
gender identity, 237
gender identity disorder (GID), 142–43
gender-neutral language, 241
gender role, 237
General Psychopathology (Jaspers), 184, 357
geneticization, 292–93
genitalia, 240
Ghaemi, S. Nassir, 44
GID. *See* gender identity disorder
Gill, Merton, 185
Gillick case, 150
Gilligan, Carole, 154, 241
Goldman, Alan, 56
Gordon, L.R., 250
Graham, George, 38–39, 42, 44, 50n.2
Great Britain. *See* United Kingdom
Grier, W.H., 247
Griew, E., 299, 301, 302
group neurosis, 317–18

Häberlin, Paul, 342, 345
Habermas, Jürgen, 185, 361
habit, 376
Hacking, Ian, 67–68, 70, 137, 165, 396, 401, 427
hallucination, 23
Hare, R.M., 210
Harrell, C.J.P., 247
Herbart, J.F., 348n.17
hermeneutics
    definition of, 181, 186
    development of, 184
    and interpretation, 187n.3
    and phenomenology, 356–61
    and psychoanalysis, 188n.5
    psychopathology and psychotherapy, 361–62
    Schafer's work in, 185
    and understanding, 353–56, 358
    and values, 220

hidden observer experiments, 109
histrionic personality disorder, 334
Hodges, Geoffrey, 273–76
Homicide Act (Great Britain), 298, 299
homosexuality
    and depression, 47–48
    gender identity disorder as precursor of, 143
    sex/gender value system, 239
    treatment in *Diagnostic and Statistical Manual of Mental Disorders*, 54–55, 56, 58, 59, 239
Hood, John, 312
Hopkins, Gerard Manley, 38–39
Human Genome Project, 293
humanism, 249
Hume, David, 41–42, 229n.11, 303, 368, 378n.2
Humphrey-Durham amendment, 428
Humpty Dumpty fallacy, 113–16
Husserl, Edmund, 40, 254, 356, 357
hyperreflexivity, 126
hypnosis, 113
hypnotic anesthesia, 108
hypochondria, 410
hysteria, 137, 154, 239, 338, 341, 345–47, 397, 399, 400

identity, 133–46
identity politics, 142
imprisonment, 280
In a Different Voice (Gilligan), 154, 241
inclusivity position, 112–13
incoherent thought, 24
infertility, 429
informed consent, 290, 291
insanity, 140, 298
insight, 27, 33–34
intentionality, 356
internalization, 26
International Classification of Diseases, 352, 423n.1
interpretation, 181, 357–58, 359–60
intersubjectivity, 25, 26
Invisible Man, The (Ellison), 252–53
involuntary action, 121

irrationality, 31–32
irresistible desires, 79–82

Jackson, Hughlings, 343
Jackson, Michael, 315, 316
James, William, 314–15, 316, 317, 343
Jamison, Kay, 50
Janet, Pierre, 107
Jaspers, Karl, 184–85, 188nn.4–5, 356–61
Jellinek, E.M., 374
John Doe v. Dept. of Public Safety, 278
Julian of Norwich, 314
Jung, Karl, 318

Kahn, Abraham, 40
Kansas Petitioner v. Michael T. Crane, 279
Kansas v. Hendricks, 279
Kant, Immanuel, 31–32, 41, 249, 303, 338–47, 418
Kefauver-Harris amendments, 428
Kendell, R.E., 418
Kierkegaard, Soren, 40
Klagsbrun, Samuel, 317, 318
Klein, George, 185
Klein, Melanie, 40
Klerman, Gerard, 43
knowledge, 153, 187n.1, 220–21
Kraepelin, Emil, 317, 428
Kramer, Peter, 38, 41, 42
Kristeva, Julia, 45–46, 47
Kuhn, Thomas, 185–86

labeling, 171–72
Lacan, Jacques, 340
Laing, R.D., 25, 154
Lamarckianism, 342, 343
language
   and gender, 241–42
   and thought, 28
   and values, 218, 219
language games, 25
Lawson, W.B., 246
Lee, C., 388
Leibniz, Gottfried, 341
Lesser, Harry, 287
Levine, Michael, 339

liability, 275–79
life-story perspective, 185
Lindley, Richard, 284
Lipps, T., 341
Listening to Prozac (Kramer), 41
lithium, 209, 211, 214–15, 217, 225–26
Littlewood, Roland, 315, 316
Locke, John, 153, 378n.2
loosening of associations, 23–25, 27
Luhrman, T.M., 312
Luria, A.R., 25, 28, 29

Macarthur Study of Mental Disorder and Violence, 272
madness. *See* mental disorder(s)
Mahoney, Michael, 382
maleness, 238, 239
mania, 43, 50
manic depression, 138–39
Manichean Psychology: Racism and the Minds of People of African Descent (Harrell), 247
manipulativity, 240–41, 334, 387
Marcuse, Herbert, 251
Marks, I.M., 331–32
Martin, Mike, 38
Marx, Karl, 254
Marxism, 251–53
masochism, 239
masturbation, 240
McDowell, John, 201
McGhie, A., 28, 29
McGuire, M., 335–36
Mealey, L., 335–36
meaningful behavior, 354–55, 357
medicalization, 172, 248, 430
medication. *See* pharmacology
Megan's Law, 277–78
Megone, C., 195–96
melancholia. *See* depression
"Melancholic Epistemology" (Graham), 38
memory, 106–17, 137–38
men, 238–39, 346
   See also maleness
mens rea, 297
menstruation, 240

mental disorder(s)
   and characterization identity, 142–43
   of children and youth, 147–60
   and criminal responsibility, 296–311
   definition of, 415–25
   and personal identity, 133, 135–36
   and racism, 247
   and reductionism, 194–97
   relationship with self, 164–65
   and religion, 317–19
   social construction of, 393–406
   stigma of, 164, 283, 430
   upsurge in, 426–32
   valuation of, 165
microreduction, 192
Mill, John Stuart, 42
Miller, G.H., 303–4
Millikan, R.G., 195, 196, 200
mind, 330–31, 367, 378n.12
Mind and World (McDowell), 201
M'Naghten Rules, 298
Morris, Herbert, 280
movement, 119–20, 125, 126
mRNA, 365–66
multiperspective approach, 217
multiperspective skills, 224, 225
multiple personality disorder, 135, 399,
   400, 427
multiplicity, 136–38, 141
mutual comprehension, 25

narrative self, 29–31, 33
National Bioethics Advisory Commission
   (NBAC), 290
National Institute of Mental Health, 428
natural conglomerates, 404n.8
naturalism, 193, 194, 197, 201–3
natural kinds, 67–68, 404n.8
natural sciences, 180–81, 341
nature, 193, 201–2, 341
NBAC. *See* National Bioethics Advisory
   Commission
Neely, Wright, 79, 80
negative hallucinations. *See* systematized
   anesthesia
Neisser, Ulrich, 22
Nelson, Hilde Lindeman, 143

nervous system, 332
Nesse, R., 331–32
neural models, 364–80
neurobiology, 351
neuroscience, 186
neurosis, 317–18
New Yorker, 41
Nietzsche, Friedrich, 248, 341
noema, 356
noesis, 356
nonuniqueness assumption, 108

objective self-consciousness, 122
observation, 168
obsessive-compulsive disorder, 429, 432
*Of Two Minds: The Growing Disorder in
   American Psychiatry* (Luhrman),
   312
ontology, 254
Oppenheim, P., 192, 203
opposites, 358–59
Othello delusion, 22
ownership assumption, 109

panic disorder, 429
parallelism, 344
paranoid irrationality, 31–32
paranoid thinking, 33
paraphilias, 54–63, 423n.2
Parsons, Talcott, 164
partition response, 137
*Pathology and Identity: The Work of
   Mother Earth in Trinidad*
   (Littlewood), 316
patient-centered practice, 213–16
patient-perspective skills, 223–24, 225
perception, 22, 100–101, 119
personal identity, 133–46
   and advance directives, 139–40
   and mental disorder, 135–36
   multiplicity and dissociative identity
      disorder, 136–38
   and responsibility for past deeds, 140
   successive selves and manic depression,
      138–39
   and therapeutic goals, 141

personality disorder(s), 64–77, 334, 395
  brief history of, 65–66
  definition of, 66, 72–73
  in *Diagnostic and Statistical Manual of Mental Disorders*, 65–67, 69, 70
  distinction from mental illnesses, 307
  as evolutionarily stable strategy, 335
  as interactive moral kinds, 67–69
  moral treatment, 71–72, 74
  problems with treatment, 69–71
perversions, 54
pharmacology
  for children and youth, 148–49
  for depression, 38, 40–43
  FDA control, 428
  for personality disorders, 69–70
  pharmaceutical industry, 431–32
  for schizophrenia, 369–71
phenomenology
  of delusion, 229n.11
  and embodiment, 119–21
  and hermeneutics, 356–61
  of thought insertion, 95–98, 101
  transcendental, 254
  and Values-Based Medicine, 220
phenothiazines, 370
philosophical field work, 219
philosophical naturalism, 193
philosophy
  Freud's debt to, 338–50
  of mental content, 197–200
  of passions, 345–47
  and psychopathology, 153–54
  transcendental, 338, 342
  and Values-Based Medicine, 207
phobia, 80, 332–33, 417, 419–20
Pies, Ronald, 372
Plato, 79, 84, 116
poetry, 42
posttraumatic stress disorder, 420, 427, 432
power, 173–74
pressure of speech, 24
principle of ascription immunity, 92–94
principle of compositional reversibility (CR principle), 114–16
principle of noncontradiction, 94

Prinz, Jesse, 153
privilege, 169
Problemata (Aristotle), 41
promiscuity, 239
Protagoras (Plato), 79
Proudfoot, Wayne, 315
Prozac, 38, 41, 42, 401, 431, 432
"Prozac and the American Dream" (Elliott), 40
psychiatric wills. *See* advance directives
psychiatry
  benchmarks for concepts, 409–14
  diagnoses, 163–79
  mindless/brainless debate, 372
  neural models in, 364–80
  power of, 165–66, 173–74
  psychopathology and psychotherapy in, 351–53
  raciation in, 245–53
  reductionism in, 191–200, 371
  and religion, 312–26
  transcendental phenomenology as underpinnings of, 254
  treatment and research ethics, 282–95
  understanding and explanation in, 180–90
  and Values-Based Medicine, 227
  without reductionist naturalism, 201–3
  See also mental disorder(s)
psychoanalysis, 154, 185, 188n.5, 318, 320, 340–43, 344
psychoanalytic Marxism, 252–53
Psychoanalytic Marxism (Wolfenstein), 251, 252
psychoanalytic models, 338–50
psychology, 340, 344, 355
psychopathology
  Darwinian models of, 329–37
  Hacking on, 427
  hermeneutic, 361–62
  and meaningful behavior, 355
  in present-day psychiatry, 351–53
  and theories of child development, 153–54
psychopaths, 335–36
psychopharmacological Calvinism, 38, 43–44

psychopharmacology, 41, 42, 43, 186, 351
Psychosemantics (Fodor), 197
psychoses, 21–34, 188n.4
psychotherapy, 351–53, 355, 361–62, 372
psychotropic medication, 148–49
punishment, 280, 297, 304
Putnam, H., 192, 203

quasi-legal ethics, 219, 222, 225–26, 230n.14
Quine, V.W.O., 193

race, 244–57
Racism and Psychiatry (Thomas and
     Sillen), 246
Radden, Jennifer, 39
rationality. *See* reasoning
Ravizza, Mark, 80, 81
reality, 32, 356
reasoning
    and competence, 265–67
    diagnosis as rationality, 169–70
    and gender, 240
    about values, 221–23
reasons-receptivity, 80
reductionism, 173, 191–204
    and mental disorder, 194–97
    and philosophical naturalism, 193
    in philosophy of mental content, 197–
       200
    in psychiatry, 191–200, 371
    psychiatry without reductionist
       naturalism, 201–3
    and unity of science, 192
reflective techniques, 26
regular reasons-receptivity, 80
Reich, Wilhelm, 251
Reitman, D., 388
reinforcement, 384
religion, 312–26
repression, 109–10
reproductive medicine, 228n.10, 429
research, 290–92
responsibility, 80, 81, 140–41, 375
    See also criminal responsibility
reward, 82–84
Ricoeur, Paul, 185, 357
Ritalin, 148, 401, 429, 431

ritual, 170–71
Riviere, Joan, 246
Rorty, Richard, 186
Rose, Gillian, 46–47
Roth, Philip, 61n.22

St. Paul, 314
Sartre, Jean-Paul, 249
Scarman, Lord, 150
Schafer, Roy, 185
schizoid gap, 28
schizophrenia
    and attention, 28, 29, 378n.11
    and benchmark problem, 410–11
    case study, 273
    and embodiment, 124–27
    and genetics, 399
    hyperreflexivity, 126
    Laing on, 154
    and loosening of associations, 24, 27
    and personal identity, 135
    psychopharmacology of, 369–71
    Stevens and Price on, 333
    subjectivity of, 369
    and thought insertion, 90, 99, 126
Schopenhauer, A., 341
Schor, Naomi, 46
science, 192–93, 212–13, 214, 352
Sedgwick, Peter, 418
selection, 387
self-ascription, 89–105
self-control, 81–85, 279
self-identity, 142
self-knowledge, 26–29
self-reflexive thought, 26
Sellars, W., 368, 378nn.2–4
sense of agency, 120–21, 126, 128n.6
sense of ownership, 120–21, 122, 128n.6
sensus communis, 31, 33
sex/gender system, 238
sexual dysphoria, 239
sexuality
    child sexual abuse, 241
    and gender, 239
    paraphilia and distress in DSM-IV, 54–
       63
    and race, 248

sickle-cell anemia, 333
Silberstein, Eduard, 340, 341, 347n.7
Sillen, S., 246
Skinner, B.F., 381, 382, 384, 385, 387
Smith and Jones v. United States, 275–76
social anxiety disorder, 429, 432
social construction
  epistemology of, 398–401
  ethics of, 401–3
  metaphysics of, 394–98
  models, 393–406
social Darwinism, 342, 343
socialization, 30
sociopaths, 335
Socrates, 79, 314
soma, 364–65, 367–68, 371, 378nn.3–4
somatic residues, 344
Spengler, Oswald, 342
spirituality, 323n.3
Spitzer, M., 24
split-brain behavior, 124
Stahl, Stephen, 371
Starobinski, Jean, 43
stigma, 164, 283, 430
stigma plus test, 277, 278
Stone, Michael, 319
Structure of Scientific Revolutions, The
  (Kuhn), 185–86
Styron, William, 39–40
subconscious denial, 110
subjective experience, 354
successive selves, 138–39
suicide, 48, 50n.1
support groups, 430
suppression, 110
Sykes, Richard, 409
systematized anesthesia, 106, 108
Szasz, Thomas, 68, 170, 194, 304, 319, 417

Tarasoff case, 320
teleological theories of content, 199–200
Teresa of Avila, 314
therapeutic relationship, 289
Thomas, A., 246
thought
  disorder, 21–34
  experiments, 300–308

influence/control, 91
as motor activity, 98–99
See also mind; thought insertion
thought insertion, 89–105, 126
  compatibility with ascription
    immunity, 94–95
  definition of, 90–91
  misidentification puzzle, 91–94
  phenomenology of, 95–98, 101
  toward complete theory of, 98–103
Tourette's syndrome, 300, 413
traits, 333–34
transcendental logic, 343
transcendental phenomenology, 254
transcendental philosophy, 338, 342
transcendental psychology, 344
trauma, 107
treatment
  advocacy, 289–90
  in community, 287–89
  ethical issues surrounding, 285–90
  justification of compulsory, 286
  right to refuse, 286–87
  therapeutic relationship, 289
  troubling, 287
Troisi, A., 335–36
trust, 242
Tuke, William, 74

Ulysses contracts. *See* advance directives
unconscious, 109–10, 341, 342, 344, 345,
  348n.16
unconscious denial, 110
understanding, 180–90, 260
  and closure, 359
  and hermeneutics, 353–56, 358
  as illumination and unmasking, 360–61
  and interpretation, 357–58, 359–60
  Jaspers on, 357–61
  and opposites, 358–59
unilateral neglect, 123, 127
United Kingdom, 230–31n.18, 288, 304–5

values, 205–34
  awareness of, 218–20
  and clinical decision making, 208–9,
    224–26

and diagnosis, 174–76
diversity of, 210, 213, 216, 229n.11,
   230n.14
in health care, 212–13
knowledge of, 220–21
particular versus universal, 421–23
reasoning about, 221–23
and reductionism, 194, 196
scale of, 210
and science, 212–13
and understanding/explanation, 187
visible and invisible, 209–12
See also Values-Based Medicine
Values-Based Medicine (VBM)
  compared with Evidence-Based
    Medicine, 208
  and philosophy, 207
  practice of, 206, 218–26
  and quasi-legal ethics, 219, 222, 225–26,
    230n.14
  ten principles of, 205–34
  theory of, 206, 207–17
values blindness, 218
values myopia, 220
VBM. *See* Values-Based Medicine
verbal hallucinations, 23
victim blaming, 245

violence, 272
volitional disorders, 78–88

Wakefield, J.C., 194–95, 196, 418, 420,
   421
Walker, Nigel, 280
weak reasons-reactivity, 80–81
Weber, Samuel, 339
Weininger, Otto, 342
Weisberger, A.M., 42
Weltanschauung, 341, 342
Winnicott, D.W., 318
Wittgenstein, L., 32
Wolfenstein, E.V., 251–53
Wolpe, Joseph, 381, 382
women
  and depression, 48–49
  exclusion of, 238
  Gilligan on, 241
  and hysteria, 154, 239, 346, 399
  sexuality, 239
  See also femaleness
worldview, 341

York Retreat, 74

Zerfahrenheit, 24, 33

CPSIA information can be obtained at www.ICGtesting.com
Printed in the USA
LVOW11s1049070913

351387LV00010B/21/P